DATE DUE

MAY 13 1986			
JUN 16 1997			
MAR 09 2001			
GAYLORD			PRINTED IN U.S.A.

Contemporary Topics in Molecular Immunology

Volume 10

The Interleukins

Contemporary Topics in Molecular Immunology

A Continuation Order Plan is available for this series. A continuation order will bring delivery of each new volume immediately upon publication. Volumes are billed only upon actual shipment. For further information please contact the publisher.

Contemporary Topics in Molecular Immunology

Volume 10
The Interleukins

EDITED BY

STEVEN GILLIS
Immunex Corporation
Seattle, Washington

and

F. P. INMAN
Quillen-Dishner College of Medicine
East Tennessee State University
Johnson City, Tennessee

PLENUM PRESS • NEW YORK AND LONDON

The Library of Congress cataloged the first volume of this title as follows:

Contemporary topics in molecular immunology. v. 2–
New York, Plenum Press, 1973–

v. illus. 24 cm.

Continues Contemporary topics in immunochemistry.

1. Immunochemistry—Collected works. 2. Immunology—Collected works.

QR180.C635 574.2′9′05 73–648513
ISSN 0090–8800 MARC–S

Volume 1 of this series was published under the title *Contemporary Topics in Immunochemistry*

Library of Congress Catalog Card Number 73-648513

ISBN 0-306-41776-6

A Division of Plenum Publishing Corporation
233 Spring Street, New York, N.Y. 10013

Printed in the United States of America

Contributors

R. Chris Bleackley — *Department of Biochemistry*
University of Alberta
Edmonton, Alberta, Canada

Colin G. Brooks — *Program in Basic Immunology*
Fred Hutchinson Cancer Research Center
Seattle, Washington

Ian Clark-Lewis — *Immunoregulation Laboratory*
The Walter and Eliza Hall Institute of Medical Research
Royal Melbourne Hospital
Victoria, Australia

Martin A Cheever — *Division of Oncology*
University of Washington School of Medicine and the Fred Hutchinson Cancer Research Center
Seattle, Washington

Richard M. Crapper — *Immunoregulation Laboratory*
The Walter and Eliza Hall Institute of Medical Research
Royal Melbourne Hospital
Victoria, Australia

Richard W. Dutton — *Department of Biology*
University of California, San Diego
La Jolla, California

Warner C. Greene — *Metabolism Branch*
National Cancer Institute
Bethesda Maryland

Philip D. Greenberg — *Division of Oncology*
University of Washington School of Medicine and the Fred Hutchinson Cancer Research Center
Seattle, Washington

Toshiyuki Hamaoka — *Institute for Cancer Research*
Osaka University Medical School
Fukushimaku, Osaka, Japan

Delsworth G. Harnish *Department of Biochemistry*
University of Alberta
Edmonton, Alberta, Canada

Christopher S. Henney *Immunex Corporation*
Seattle, Washington

Eugene W. Holowachuk *Department of Biochemistry*
University of Alberta
Edmonton, Alberta, Canada

Maureen Howard *Laboratory of Microbial Immunity*
National Institute of Allergy and Infectious Diseases
National Institutes of Health
Bethesda, Maryland

James N. Ihle *Basic Research Program-LBI*
NCI-Frederick Cancer Research Facility
Frederick, Maryland

Peter E. Lipsky *Rheumatic Diseases Unit*
Department of Internal Medicine
University of Texas Health Science Center
Southwestern Medical School
Dallas, Texas

Malcolm A. S. Moore *Department of Developmental Hematopoiesis*
Sloan-Kettering Institute for Cancer Research
New York, New York

Verner Paetkau *Department of Biochemistry*
University of Alberta
Edmonton, Alberta, Canada

Denis Riendeau *Department of Biochemistry*
University of Alberta
Edmonton, Alberta, Canada

Richard J. Robb *Central Research and Development Department*
E. I. du Pont de Nemours and Company
Glenolden Laboratory
Glenolden, Pennsylvania

John W. Schrader *Immunoregulation Laboratory*
The Walter and Eliza Hall Institute of Medical Research
Royal Melbourne Hospital
Victoria, Australia

Sabariah Schrader *Immunoregulation Laboratory*
The Walter and Eliza Hall Institute of Medical Research
Royal Melbourne Hospital
Victoria, Australia

Susan L. Swain *Department of Biology*
University of California, San Diego
La Jolla, California

Grace H. W. Wong *Immunoregulation Laboratory*
The Walter and Eliza Hall Institute of Medical Research
Royal Melbourne Hospital
Victoria, Australia

Yee-Pang Yung *Department of Developmental Hematopoiesis*
Sloan-Kettering Institute for Cancer Research
New York, New York

Preface

Investigations of the activation, proliferation, and, in some cases, differentiation of mononuclear cells involved in the immune response are proceeding rapidly. These studies have resulted in the discovery of several factors that promote these cellular events, some of which have been characterized biochemically to various extents. Because of the considerable interest in understanding these cellular changes at the molecular level, we chose to produce the first thematic volume for *Contemporary Topics in Molecular Immunology;* the theme deals with certain regulatory factors that promote proliferation and differentiation. We have compiled contributions from numerous scientists well known for their work with several regulatory factors. In the following paragraphs, the reader will find an overview of the contents of this volume.

Greene and Robb review data they have generated over the past 2–3 years with respect to characterization of hormone-specific Interleukin-2 (IL-2) receptors on the surface of activated T cells. Their chapter traces the development of a quantitative assay for assessment of IL-2 receptors based on the preparation and use of radiolabeled IL-2 prepared biosynthetically with the aid of IL-2-producer leukemic cells. The authors then describe an alternate approach, the preparation of a monoclonal antibody previously determined to be directed against a T-cell-activation antigen. This so-called anti-Tac antibody was later found to recognize a determinant on or near the IL-2 receptor. The interplay of these assays (anti-Tac binding and radiolabeled IL-2 binding) have led to the conclusion that IL-2 receptors (in the range of 10,000–100,000 sites/cell) are generated rapidly after T cells are activated either by antigen or mitogen.

The authors describe the use of the anti-Tac antibody in experiments demonstrating its capacity to suppress immune responses via blocking of IL-2 binding to IL-2 receptors. In the final part of their chapter the authors discuss what has been an appealing possibility for many investigators, namely, the IL-2 and IL-2-receptor triggering may have something to do with the proliferation of leukemic T cells. Greene and Robb use their techniques to locate IL-2 receptors in cells from some patients with cases of acute T-cell leukemia. The recent demonstration that the epidermal growth factor receptor bears homology to several previously identified *onc* genes may lead to the eventual realization that the T-cell growth-factor receptor (IL-2 receptor) may be a product of viral transformation.

Paetkau was one of the original investigators to describe IL-2 activity (previously referred to in his laboratory as costimulator). He has continued to keep pace with lympokine investigation as it progressed from phenomenology into biochemistry and now into molecular biology. Paetkau and colleagues examined biochemical and biological characteristics of primate and rodent IL-2. Purification methods are compared and in doing so it becomes clear that IL-2 is a partially defined set of proteins and is relatively heterogeneous. They describe experiments detailing the isolation of poly A^+ messenger RNA from various IL-2-producer cell lines and the translation of these RNAs *in vitro* to yield biologically active IL-2. Systems for such message translation and initial results on posttranslational processing are described. In addition, these scientists provide for the student of lymphokine biology a rational approach to the molecular biology of products of activated T lymphocytes. In essence they have summarized the molecular properties of IL-2 and have pointed out new directions for research which should be useful in unraveling the molecular mechanisms by which lymphokines regulate cell-mediated immune responses.

Brooks and Henney initially detailed the capacity of lymphokine-containing conditioned medium to promote the long-term growth and differentiation of natural killer (NK) cells. The capacity of IL-2 to boost natural killer cell responses even in the presence of exogenous interferon has led to increasing pressure upon the research community to provide IL-2 in significant quantities for use in clinical trials. Brooks and Henney have carefully reviewed the state of the art conditions for the culture and propagation of NK cells *in vitro* and have dramatically shown that IL-2 may not be uniquely sufficient for the growth of such cells *in vitro*. According to the authors, at least two distinct pathways have been identified for the mechanism behind the capacity of IL-2 to boost *in vitro* and *in vivo* NK cell responses. It would appear that via a complex series of cell interactions, IL-2 can lead to elaboration of gamma-interferon (γ-IFN) which itself enhances cytolysis by natural killer cells. Second, it would appear that IL-2 can induce the expression of promiscuous NK-like cytotoxicity in cells previously belonging to the cytotoxic T-lymphocyte (CTL) lineage by a process probably more akin to hematopoietic differentiation than activation per se. Clearly, these results may place NK cells as firm residents of the T-cell family in marked contradiction to investigators who have previously claimed that NK cells in fact are derived from the monocytic series. The data reviewed in this chapter together with those of additional investigators who have shown a similar capacity of IL-2 to boost the natural killing activity of large, granular lymphocytes clearly establish that this lymphokine may play an important role in controlling natural host defenses *in vivo*.

Ihle reports that conditioned media from activated T cells contain a factor that induces 20-alpha-hydroxysteroid-dehydrogenase (20αSDH) activity in cultures of *nu/nu* splenic lymphocytes. The enzyme is uniquely allied with the T-cell lineage, and in mice it is associated predominantly with Thy 1-positive, functional T cells. Therefore, it appears that the factor in conditioned media causes a precursor cell from *nu/nu* lymphocytes to differentiate, becoming Thy 1^+, hydrocortisone resistant, and 20αSDH-positive. On the basis of this assay as a measure of early T-cell differentiation, as well as the T-cell origin of the factor and some biochemical characteristics, the factor was named Interleukin-3 (IL-3).

In his contribution to this volume, Ihle describes the preparation of IL-3 from the culture supernatant fluid of WEHI-3 cells, and gives its amino acid composition and NH_2-terminal sequence. Several biological activities are associated with IL-3, such as its being a growth factor and a factor for differentiation and/or proliferation of mastlike cells. These activities and the sequence of differentiation promoted by IL-3 are discussed in detail. A variety of murine lymphomas were induced by IL-3, and Ihle describes the three general phenotypes observed. Finally, a sequence for the differentiation of stem cells induced by IL-3 is proposed; the scheme is supported by the information given earlier in the chapter. The scheme is provocative in proposing that mastlike cells are derived from a lineage that includes early T-cell differentiation and that another functional product of this lineage is a unique monocyte-like adherent cell characterized by the expression of Ia but lacking Mac-1.

Schrader was one of the first—if not the first—investigators to describe a unique lymphokine produced by mitogen-activated T cells and later by particular murine T-cell hybridomas. This factor was first called P-cell stimulating factor, as it gave rise to a population of lymphokine-dependent progenitor cells from murine splenocytes *in vitro*. P cells could be made to differentiate into basophil-like cells and eventually into mast cells. It became clear from Schrader's work that P-cell growth factor or P-cell stimulating factor, mast-cell growth factor, and IL-3 were, if not molecularly similar, clearly members of a closely related family of molecules. In their chapter, Schrader and his colleagues detail the biochemical characteristics of P-cell stimulating factor and describe its assay. They review their recently published work, which uses biochemical protocols to separate P-cell factors from either IL-2 or T-cell-derived granulocyte macrophage colony-stimulating factor (CSF). Their work hints at a molecular characterization of P-cell stimulating factor, as the chapter contains additional experimentation detailing the translation of P-cell stimulating factor mRNA by *Xenopus* oocytes into a protein exhibiting biological activity. While discussing the relationship of P-cell stimulating factor to various other lymphokines, the authors keep an eye on the *in vivo* physiological relevance of this factor and discuss its potential use *in vivo* as well as experimentation aimed at demonstrating an *in vivo* effect for the factor. Finally, as is the case with the Greene and Robb contribution, Schrader *et al.* discuss P-cell factor and its potential role in tumorigenesis. The association between activation by lymphokines and uncontrolled growth of malignant white blood cells becomes clear in their analysis of the capacity of P-cell stimulating factor-dependent cell lines to become autonomous in their growth due to concomitant production of the same growth factor for which they were once dependent.

Mast cells can now be grown in culture. Yung and Moore review recent developments in *in vitro* growth of mast cells and especially suitable sources of growth factor. A variety of lymphokines is present in mitogen-activated murine leukocyte conditioned medium and in medium conditioned by the WEHI-3 cell line. Yung and Moore consider it important to establish mast-cell growth factor (MCGF) as unique for mast cells and different from the other known factors. Thus, a partial biochemical characterization of MCGF is undertaken and the results are described. A biochemical and biological comparsion of MCGF and colony-stimulating factor is made, as these factors have several characteristics in common. Differentiation factor, stem-cell stimulating factor, and IL-3 also are examined in the context of their relationship with MCGF. Finally, the authors discuss the origin and the maturation of mast cells, as well as the role of MCGF in the differentiation and proliferation of mast cells or mastoblasts from the precursors.

Howard provides evidence to support the hypothesis that soluble proliferation factors stimulate antigen-activated B cells to proliferate. Using a low-cell-density B-cell costimulator assay, she and her co-workers found that antibodies specific for the B cell's Ig receptors, a T-cell-derived B-cell growth factor (BCGF-1), and IL-1 are required to cause murine Lyb-5$^+$ B lymphocytes to enter S phase. The data support the notion that BCGF and IL-1 are B-cell-specific proliferation cofactors. The biochemical and biological nature of B-cell growth factor is explored. In addition, Howard considers what is known of its role in B-cell activation and development. B cells activated with anti-IgM, BCGF-1, and IL-1-synthesized DNA but did not differentiate into antibody-forming cells unless two additional growth factors were present. A scheme of the events from activation of a G_0 B cell to differentiation into an antibody-forming cell is given; the reader will find that it summarizes the hypothesis mentioned above very clearly.

Although the role of IL-1 in augmenting T-cell proliferation is well known, Lipsky describes the role of IL-1 in the generation of Ig-secreting cells. In the presence of macrophages and T cells, purified IL-1 augments the formation of Ig-secreting cells stimulated with pokeweed mitogen. What is the mechanism of this activity? Early supernatants of culture macrophages enhanced the generation of Ig-secreting cells, as did purified IL-1 when added to supernatants of preincubated macrophages that contained no augmenting activity. Antibodies to IL-1 removed the active principle from supernatants. The conclusion reached by Lipsky, based on an extensive series of experiments, is that the major role of IL-1 in the generation of Ig-secreting cells in humans may not be to facilitate the generation of helper T-cell factors, but rather to provide a necessary signal to B cells. IL-1 plays a role only during the first few hours of B-cell activation, whereas helper T-cell factors are found to be required later.

Swain and Dutton review data they have generated regarding the capacity of factors produced by T cells to control both B-cell growth and differentiation into antibody-secreting cells. Their work revolves around the description and characterization of two particular factors: (1) a differentiation-inducing factor, or T-cell replacing factor (TRF), which is a T-cell derived signal to B lymphocytes to produce and secrete immunoglobulin; and (2) a factor that this laboratory believes controls B-cell activity, which is a B-cell growth factor, one that acts in an analogous fashion to the way that IL-2 works on T cells. The authors detail assays for both factors and discuss the experimentation that clearly distinguishes between their effects. BCGF acts directly on B cells and does not mediate its effects through any other accessory cell. This chapter establishes itself as a fitting summary of the lymphokine work currently being conducted in one of the world's most productive and insightful cellular immunology laboratories.

Like the previously detailed chapter by Swain and Dutton, Hamaoka's chapter addresses the production and action of T-cell replacing factor (TRF). He traces the work that has been conducted over the past 4 years in his laboratory, which clearly established procedures for producing T-cell hybridomas that had the capacity to secrete TRF spontaneously. Hamaoka uses such cell lines to conduct initial biochemical experimentation, and he describes the preliminary biochemical characterization of the TRF molecule.

By the use of an interesting inbred mouse, the DBA2/Housa strain, Hamaoka describes an X-linked recessive gene that controls defective expression of TRF receptors on B cells in these mutant mice. His experiments took advantage of these mice to generate monoclonal antibodies directed against the TRF receptor on such B cells. The antibody itself has the capacity to block TRF action via competition for the TRF receptor. In the absence of TRF, however, various concentrations of the antireceptor monoclonal antibodies have the ability to trigger B cells. Thus it would appear that the antibody can act both in an antagonistic and an agonistic fashion. Hamaoka has used monoclonal antibodies directed against the TRF receptor to begin physiochemical characterization of the receptor. Through the use of hybridization technology both for the production of large quantities of TRF and for the production of the monoclonal antibody directed against the TRF receptor, it would appear that his group is well on the way to understanding how this T-cell-derived, differentiation-induced lymphokine acts to control immunoglobulin production by B cells.

Cheever and Greenberg's contribution to this volume is an appropriate final chapter, since it explores the use of exogenously administered lymphokines to alter immune responses *in vivo*. Cheever and Greenberg were among the first investigators to show that exogenously administered IL-2 has the ability to boost T-cell growth *in vivo*. In so doing, it significantly augments antitumor immune reactivity. Data detailed in their contribution reviews their initial provocative results and describes in some depth the pharmacokinetics of IL-2 administration. They address some of the key questions that will have to be faced by investigators hoping to use any lymphokine *in vivo*, such as potential inhibitors of lymphokine function and various biological effects and toxicities that may limit the ability of exogenously administered lymphokines to significantly alter immune responses *in vivo*. Nevertheless, the initial data from this laboratory are quite compelling and bode well for the eventual use of IL-2 in various therapeutic settings. The authors use their previously generated data as a base from which to identify several immunodeficient states both in mouse and in humans that would potentially be responsive to IL-2 exogenously applied.

We thank the authors for their fine contributions. We anticipate that our readers will find the information timely and that it will stimulate even greater interest in research on the regulation of immune responses.

Steven Gillis

Immunex Corporation
Seattle, Washington

F. P. Inman

East Tennesee State University
Johnson City, Tennesee

Contents

Toward the Molecular Biology of IL-2

Verner Paetkau, R. Chris Bleackley, Denis Riendeau, Delsworth G. Harnish, and Eugene W. Holowachuk

Interleukin-2 and the Regulation of Natural Killer Activity in Cultured Cell Populations

Colin G. Brooks and Christopher S. Henney

Biochemical and Biological Properties of Interleukin-3: A Lymphokine Mediating the Differentation of a Lineage of Cells that Includes Prothymocytes and Mastlike Cells

James N. Ihle

P-Cell Stimulating Factor: Biochemistry, Biology and Role in Oncogenesis

John W. Schrader, Ian Clark-Lewis, Richard M. Crapper, Grace H. W. Wong, and Sabariah Schrader

Mast-Cell Growth Factor: Its Role in Mast-Cell Differentiation, Proliferation, and Maturation

Yee-Pang Yung and Malcolm A. S. Moore

Soluble-Factor Induction of B-Cell Growth

Maureen Howard

Role of Interleukin-1 in Human B-Cell Activation

Peter E. Lipsky

T-Cell Factors That Promote Cell Proliferation and Differentiation

Susan L. Swain and Richard W. Dutton

T-Cell-Replacing Factor and Its Acceptor Site on B Cells: Molecular Properties and Immunogenetic Aspects

Toshiyuki Hamaoka

***In Vivo* Administration of Interleukin-2**

Martin A. Cheever and Philip D. Greenberg

Receptors for T-Cell Growth Factor: Structure, Function and Expression on Normal and Neoplastic Cells

Warner C. Greene

Metabolism Branch
National Cancer Institute
Bethesda, Maryland 20205

and

Richard J. Robb

Central Research and Development Department
E. I. du Pont de Nemours and Company
Glenolden Laboratory
Glenolden, Pennsylvania 19036

I. INTRODUCTION

During the years since its discovery (Morgan *et al.*, 1976), the preception of T-cell growth factor (TCGF), also called Interleukin-2 (IL-2), as an *in vitro* novelty has given way to an appreciation of its crucial role both in the immune response and in the etiology and potential therapy of a number of diseases. In addition to playing a pivotal role in the culturing and cloning of T cells (Gillis and Smith, 1977; Schreier *et al.*, 1980), TCGF potentiates the release of a number of other important lymphokines, including γ-interferon (γ-IFN) (Farrar *et al.*, 1981; Kasahara *et al.*, 1983), B-cell growth factor (BCGF) (Howard *et al.*, 1983), and B-cell differentiation factor (BCDF) (Inaba *et al.*, 1983). Moreover, TCGF or defects in its production or function have been implicated in such pathological states as congenital and acquired immunodeficiency (Palladino *et al.*, 1984; Flomenberg *et al.*, 1983; Harel-Bellan *et al.*, 1983; Stötter *et al.*, 1980; Thoman and Weigle, 1982), autoimmunity (Altman *et al.*, 1981; Dauphinée *et al.*, 1981; Linker-Israeli *et al.*, 1983), and cancer (Gootenberg *et al.*, 1981; Rey *et al.*, 1983). Indeed, the receptor for this growth factor is expressed on the cells of several types of neoplasms (see Section VII), raising the question of whether its presence in such instances is fortuitous or physiologically significant. From the viewpoint of clinical therapy, several reports have appeared demonstrating the efficacy of TCGF in promoting *in vitro* and *in vivo* activity of alloreactive (Kern *et al.*, 1981) and tumor-reactive T-cells as well as natural and lymphokine-activated killer populations (Lotze *et al.*, 1980, 1981; Wagner *et al.*, 1980; Gillis and Watson, 1981; Cheever *et al.*, 1982; Hefeneider *et al.*, 1983; Eberlein *et al.*, 1982; Rosenberg *et al.*, 1983; Paetkau *et al.*, 1982; Merluzzi *et al.*, 1983; Henney *et al.*, 1981, Donohue *et al.*, 1984; Grimm *et al.*, 1983). This review discusses various aspects of the structure, function, and selective cellular expression of the receptor for TCGF. An understanding of such ligand–receptor interactions should provide a foundation for the clinical manipulation of the immune system using this lymphokine.

T-cell proliferation in response to foreign antigen or lectin involves a variety of cell types and soluble mediators (Fig. 1). Indeed, TCGF is but one element in a cascade of lymphokines formed during an immune response (Farrar *et al.*, 1982). Although questions remain as to which and how many different cell types are involved in the production of and response to TCGF (broken arrows, Fig. 1) some aspects of the model are nearly universally accepted (solid arrows, Fig. 1) (Smith, 1980; Smith *et al.*, 1980; Anderson *et al.*, 1979; Larsson, 1981; Larsson and Coutinho, 1979; Larsson *et al.*, 1980; Wagner and Rollinghoff, 1978). TCGF secretion and receptor expression require antigen presentation to T cells in a major histocompatibility complex (MHC)-restricted form. T cells recognizing antigen in turn become responsive to a macrophage-derived lymphokine termed Interleukin-1 (IL-1). A specific membrane receptor for IL-1 (Gillis and Mizel, 1981) is depicted in Fig. 1, although its existence has not yet been formally demonstrated. Appropriate T cells that have interacted with both antigen and IL-1 are then triggered to synthesize and secrete TCGF (Smith, 1980). These same or other signals may be involved in the expression of TCGF receptors. Although some investigators have shown that cytotoxic/suppressor T cells as well as helper T cells can produce TCGF under appropriate conditions (Andrus *et al.*, 1981; Luger *et al.*, 1982; Meuer *et al.*, 1982; Glasebrook *et al.*, 1982), several studies at the single-cell level indicate that helper T cells are the major source of TCGF (Kelso and MacDonald, 1982; Ceredig *et al.*, 1982). Similarly, although helper, cytotoxic, and suppressor T cells have been grown in TCGF (Schreier *et al.*, 1980; Kurnick *et al.*, 1981), some investigators maintain that responding, receptor-positive cells are virtually all members of the cytotoxic/suppressor subclasses (Gullberg and Larsson, 1983).

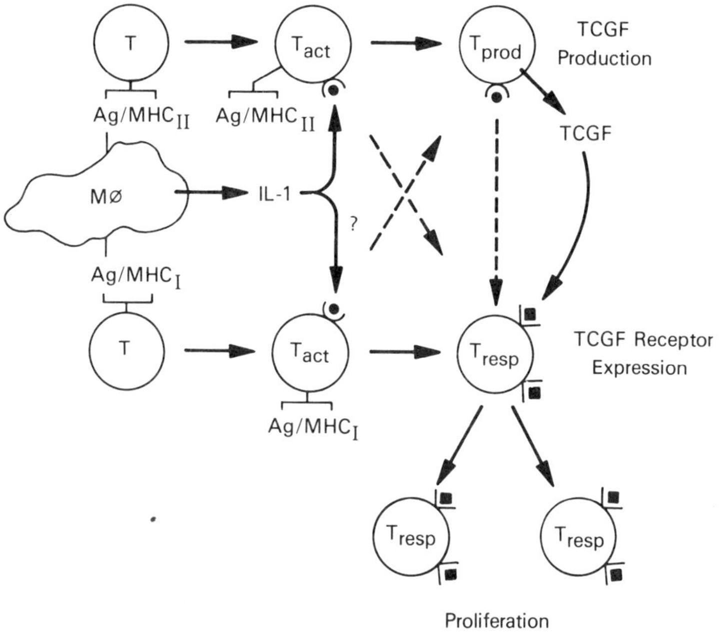

Figure 1. Model of lymphokine and receptor interactions involved in T-cell proliferation. MHC_I and MHC_{II} refer to type 1 and 2 antigens located in the major histocompatibility complex. Broken arrows signify that under some conditions T cells activated to MHC_I can become TCGF producers and those activated to MHC_{II} can become TCGF responders. In at least some instances, producer cells also express receptors and proliferate. Ag, antigen; MHC, major histocompatibility complex; TCGF, T-cell growth factor.

Irrespective of the details of cell types and numbers, T-cell proliferation depends on two basic requirements: a source of TCGF and the expression of receptors for the factor. The factor itself is antigen nonspecific; it will lead to proliferation of any receptor-positive T cell. The specificity of the immune system is instead maintained at the level of receptor expression. Only cells reactive with the particular antigen introduced will be rendered capable of responding to TCGF. The availability of TCGF and the expression of TCGF receptors are likely to be modulated in a number of ways:

1. Dissemination of secreted TCGF may be limited by the high affinity of the cellular receptor (Robb *et al.*, 1981). Thus, small amounts of the factor may be rapidly absorbed by nearby responding cells.
2. There is evidence of a serum inhibitor that could neutralize the factor as its concentration declines with dispersion (Hardt *et al.*, 1981).
3. TCGF is apparently rapidly cleared from the circulation by a non-T-cell mechanism(s) (Mühlradt and Opitz, 1981). Secretion may also be self-limiting if, as some believe (Larsson *et al.*, 1981; Gullberg and Larsson,

1983; Steinmann *et al.*, 1983), the producer cells do not normally respond and divide.

4. Secretion may also be downregulated by suppressor cells (Gullberg *et al.*, 1981; Gullberg and Larsson, 1982; Northoff *et al.*, 1980; Malkovsky *et al.*, 1982) and other mechanisms (Chouaib and Fradelizi, 1982).
5. Expression of TCGF receptors following stimulation is a transient phenomenon (Cantrell and Smith, 1983; Andrew *et al.*, 1984; Robb, 1984; Depper *et al.*, 1984). After the first few rounds of division, stimulation by antigen or lectin is necessary to elicit receptor reappearance (Andrew *et al.*, 1984).

The level of proliferation, and thus the degree of immunity, will depend on the interplay of all these parameters.

II. THE STRUCTURE OF TCGF–IMPLICATIONS FOR RECEPTOR INTERACTIONS

The availability of pure TCGF and a detailed description of its molecular structure are prerequisites for a complete understanding of the interaction of the factor with its cellular receptor. Efforts to purify TCGF were hampered for years both by the minute quantities secreted by stimulated normal peripheral blood cells and by the tendency of this hydrophobic protein to adsorb to various surfaces as its purity approached homogeneity. Two developments provided the key to overcoming these difficulties and made possible, within a very short period of time, the nearly total elucidation of the factor's structure.

The first development, by Gillis and Watson (1980), was the discovery that a human T-leukemia cell line, named Jurkat, was capable of releasing 100 times more TCGF after stimulation than normal lymphocytes. With this cell line, the preparation of milligram quantities of the factor became feasible (Robb, 1982a; Robb *et al.*, 1983a). As the amount of TCGF subjected to various purification steps increased, the adsorptive losses that had plagued early attempts rapidly became negligible. The first quantitative description of the interaction of TCGF with its cellular receptor was largely dependent on the exceptional productivity of the Jurkat line and the ease with which TCGF could be purified from the highly enriched cell supernatant (Robb *et al.*, 1981).

The second key development was the cloning of a cDNA corresponding to TCGF mRNA. This feat was first reported by Taniguchi *et al.* (1983) with cDNA prepared using stimulated Jurkat cells, and more recently by Devos *et al.* (1983) using stimulated human splenocytes. Together with protein sequence information obtained from purified TCGF, the cDNA data provided the primary amino acid sequence of the entire molecule. Moreover, restriction enzyme mapping of genomic DNA from various cell types indicated only a single copy of the structural gene for the factor (Maeda *et al.*, 1983; Seigal *et al.*, 1984). Thus, the potential for distinct forms of TCGF, each acting on different T-cell subsets, was finally eliminated.

All that remained to be examined was the extent, if any, to which posttranslational modification of the polypeptide chain occurred.

The structure of TCGF, depicted in Fig. 2 using an arbitrary folding pattern, provides the basis for description of the interaction of the factor and its receptor in molecular terms. Each of the 133 amino acids predicted by the cDNA data has been confirmed by automated Edman degradation of isolated peptides (Robb *et al.*, 1984). The molecule has three crysteine residues. Quantitative reduction and alkylation experiments indicate that two of the three cysteines (positions #58 and #105) form an intramolecular disulfide bridge which is important for maintaining a biologically active conformation of the molecule (Robb *et al.*, 1983a; Robb *et al.*, 1984).

Extensive data also exist concerning posttranslational modification of the molecule. Several laboratories have demonstrated heterogeneity in the size and charge of human TCGF prepared from normal cells and from the Jurkat cell line

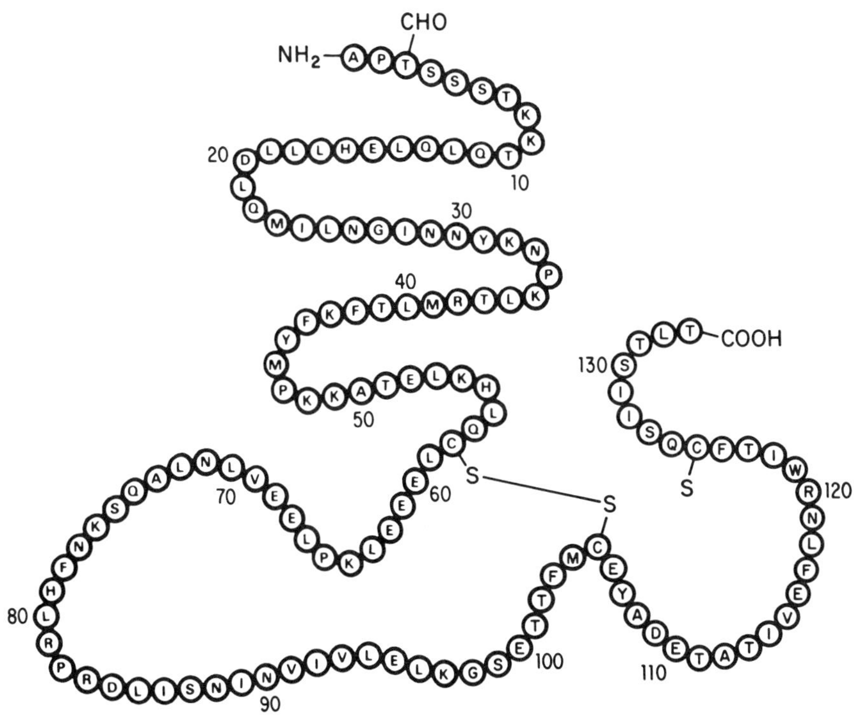

Figure 2. Amino acid sequence of the TCGF molecule based on the cDNA data of Taniguchi *et al.* (1983). Each of the residues has been confirmed by automated protein sequence analysis of peptide fragments. As indicated, threonine #3 represents one known site of glycosylation. Cysteines (#58 and #105) form an intramolecular disulfide bridge. CHO, carbohydrate. Reprinted from Robb (1984), by permission of Elsevier Science Publishers B.U.

(Mier and Gallo, 1980; Gillis *et al.*, 1980; Robb and Smith, 1981; Welte *et al.*, 1982). For example, TCGF from normal cells was separated into three distinct major forms by isoelectric focusing (Robb and Smith, 1981). On the basis of experiments employing glycosidases, this heterogeneity appeared to be largely attributable to a variable sialic acid content. A preliminary indication (Robb and Smith, 1981) that the carbohydrate was attached via asparagine, however, was erroneous, since no appropriate site for such modification exists in the primary sequence. This fact, together with difficulties in demonstrating binding of the molecule to lectin columns (Mier and Gallo, 1980; Robb and Smith, 1981), raised doubts about the existence of covalently linked carbohydrate. Recent sequence data, however, indicate that TCGF from Jurkat cells is often modified at the third residue in the polypeptide chain (Robb *et al.*, 1983a). Compositional analysis and mass spectrometry of the NH_2-terminal tryptic octapeptide demonstrates that one form of this modification is the addition of a single residue of *O*-linked *N*-acetyl-*D*-galactosamine while another form involves the attachment of *N*-acetyl galactosamine, hexose, and sialic acid (Robb *et al.*, 1983b; Robb *et al.*, 1984). In addition to glycosylation, some investigators suggested that other types of modification might contribute to the unexpectedly high hydrophobicity of the molecule (Henderson *et al.*, 1983). No evidence for such modification, however, was found using Jurkat-derived TCGF (Robb *et al.*, 1984).

Now that TCGF is available in a pure form and its structure is largely known, future research is likely to concentrate on defining the site(s) involved in the molecule's bioactivity. One approach to this problem involves modification of particular components of the factor. To the extent that the carbohydrate component could be removed enzymatically, it did not appear necessary for *in vitro* bioactivity (Robb and Smith, 1981). Moreover, the presence of various amounts of sialic acid had only a marginal effect on the factor's high-affinity binding to its cellular receptor (Robb *et al.*, 1981). A similar conclusion concerning the apparent lack of involvement of posttranslational modification is suggested by the potent bioactivity of the *Escherichia coli*-expressed product (Devos *et al.*, 1983). In the latter case, however, a direct comparative investigation of specific activities of bacterial and mammalian products remains to be performed. In contrast to the experience with the carbohydrate, generalized modification of amino acids by various reactions (e.g., lactoperoxidase and chloroglycoluril iodination, Bolton–Hunter reagent, carbodiimide) usually resulted in partial or total loss of activity, suggesting that if a limited and specific modification could be made, it would aid in defining the active site of the molecule.

Another approach to finding the active site(s) is examination of fragments of molecule for bioactivity or binding to the receptor. Although cleavage of TCGF by a number of proteolytic and chemical means has thus far failed to generate an active fragment (R. J. Robb, unpublished data), the amino acid sequence will be useful in repeating this type of analysis using synthetic peptides. Finally, a number of monoclonal antibodies have been prepared against TCGF (Gillis *et al.*, 1981; Stadler *et al.*, 1982; Robb *et al.*, 1983; Robb and Lin, 1984), some of which directly block bioactivity and receptor binding. Mapping of their binding sites should provide clues to the site of receptor recognition.

III. INTERACTION OF TCGF WITH ITS CELLULAR RECEPTOR

A. Radiolabeled TCGF Binding Assay

The first evidence for the existence of a receptor for TCGF came from studies of cellular absorption of the biological activity (Bonnard *et al.*, 1979; Smith *et al.*, 1979; Coutinho *et al.*, 1979). Lectin or alloantigen-activated T cells, but not unstimulated T cells or a variety of non-T cells, were capable of removing TCGF bioactivity from crude conditioned medium. In addition, the absorbed factor could be recovered from the cells in an active form by treatment with an acidic buffer (Gootenberg *et al.*, 1981).

Although such experiments were suggestive of a cell membrane receptor, it was not until a highly purified, radiolabeled TCGF became available that a quantitative description of the interaction could emerge (Robb *et al.*, 1981). A particularly high-producing subclone of the Jurkat line made possible the preparation of biosynthetically labeled factor of reasonably high specific radioactivity (20×10^6 dpm/μg), as well as its purification to homogeneity by gel filtration and isoelectric focusing. Using this material, Robb and co-workers demonstrated that TCGF-dependent cells rapidly bound the factor in a saturable manner. The receptors possessed a high affinity for TCGF (apparent $K_d \sim 10^{-11}$-10^{-12} M) and were present in relatively low numbers (5000–15,000 sites per cell as a population average). In fact, the number of high-affinity receptors originally reported (Robb *et al.*, 1981) may have been overestimated twofold due to a reliance on a particular protein assay that underestimated the specific activity of the labeled factor (Robb *et al.*, 1983). A survey of various cell types indicated that the binding was largely restricted to lectin or alloantigen-activated T cells, TCGF-dependent T-cell lines, and certain TCGF-independent T-cell lines. In fact, TCGF-dependent lines of the cytotoxic, suppressor, and helper phenotypes all expressed similar receptor capabilities (Robb, 1982b).

Typical binding curves of radiolabeled TCGF for human phytohemagglutinin (PHA)-blast cells and the HUT-102B2 cell line are illustrated in Fig. 3. The HUT-102 line was originally isolated from a lymph node of a patient with a cutaneous T-cell lymphoma by culturing cells in TCGF-containing medium (Poiesz *et al.*, 1980a). This T-cell line displays 2–5 times more receptor sites than the average

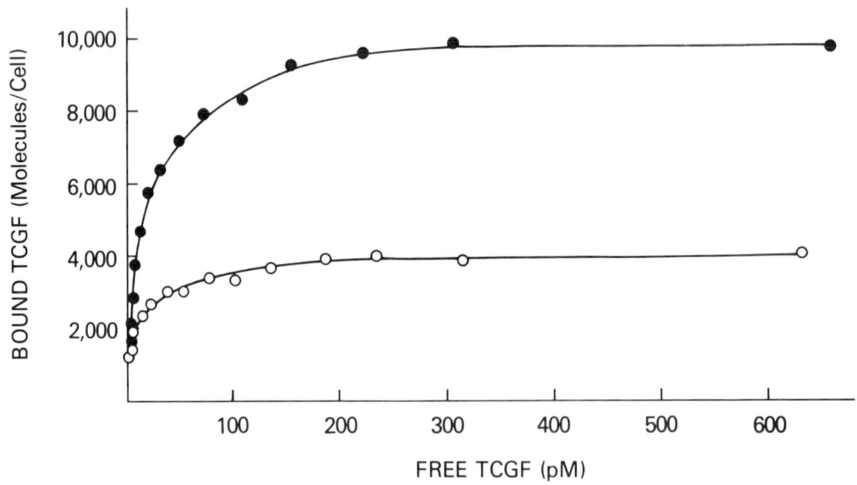

Figure 3. Curves of the high-affinity binding of [^{3}H]-Leu, Lys TCGF to HUT-102B2 (•) and 72-hr human PHA-blast cells (○). The assay was performed as previously described (Robb *et al.*, 1981) using biosynthetically radiolabeled TCGF (23.4 × 10^6 dpm/μg) purified on an immunoaffinity column (Robb *et al.*, 1983a).

PHA-blast cell and a similar affinity. Scatchard plots of such binding data generally formed straight lines (Robb *et al.*, 1981), suggesting that a single class of binding sites was present on each cell type. A combination of the high affinity of the receptor and the limited specific radioactivity of the TCGF ligand, however, made it impossible to measure binding accurately at concentrations much below the apparent dissociation constant. Thus, additional binding measurements at low TCGF concentrations are necessary to determine if extrapolation of the Scatchard plots was justified. Another shortcoming of the original analysis was that it employed low concentrations of radiolabeled TCGF. Although the high-affinity receptors thus detected are probably responsible for the physiological response (Section III.C), the original assay would have failed to detect exceptionally low-affinity receptors. In fact, recent preliminary experiments, employing high levels of radiolabeled TCGF, indicate that there may indeed be a pool of such low-affinity binding sites (Section IV.B.).

B. Postbinding Fate of TCGF

Early observations indicated that, after binding to the high-affinity receptor, the factor went through a degradative process that was sensitive to the lysomotropic agents, NH_4Cl and chloroquine (Robb *et al.*, 1981). As cell surface-bound ligand can often be dissociated by a brief treatment with low pH (Haigler *et al.*, 1980; Olefsky and Kao, 1982), a similar technique was employed for TCGF (Robb and Lin, 1984). When the binding of radiolabeled TCGF was carried out at 0°C to prevent internalization, virtually all the cell-bound factor could be recovered in an intact form using a 30-sec treatment at pH 4. The viability of the cells (murine TCGF-dependent line, human PHA-blast cells) was only marginally lowered. When the cells with surface-bound TCGF were warmed to 37°C in the presence of chloroquine, the fraction of labeled factor that could be eluted gradually declined. Assuming that, as with other polypeptide factors (Olefsky and Kao, 1982), this process represented internalization, the half-time of entry into the cell was about 25–30 min. A similar approach was used to examine TCGF degradation. Cells with bound factor were warmed to 37°C in the absence of chloroquine, and aliquots were sequentially removed for measurement of the TCA precipitability of radiolabeled factor. There was a lag period of about 30 min, during which the factor remained intact, followed by a gradual conversion ($T_{1/2} \sim 80$ min) to a TCA-soluble form. The time courses of internalization and degradation of labeled TCGF (high-affinity receptors only) were similar to those of other polypeptide factors and hormones (Olefsky and Kao, 1982; Hizuka *et al.*, 1981; Gorden *et al.*, 1978).

Another postbinding event commonly observed with other polypeptide growth factors is the stimulation of tyrosine-specific (auto-) phosphorylation of their receptors (Ushiro and Cohen, 1980; Ek *et al.*, 1982; Zick *et al.*, 1983). Repeated attempts have been made, using whole cells and solubilized membranes, to induce phosphorylation of the TCGF receptor with exogenous TCGF (W. C., Greene, unpublished data; R. J., Robb, unpublished data). Although the experiments were hampered by the relatively low level of receptors and potential complications from endogenous TCGF, no evidence of inducible phosphorylation of the 55,000 M_r receptor protein was detected (but see Section V.B). Nevertheless, TCGF might induce phosphorylation of an as yet undetected subunit of the receptor if the receptor consists of a molecular complex.

C. Role of TCGF in the Cell Cycle: Physiological Significance of High-Affinity Binding

Several lines of evidence indicate that the signal provided by TCGF for T-cell proliferation is delivered in the late G_1 phase of the cell cycle. After stimulation with lectins, TCGF and the ability to absorb TCGF bioactivity were first detected once the cells had entered the late G_1 phase (Stadler *et al.*, 1981). Actual utilization of the factor appeared to occur as the cells progressed from G_1 to S. TCGF clearly played a crucial role in this transition, since removal of the factor caused an arrest of the activated cells at the G_1/S interphase (Maizel *et al.*, 1981; Sekaly *et al.*, 1982; Walker *et al.*, 1983; R. L. Brown *et al.*, 1982). Readdition of TCGF to these cells resulted in S phase entry after a 10–12-hr lag period. Furthermore, the proportion of cells making the transition was dependent on the TCGF concentration (Sekaly *et al.*, 1982). Recently, Neckers and Cossman (1983) demonstrated that the interaction of TCGF with its cellular receptor during G_1 phase caused the induction of receptors for transferrin. The subsequent binding of transferrin by these cells was an obligatory step for the initiation of DNA synthesis. Thus, the binding of TCGF to its receptor appears to be only one of a series of signals involved in triggering the proliferative response in T cells.

Two pieces of evidence indicate that the high-affinity receptor sites originally detected using radiolabeled TCGF are responsible for mediating the physiological response to the factor, i.e., entry into the S phase. First, the apparent dissociation constant of the high-affinity binding was very close to the concentration of TCGF necessary to sustain proliferation, as measured by [^{3}H]thymidine incorporation. Further, maximal TCGF induced proliferation occurred at a factor concentration at which the high-affinity receptors were nearly saturated. Of course, the precise relationship of the proliferative and receptor binding phenomena is determined by the role of any second messenger involved in transmitting the signal of ligand binding (Strickland and Loeb, 1981). Considering the intermediary role of the transferrin receptor (Neckers and Cossman, 1983), the dissociation constants of a number of processes and potential second messengers are likely to be important in the juxtaposition of the TCGF binding and cellular proliferation curves.

A second piece of evidence that the high-affinity binding is physiologically significant comes from studies employing monoclonal antibodies. A murine monoclonal antibody prepared to Jurkat-derived TCGF was found to directly block the *in vitro* bioactivity of TCGF derived from lectin-stimulated Jurkat cells, normal human lymphocytes, murine splenocytes, and a gibbon ape cell line, MLA-144 (R. Robb, 1984). Excess TCGF could overcome the effect of the antibody, suggesting that the inhibition was due to blockade of receptor binding. Indeed, addition of the antibody to the receptor binding assay showed that the antibody directly inhibited the binding of labeled TCGF in a dose-dependent manner. In fact, antibody concentration curves for inhibition of proliferation and receptor binding, using the same amount of TCGF, were essentially identical (Robb and Lin, 1984). Similar data have been derived using the anti-Tac (T-cell activation antigen) antibody, which is directed toward the receptor rather than the growth factor. Inhibition of cellular proliferation for TCGF-dependent cells occurred at an anti-Tac antibody concentration (Depper *et al.*, 1983a) close to that needed to block high-affinity TCGF binding (Robb and Greene, 1983). Thus, the high-affinity binding of TCGF, which each antibody blocked directly, was apparently responsible for the physiological effect.

IV. MONOCLONAL ANTIBODIES TO THE TCGF RECEPTOR

A. Preparation of Antibodies to the Receptor

The radiolabeled TCGF binding assay provided a means to detect receptors, estimate their number and relative affinity, and examine the fate of the factor after receptor interaction. It also proved useful for quantitation of the level of unlabeled TCGF (Robb *et al.*, 1981) and for testing analogs of the factor. The method was limited, however, by the fact that the number of receptors measured represented an average for the whole cell population. It thus gave no information on the variability of receptor expression or the presence of positive and negative subpopulations. The latter shortcoming was particularly troublesome in trying to determine whether non-T-cell populations possessed low levels of receptor, as it was difficult to eliminate the potential for small numbers of contaminating, receptor-positive T cells. The ideal tool for overcoming the limitations of the TCGF binding assay would be a monoclonal antibody specific for the receptor. Within a remarkably short period of time, several such antibodies, reacting with TCGF receptors from different species, have been identified. These antibodies have provided the key to the rapid structural characterization of the receptor and to the detection of the receptor in complex populations of normal and neoplastic cells (see Sections V and VII).

The first report of a monoclonal antibody to the TCGF receptor described an antibody, termed anti-Tac, that was prepared by immunization of mice with a TCGF-dependent, human T-cell line (Uchiyama *et al.*, 1981). The antibody reacted with a portion of normal human T cells that had been activated by lectins or alloantigen, but not with resting T cells, B cells, or monocytes. In discussing their results, Uchiyama and co-workers suggested that the receptor for TCGF was one candidate for the molecule recognized by anti-Tac. Direct evidence for anti-Tac recognition of the TCGF receptor was then provided by Leonard *et al.* (1982), who demonstrated that the antibody could block the binding of radiolabeled TCGF to receptor-positive cells and directly inhibit the proliferative response of TCGF-dependent cells. Similar supporting data were independently provided by Miyawaki *et al.* (1982), who demonstrated the ability of anti-Tac to block absorption of TCGF bioactivity. The anti-Tac antibody was capable of reacting with the activated T-cells of human origin as well as cells from rhesus and marmoset monkeys and the gibbon ape. In contrast, the antibody did not react with activated cells of guinea pig, mouse, and rat origin. A second murine monoclonal antibody, termed B1-49.9 (prepared by B. Malissen and C. Mawas), also appears to recognize the human TCGF receptor (Cotner *et al.*, 1981, 1983). Like anti-Tac, B1-49.9 was found to inhibit TCGF bioactivity and radiolabeled TCGF and anti-Tac binding (W. C. Greene, and R. J. Robb, unpublished observations). Recently, two additional antibodies were described that appear to react with the receptor on rat and mouse cells. Osawa and Diamantstein (1983) immunized mice with phorbol ester-activated rat T cells and produced a monoclonal antibody specific for rat cells that was capable of blocking TCGF-dependent proliferation and absorption of bioactivity. Likewise, Malek *et al.* (1983) reported the preparation of a rat monoclonal antibody against a TCGF-dependent murine cell line that blocked proliferation of activated murine T cells. The antibody was relatively ineffective in directly blocking the binding of radiolabeled TCGF to receptor-positive cells. Nevertheless, it was capable of binding a noncovalent complex formed between detergent-solubilized receptor and radiolabeled factor. The molecular characteristics of the putative murine receptor were similar to those of the human receptor recognized by anti-Tac (see Section V).

B. Demonstration That Anti-Tac Recognizes the Human TCGF Receptor

The demonstration that the anti-Tac antibody blocked the binding of radiolabeled TCGF to receptor-positive cells (Leonard *et al.*, 1982) provided a strong indication that the Tac antigen represented the TCGF receptor. The antibody was shown to bind a glycoprotein of 47,000-53,000 M_r (termed p50) as well as one or two minor components from detergent-solubilized, biosynthetically radiolabeled cells of the HUT-102B2 cell line. In normal PHA-activated lymphoblasts, anti-Tac reacted with a slightly larger glycoprotein with an M_r of 52,000–58,000 (Leonard *et al.*, 1983b). However, it was not clear as to which component(s) actually contained a TCGF binding site or whether these molecules were simply associated with the TCGF receptor on the cell surface.

Two experimental approaches have since been used to demonstrate directly that the p50 Tac glycoprotein contains a TCGF binding site. In the first approach, Leonard *et al.* (1983a) chemically crosslinked and surface-iodinated cellular proteins after the cells (HUT-102B2) had been incubated with TCGF. In crosslinked samples, anti-Tac bound both the expected p50 component (uncrosslinked) plus a molecule that was 12,000–14,000 daltons larger. The larger molecule was also bound by monoclonal antibodies to TCGF and thus appeared to consist of a crosslinked complex of p50 and TCGF. In the second approach (Robb and Greene, 1983), radiolabeled cellular proteins from PHA-blasts were incubated with affinity supports coupled with either anti-Tac antibody or TCGF. Both supports bound molecules of identical size (Fig. 4), suggesting that the Tac antigen actually interacted directly with TCGF. More importantly, Robb and Greene (1983) demonstrated that incubation of the mixture of cellular proteins with either the TCGF-coupled support or the anti-Tac-coupled support effectively removed molecules reactive with the alternative support (Table I). Thus,

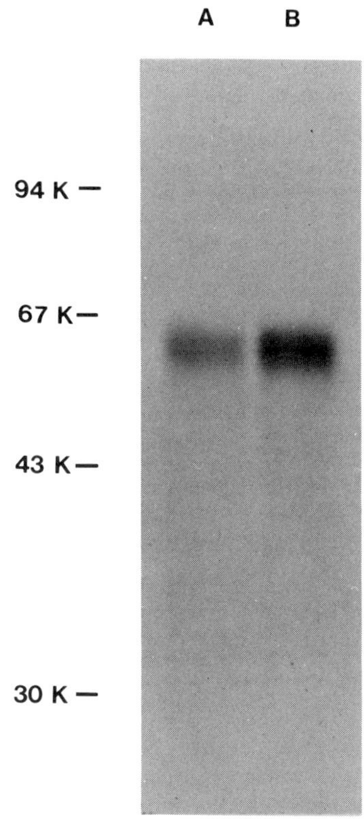

Figure 4. SDS-PAGE (8.75% acrylamide, with 2-mercaptoethanol) analysis of ^{35}S-methionine-labeled cellular proteins (solubilized in NP-40) from human PHA-blast cells bound to TCGF-coupled Affigel (A) and anti-Tac-coupled Sepharose (B). The bands were visualized by fluorography. Negligible binding occurred with control-IgG-coupled Sepharose or Affigel.

Table 1. Sequential Binding of Radiolabeled Cellular Proteins to TCGF-Coupled Affigel and Anti-Tac-Coupled Sepharose[a, b]

	Incubation #1		Incubation #2		Incubation #3	
Sample	TCGF Affigel	Anti-Tac Sepharose	TCGF Affigel	Anti-Tac Sepharose	TCGF Affigel	Anti-Tac Sepharose
1	15,200 (79)	–	3,100 (16)	–	–	900 (5)
2	–	20,100 (96)	–	580 (3)	350 (1)	–

[a]Two identical samples of NP-40-solubilized molecules from [^{3}H] glucosamine-labeled PHA-blast cells were sequentially incubated with TCGF-Affigel and/or anti-Tac-Sepharose. The results are given in disintegrations per minute ^{3}H-radiolabel and percentage (in parentheses) of the total bound radiolabel.

[b]From Robb and Greene (1983), by permission of the *Journal of Experimental Medicine*, Rockefeller University Press.

under the particular conditions used, all anti-Tac-reactive molecules appeared capable of binding TCGF, and the ability to bind TCGF was limited to the Tac protein.

Although the 47,000–53,000-M_r (HUT-102B2; 52,000–58,000 M_r on PHA-blasts) component appeared to contain a TCGF binding site, some discrepancies remained between measurements of anti-Tac binding and the high-affinity binding measured with radiolabeled TCGF. For example, although PHA-blasts and HUT-102B2 cells, on the average, were capable of binding about 60,000 and 200,000 molecules of anti-Tac, respectively (Depper *et al.*, 1983b and unpublished data), they had only about 4000 (PHA-blasts) and 10,000 (HUT-102B2) high-affinity sites for TCGF (Fig. 3). In addition, although the ratio of anti-Tac binding to high-affinity TCGF binding was reasonably similar for some cell types, it was markedly different for others (R. J. Robb, L. O. Gehman, F. S. Ligler, and M. Schlam unpublished observations). Finally, whereas a 50-fold molar excess of anti-Tac was required to reduce high-affinity TCGF binding by one-half (Robb and Greene, 1983), a similar excess of TCGF was necessary to block anti-Tac binding (Leonard *et al.*, 1983a). Thus, in one case, TCGF appeared to have a higher affinity for the receptor, while in the other case, the antibody, anti-Tac, seemed to have the higher affinity.

Several explanations could account for some or all of the discrepancies in the two assays for the TCGF receptor:

Model 1. Involvement of Fc receptors could have led to an overestimation of anti-Tac binding. This possibility was ruled out, however, in binding assays using radiolabeled Fab fragments of the antibody.

Model 2. The number of high-affinity receptors for TCGF could have been underestimated due to occupancy by endogenously produced TCGF. This possibility was also largely eliminated by washing the cells at pH 4 before performing the radiolabeled TCGF assay (Section II.B.).

Model 3. The discrepancies could arise if there are two or more classes of TCGF receptors having markedly different affinities. Just such a multiplicity of affinities was recently reported for the receptor for epidermal growth factor on epidermoid carcinoma cells (Kawamota *et al.*, 1983). If such is the case for the TCGF receptor, the original binding assay, which was performed at picomolar levels of TCGF, would not have detected low-affinity binding sites. By contrast, anti-Tac might recognize the same epitope on each receptor class. Differences in the ratio of high- and low-affinity sites between different cell types would then explain the variation in the ratio of anti-Tac and high-affinity TCGF binding. Likewise, an excess of anti-Tac would be needed to block the high-affinity TCGF binding sites, while an excess of TCGF would be needed to block anti-Tac binding to the low-affinity receptors. Although this model is only hypothetical, preliminary results (R. J. Robb, unpublished data) of binding assays with very high TCGF concentrations (20–200 nM) indicates the presence of a sizable pool of potential receptor sites having an affinity 1,000–2,000 times lower than that of the high-affinity sites originally detected (Robb *et al.*, 1981). Further analysis will be necessary to determine if such receptor sites are genuine or an artifact of the assay methodology and what role, if any, they may play in the physiological response to TCGF. With respect to the latter point, the extremely high levels of TCGF necessary for low-affinity binding are unlikely to occur *in vivo*. Moreover, the relationship of these binding sites to the Tac protein remains to be determined.

V. BIOCHEMICAL CHARACTERIZATION OF THE HUMAN TCGF RECEPTOR

A. Presence of Intrachain Disulfide Bonding

Both anti-Tac and TCGF, covalently linked to bead supports, specifically reacted with a 52,000–58,000-M_r protein p55 from PHA-activated T lymphoblasts (Robb and Greene, 1983) (see Section IV.B and in Fig. 4). When the electrophoretic analysis was instead performed under nonreducing conditions, this protein migrated with an apparent M_r of 47,000–52,000 (Leonard *et al.*, 1983a). This difference suggested the presence of intrachain disulfide bonding, with reduction leading to greater protein unfolding and slower migration. Intact disulfide bonding appeared to be required for recognition of the receptor by anti-Tac. This was indicated by the finding that electrophoretic separation of cellular proteins and transfer to nitrocellulose by Western blotting (Towbin *et al.*, 1979; Burnette, 1981) was followed by reaction between anti-Tac and the TCGF receptor only if the initial electrophoresis was performed under nonreducing conditions (Leonard *et al.*, 1983b).

Although the Tac protein was clearly not linked to other molecules via disulfide bridges, noncovalent association with additional subunits has not been ruled out. Indeed, two other proteins, of 113,000 and 180,000 M_r, often appeared as minor components of anti-Tac immunoprecipitates and may be part of a receptor complex. In addition, p55 always migrated as a broad band on sodium dodecylsulfate-polyacrylamide gel electrophoresis (SDS-PAGE), raising the question of whether it represented multiple subunits. Although the latter possibility has not been eliminated, it seems unlikely, since amino acid sequence analysis suggests that p55 has a single amino-terminal sequence (W. J. Leonard, S. Rudikoff, and W. C. Greene, unpublished data).

B. Posttranslational Processing of the Receptor

Pulse-chase labeling studies employing [^{35}S]methionine were used to investigate potential precursor forms of the mature TCGF receptor (Leonard *et al.*, 1983a). As shown schematically in Fig. 5, the TCGF receptor appeared to be composed of a 33,000-dalton polypeptide chain (p33) that was sequentially processed to a densely glycosylated, sulfated, and phosphorylated mature form. Initially, p33 was modified by *N*-linked glycosylation, yielding two slightly larger glycoprotein precursors of 35,000 and 37,000 M_r, p35 and p37, respectively. This transition was due to the addition of *N*-linked carbohydrate, as indicated by tunicamycin blockade of the conversion of p33 to p35/p37 and endoglycosidase F digestion of p35/p37 to p33. The transition of p33 to p35 or p37 occurred very rapidly, since p33 was normally (in the absence of tunicamycin) undetectable after very short labeling periods (5 min). After approximately 30–60 min of chase, p35/p37 disappeared, concomitant with the appearance of the mature 55,000-dalton receptor (p55, Leonard *et al.*, 1983a). This large saltatory increase in receptor size involved the introduction of *O*-linked sugars and addition of sialic acid. Digestion of p55 with neuraminidase produced a 4000–6000-dalton decrease in receptor size indicating the addition of sialic acid. In contrast, the migrations of p35 and p37 were not altered by neuraminidase digestion. The presence of *O*-linked sugars on p55 was indirectly demonstrated by a progressive decline in receptor size following sequential digestion with endoglycosidase F (removal of *N*-linked sugars) and neurmaminidase (removal of sialic acid). Thus, these data indicated that some of the sialic acid resided on non-*N*-linked (presumably *O*-linked) carbohydrate structures.

Processing of the TCGF receptor was also studied using the carboxylic ionophore, monensin, which appears to interfere with Golgi-associated, posttranslational modification of protein (Tartakoff *et al.*, 1977, Strous and Lodish, 1980; Jacobs *et al.*, 1983; M. S. Brown *et al.*, 1983). Treatment of T lymphoblasts with noncytotoxic concentrations of monensin (10^{-5}–10^{-6} M) produced an accumulation of p37 in the absence of detectable amounts of p35 or p55. These data suggested that late processing of the receptor (p37 to p55) occurred in the Golgi apparatus and that p35 was probably processed to p37 before being converted to p55. Although *O*-linked glycosylation and sialic acid addition were involved in the conversion of p37 to p55, a covalent association of a second protein with p37, perhaps by transglutamination (Folk, 1980), has not been completely excluded.

In addition to glycosylation, the TCGF receptor was found to be modified by posttranslational sulfation (W. C. Greene, and W. J. Leonard, unpublished

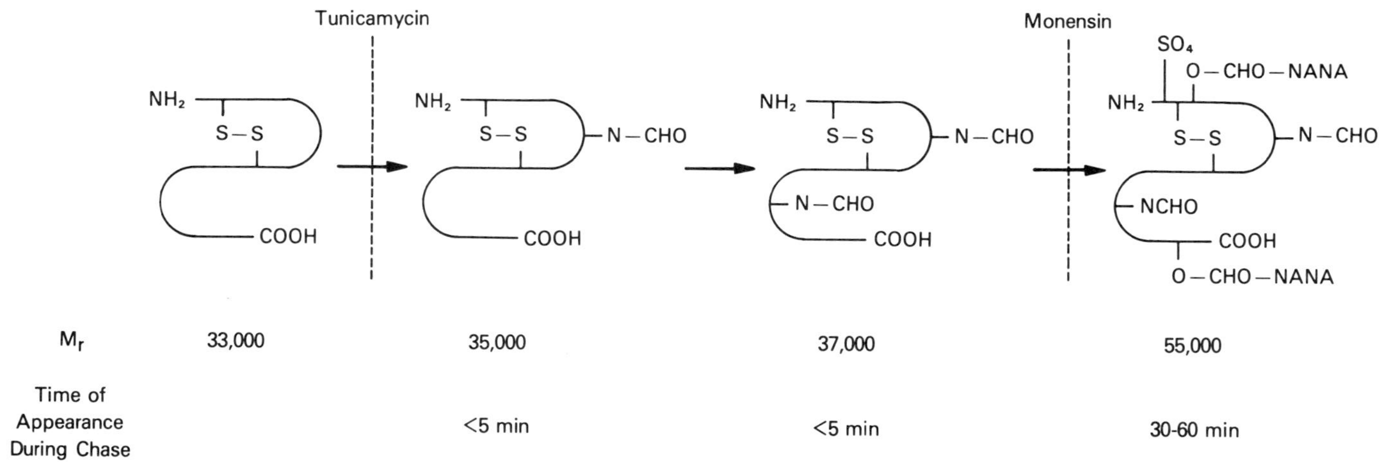

Figure 5. Schematic representation of posttranslational processing of the T-cell growth factor (TCGF) receptor. Apparent size (M_r) and time of appearance of each precursor during the chase period are indicated. Dotted lines indicate proposed sites of drug inhibition of processing.

data). It is not yet known, however, at what processing step the sulfate group(s) was introduced or where this modification(s) occured on the molecule. In recent studies, phosphorylation of the TCGF receptor has also been demonstrated (W. J. Leonard, J. M. Depper, and W. C. Greene, unpublished observations). Convincing evidence for induction of receptor phosphorylation by TCGF, however, has not yet been obtained, nor have the phosphorylated amino acids been identified. In contrast to the transferrin receptor (Omary and Trowbridge, 1981), the TCGF receptor did not appear to be covalently associated with palmitic acid.

Recently, we demonstrated that TCGF also binds to the precursor forms (p33, p35, and p37) of the mature TCGF receptor (R. J. Robb, and W. C. Greene, unpublished data). Thus while extensive post-translational modifications of this receptor occur, these events are not obligate requirements for recognition of the receptor by TCGF or anti-Tac. Nevertheless, posttranslational processing may alter the affinity of the receptor–ligand interaction.

Despite their capacity to recognize unglycosylated precursors of the mature receptor, anti-Tac, B1-49.9, and combinations of these antibodies were unable to immunoprecipitate the primary translation product of the TCGF receptor in either the rabbit reticulocyte or wheat germ lysate cell-free translation systems (W. J. Leonard, and W. C. Greene, unpublished data). Precipitation of a primary translation product with an M_r of 34,500 was achieved however, using a rabbit heteroantiserum prepared by immunization with the mature receptor protein purified on an anti-Tac immunoaffinity column. Since the nonglycosylated TCGF receptor precursor has a M_r of 33,000, these data are consistent with a 1500-dalton signal peptide for this protein.

VI. IMMUNOREGULATORY EFFECTS OF ANTI-TAC

Depper and colleagues (1983a) studied the effects of anti-Tac on antigen- and mitogen-activated *in vitro* responses of normal human T and B cells. These workers demonstrated that anti-Tac blocked >80% of the T-cell proliferation that occurred in response to soluble, autologous, and allogeneic antigens. Furthermore, anti-Tac inhibition of antigen-induced proliferation was reversed by the addition of purified TCGF. As anti-Tac was not found to inhibit endogenous TCGF production (Depper *et al.*, 1983a), this result suggested that the antibody functioned by competition with TCGF for receptor binding. Anti-Tac also partially blocked proliferation induced with concanavalin A (Con A), pokeweed mitogen (PWM), and PHA. Furthermore, anti-Tac abrogated the maturation of cytotoxic T cells in allogeneic cell cocultures (Depper *et al.*, 1983a) and the *in vitro* induction of suppressor T cells by Con A (T. A. Waldmann, unpublished data) but had no effect on the effector function of mature cells of such subclasses. Abo *et al.* (1983) extended the analysis by demonstrating that anti-Tac blocked the TCGF induced proliferation of a subpopulation of NK cells which expressed T-cell-associated antigens (Leu 4, sheep erythrocyte rosette receptor).

Pokeweed mitogen-activated B-cell immunoglobulin synthesis was also inhibited by anti-Tac (Depper *et al.*, 1983a). As stimulation of B cells with pokeweed mitogen requires the presence of helper T cells (Broder *et al.*, 1976; Keightly *et al.*, 1976), it was unclear whether anti-Tac interfered with helper T-cell function or acted directly on B cells. In contrast, anti-Tac did not block proliferation or immunoglobulin (Ig) production by purified B cells activated with Epstein-Barr virus, a helper T-cell-independent activator of human B cells (Kirchner *et al.*, 1979). Although these findings together suggested that anti-Tac functioned by abrogating T-cell help, an interaction of anti-Tac with receptors expressed on human B cells has not been excluded (see Section VII.C). In fact, Waldmann and colleagues recently obtained data indicating that normal B cells can be induced to express receptors recognized by anti-Tac.

Depper and associates (1983b) also defined the time course of TCGF receptor expression after activation of normal peripheral blood T cells with PHA. In [^{3}H]anti-Tac-binding assays, receptor expression was detected within 6–8 hr after addition of PHA. Using flow microfluorometry, Cotner and co-workers (1983) described a similar time course of receptor expression using both monoclonal anti-Tac and B1-49.9. Neckers and Cossman (1983) reported that TCGF receptors are expressed before the appearance of receptors for transferrin and that treatment of lymphocytes with anti-Tac blocked subsequent expression of transferrin receptors (Section III.C). Similarly, Tsudo and colleagues (1982) demonstrated that anti-Tac blocked later expression of Ia antigens in T cells activated with alloantigens. Thus, anti-Tac modulated a variety of *in vitro* normal immune responses dependent on the action of TCGF. All these data are consistent with the production of a functional blockade of the TCGF receptor by anti-Tac.

VII. TCGF RECEPTOR EXPRESSION ON NEOPLASTIC CELLS

Recently, we initiated studies evaluating TCGF receptor expression in varying human lymphoid malignancies. Although immature leukemic T lymphoblasts normally lacked TCGF receptors, some of these cells could be induced with phorbol diesters to display such receptors (Greene *et al.*, 1984). In addition, Waldmann and co-workers (1984) demonstrated that mature leukemic cells obtained from patients with adult T-cell leukemia (ATL) (Uchiyama *et al.*, 1977) expressed TCGF receptors recognized by anti-Tac. In contrast, a second leukemia of mature T cells, the Sézary syndrome (Broder *et al.*, 1976) was distinguished from ATL by the lack of TCGF receptor expression. A variety of B-cell malignancies were also studied, most of which were unreactive with anti-Tac.

Korsmeyer and colleagues (1983), however, demonstrated that virtually all hairy cell leukemias (HCLs) were B-cell malignancies and expressed surface receptors recognized by anti-Tac. Similarly, select Burkitt B-cell lymphoma lines specifically reacted with anti-Tac (W. C. Greene, W. J. Leonard, J. M. Depper, S. J. Korsmeyer, T. Uchiyama, and T. A. Waldmann, unpublished data). Studies of TCGF receptors in these lymphoproliferative disorders may provide critical insights into the structure and function of these receptors as well as contribute to a greater understanding of the biology of these human leukemias.

A. Induction of TCGF Receptor Expression in Human Acute Lymphocytic Leukemia

In general, the acute T-lymphocytic leukemias (T-ALLs) are composed of malignant expansions of immature T lymphoblasts that lack immunoregulatory function. Consistent with this stage of development, T-ALL cells did not normally express TCGF receptors. After activation with phorbol myristate acetate (PMA), 50 ng/ml (Nagasawa and Mak, 1980; Ryffel *et al.*, 1982) and phytohemagglutinin (PHA), 1 μg/ml, however, both Jurkat and HSB-2 T-ALL cells displayed surface determinants recognized by anti-Tac (Greene *et al.*, 1984). In contrast, PMA and PHA did not induce MOLT-4 and CEM T-ALL cells to express receptors recognized by anti-Tac.

In fluorescent-activated cell sorting analyses, uninduced Jurkat and HSB-2 cells did not bind anti-Tac. In contrast, following activation of these cells for 18 hr with PMA and PHA, >95% of the leukemic cells were stained with a combination of anti-Tac and goat anti-mouse immunoglobulin conjugated to fluorescein isothiocyanate. Staining of induced cells with second antibody alone produced a fluorescence profile essentially identical to that of uninduced cells. As shown in Fig. 6, similar results were obtained in [^{3}H]anti-Tac radioreceptor binding assays performed with uninduced and induced Jurkat or HSB-2 leukemic cells. Uninduced T-ALL cells did not bind significant amounts of [^{3}H]anti-Tac. After PMA and PHA induction, however, marked [^{3}H]anti-Tac binding occurred, and the binding of anti-Tac was blocked in a dose-related manner by purified TCGF.

The average number of receptors displayed on induced Jurkat cells was estimated by Scatchard analysis (Rodbard, 1973) of [^{3}H]anti-Tac binding. These studies indicated approximately 7000 receptors per cell and an apparent K_d of 1.65×10^{-9} M. This receptor number was 5- to 10-fold less than that obtained with PHA-activated T lymphoblasts (30,000–60,000 receptors per cell). Studies of the time course of [^{3}H]anti-Tac binding to Jurkat cells showed the presence of receptor expression as early as 6–8 hr after addition of PHA and PMA. A similar time course of receptor expression was obtained with normal lymphocytes activated with PHA (Depper *et al.*, 1983b). Furthermore, as with PHA-blast cells,

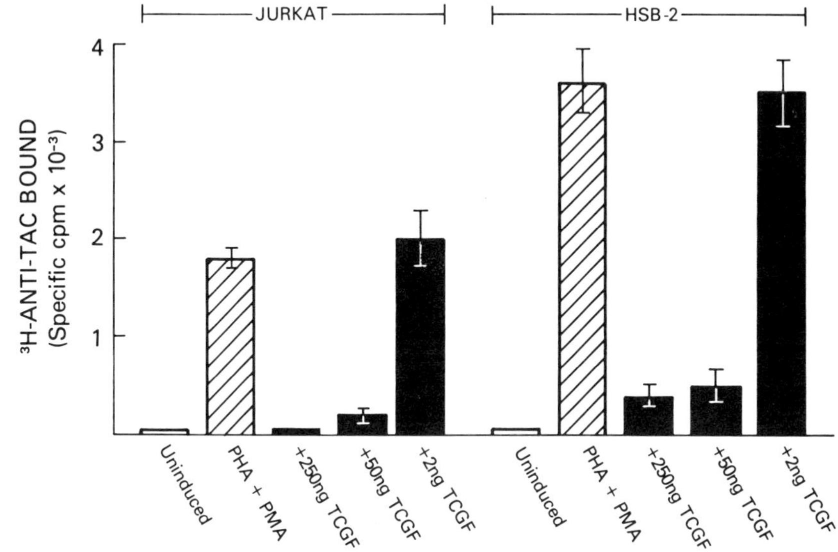

Figure 6. [^{3}H]-anti-Tac binding with uninduced and induced Jurkat and HSB-2 cells in the presence and absence of purified TCGF. Jurkat and HSB-2 cells were either used untreated or induced for 18 hr with PMA (50 ng/ml) and PHA (1 μg/ml). [^{3}H]-anti-Tac binding (10 ng/culture) with 1×10^6 cells in 200 μl binding medium (RPMI 1640, 10 mg/ml BSA, 1 mg/ml human IgG, 10 mM Hepes, pH 7.4) was measured in the presence or absence of varying quantities of immunoaffinity-purified TCGF (Robb *et al.*, 1983). Error bars indicate standard errors of the mean for triplicate determinations.

receptor induction was blocked by actinomycin D, suggesting a requirement for new mRNA synthesis.

TCGF receptors expressed by induced Jurkat and HSB-2 cells were further characterized by immunoprecipitation with anti-Tac and SDS-PAGE analysis. As expected, no receptors were identified with uninduced cells from either leukemia. After activation with PHA and PMA, receptors from both Jurkat and HSB-2 cells were detected. Although the HSB-2 receptors were similar in size to receptors present on PHA-activated T lymphoblasts, the Jurkat receptors were approximately 2000–3000 daltons smaller. As preliminary data suggested that Jurkat cells contained normal-size *N*-glycosylated receptor precursors (p35/p37), the apparent small difference in M_r may occur secondary to late receptor modifications involving the addition of *O*-linked carbohydrate and sialic acid.

Gillis and Watson (1980) reported that Jurkat cells could be induced with PMA and PHA to secrete large quantities of TCGF (see Section II). Similarly, Stadler and Oppenheim (1982) demonstrated PMA- and lectin-induced production of TCGF by HSB-2 cells. Since PMA and PHA also induced expression of

TCGF receptors in these cells, we studied the possibility that expression of the genes encoding both the growth factor and receptor was coordinately linked. To test this relationship, Jurkat cells were induced under varying conditions and the production of TCGF and receptors was measured (Greene *et al.*, 1984). As expected, dual induction with PHA and PMA induced marked TCGF secretion (100-200 U/ml) as well as TCGF receptor expression. In contrast, induction of Jurkat cells with PMA alone resulted in minimal TCGF secretion ($\leqslant$0.3 U/ml) but well-preserved TCGF receptor expression. Thus, induction of Jurkat leukemic cells with PMA alone largely uncoupled TCGF secretion and TCGF receptor expression, indicating that the genes encoding these proteins are not necessarily expressed in a coordinate manner.

B. TCGF Receptor Expression in Leukemias of Mature T Cells

Adult T-cell leukemia (ATL) (Uchiyama *et al.*, 1977; Catovsky *et al.*, 1982; Blaney *et al.*, 1983; Bunn *et al.*, 1983) and the Sézary syndrome (Broder *et al.*, 1976; Lutzner *et al.*, 1975; Broder and Bunn, 1980) each represent lymphoproliferative diseases involving mature T cells. These leukemic cells do not generally contain detectable terminal deoxynucleotidyl transferase, indicative of their mature state of differentiation (Bollum, 1979). A human type C retrovirus, human T-cell leukemia/lymphoma virus ($HTLV_I$), has been etiologically associated with ATL (Poiesz *et al.*, 1980b, 1981; Yoshida *et al.*, 1982; Gallo and Wong-Staal, 1982). In contrast, no virus has yet been identified in the Sézary syndrome.

Patients with these leukemias may be difficult to properly classify upon initial presentation. Select historical, epidemiological, and clinical features, however, often aid in the assignment of the correct diagnosis. Several salient features of the Sézary syndrome and adult T-cell leukemias are compared in Table II. Geographically, the Sézary syndrome occurs worldwide, whereas most recognized cases of ATL are clustered in discrete areas, including southwestern Japan, the Caribbean basin, and southeastern United States. With wider recognition and perhaps increased incidence of this disease, ATL is now being detected in other areas of the world as well.

The leukemic T cells in both diseases display an interesting tropism for skin. The Sézary syndrome is often associated with extensive epidermal infiltration (Pautrier's microabscesses), marked erythroderma, and exfoliation, whereas ATL often involves the dermis and may spare the epidermis. ATL, but not the Sézary syndrome, is frequently associated with a paraneoplastic syndrome consisting of hypercalcemia, osteolytic bone lesions, and histological evidence of osteoclast activation (Brigham *et al.*, 1982; Blaney *et al.*, 1983). The clinical progression of these diseases usually differs as well. The Sézary syndrome may follow a chronic, smoldering course, while ATL is often characterized by an acute illness with median survival of less than 1 year. ATL patients also frequently develop oppor-

Table II. Comparison of Two Human Mature T-Cell Leukemias

	Sèzary syndrome	Adult T-cell leukemia
Distribution	Worldwide	Clustered; (Japan, Caribbean Basin, Southeastern United States)
Viral association	?	$HTLV_I$[a]
Clinical course	Chronic	Acute, subacute
Skin involvement	Usually epidermis (Pautrier's microabscesses)	Usually dermis
Distinguishing clinical features	Marked erythroderma, exfoliation, pruritus	Hypercalcemia, osteolytic bone lesions
Cell-surface phenotype	$T3^+$, $T4^+$, $T8^-$	$T3^+$, $T4^+$, $T8^-$
Immunoregulatory function	Helper	Suppressor
Reactivity with anti-Tac	Negative	Positive

[a] Human T-leukemia/lymphoma virus, subclass I.

tunistic infections (*Pneumocystis carinii*, fungi, or protozoa) in the absence of severe leukopenia (Bunn *et al.*, 1983). The Sézary syndrome may respond to several forms of therapy, including topical alkylating agents, electron beam radiotherapy, and systemic chemotherapy. In contrast, while aggressive combination chemotherapy may produce remissions in ATL, these responses are often short lived, and recurrent disease is often resistant to further therapeutic interventions (Bunn *et al.*, 1983).

Waldmann and co-workers (1984) have compared the cell-surface phenotype of Sézary and ATL cells using monoclonal antibodies to various T-cell-associated antigens. Leukemic cells from both Sézary and ATL patients consistently expressed T3 and T4 antigens, but rarely T8 antigens. Despite the similar helper-inducer cell-surface phenotype, these leukemic cells displayed opposing immunoregulatory function in *in vitro* assays of immunoglobulin biosynthesis. As reported by Broder and colleagues (1976), Sézary leukemic cells often provided helper activity for Ig production by purified B cells. In contrast, ATL cells lacked helper cell function and often displayed potent suppressor function (Waldmann *et al.*, 1984).

The diagnosis of ATL may be secured by the detection in serum of circulating antibodies recognizing core protein determinants (p19, p24) of $HTLV_I$ (Kalyanaraman *et al.*, 1981; Robert-Guroff *et al.*, 1982) or by the demonstration of integrated $HTLV_I$ DNA sequences by liquid hybridization (Gallo *et al.*, 1982). However, these tests are neither widely available nor easily performed. Waldmann and colleagues (1984) recently demonstrated that ATL cells can be distinguished from Sézary leukemic cells by the presence of TCGF receptors.

Thus far, analysis of more than 20 long-term cultures of ATL cells has demonstrated uniform reactivity with anti-Tac. In contrast, Sézary leukemic cells from 9 of 10 patients studied did not express TCGF receptors. Furthermore, anti-Tac reactivity has been detected with all $HTLV_I$-transformed cord lymphocyte lines examined. Thus, anti-Tac provides a valuable clinical tool in the diagnosis of ATL.

Studies of [^{3}H]anti-Tac binding with $HTLV_I$-infected ATL cell lines have found high-level TCGF receptor expression by these cells (J. M. Depper, W. J. Leonard, and W. C. Greene, unpublished data). Three-day PHA-activated normal lymphoblasts express 30,000–60,000 TCGF receptors per cell measured by radiolabeled anti-Tac binding. In contrast, almost all ATL cells express greater than 200,000 receptors per cell. Tsudo and colleagues (1983) reported that anti-Tac fails to modulate TCGF receptors in ATL cells but will modulate these receptors on normal activated T cells. Thus a substantial increase in the level of receptor expression as well as diminished receptor mobility on the membrane are characteristic of ATL cells.

In addition to quantitative differences in TCGF receptor expression, some but not all ATL cells express aberrant forms of the TCGF receptor (Leonard *et al.*, 1983b). Shown in Fig. 7 are anti-Tac immunoprecipitates from the ATL T-cell line, HUT-102B2, and normal PHA-activated lymphoblasts labeled with [^{35}S]methionine. The HUT-102B2 receptor is approximately 5000 daltons smaller than the receptor present on PHA-blasts. Two-dimensional gel analysis (O'Farrell, 1975) showed a slightly more basic pI (5.5–6.0) for the HUT-102B2 receptor, as compared with the PHA-lymphoblast receptor (5.4–5.7) (Leonard *et al.*, 1983b). In studies addressing the molecular basis for this size difference, we found that HUT-102B2 cells contained the same p33, p35, and p37 receptor precursors present in normal activated T cells. Thus, the difference in receptor size was apparently generated during the late processing of p37 to the mature receptor. This processing involved addition of *O*-linked carbohydrate, sialic acid, and perhaps sulfate groups (see Section V.B). Preliminary evidence suggests that the HUT-102B2 receptors may be less heavily sulfated and sialylated than the normal PHA-lymphoblast receptor.

It is unclear whether the TCGF receptors uniformly present on ATL cells are involved in the malignant growth of these cells. Secretion of TCGF by ATL cells has been detected (Gootenberg *et al.*, 1981). The combined presence of growth factor and appropriate receptors could theoretically produce autocrine stimulation of uncontrolled growth. Interestingly, anti-Tac does not inhibit proliferation of ATL cells that grow in the absence of added exogenous TCGF. While these data are consistent with malignant growth by a mechanism independent of the TCGF–TCGF receptor axis, they do not necessarily exclude participation of this growth factor and its receptor. The affinity of TCGF for its receptor (Robb *et al.*, 1981) is approximately 100-fold greater than that for anti-Tac

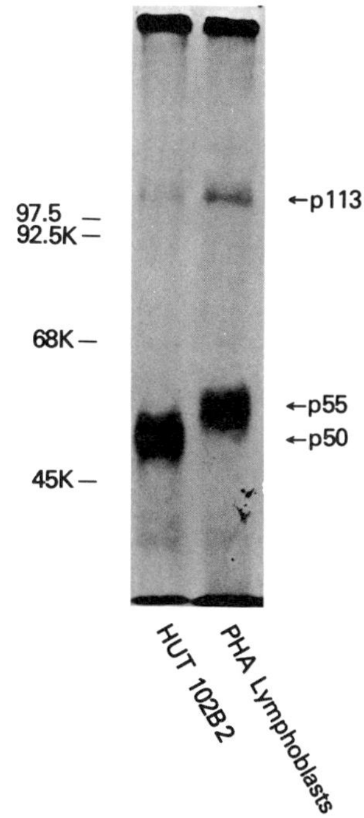

Figure 7. SDS-PAGE analysis of anti-Tac immunoprecipitations from ^{35}S-methionine-labeled HUT-102B2 cells and 72-hr PHA-activated lymphoblasts. Detergent-solubilized cellular proteins were immunoprecipitated with anti-Tac and Cowan I strain *Staphylococcus aureus* as described by Leonard *et al.* (1982). Migration of molecular weight standards is shown on the left. The position of the HUT-102B2 receptor (p50) and PHA-lymphoblast receptor (p55) is indicated. Also shown is p113, a protein routinely found in anti-Tac immunoprecipitations from ^{35}S-methionine-labeled cells, but not in surface iodinated cells.

binding (Depper *et al.*, 1983b). Thus, locally at the level of the membrane, secreted TCGF may compete successfully with anti-Tac for receptor binding sites. Furthermore, an intracellular interaction of TCGF with its receptor has not been excluded. Using cDNA probes specific for TCGF, production of TCGF mRNA by $HTLV_I$-infected T-cell lines found to grow independently of added growth factor was recently analyzed (Arya *et al.*, 1984). In many of these lines, transcription of TCGF mRNA has not been identified. Thus, these data argue against the autocrine model for malignant cell growth, but do not exclude an action of circulating TCGF *in vivo*. The possibility that the ATL receptor is activated by mechanisms independent of TCGF binding is a current focus of investigation.

Lando and co-workers (1983) recently demonstrated that the Tac antigen is not only expressed on the membrane of $HTLV_I$-infected cells, but is also present on the envelope of virions secreted by these cells. Using purified $HTLV_I$ virions, these investigators found that Tac antigen expression markedly exceeded that of other cell-surface markers, including Leu-1, HLA-Dr, T4, T9, and the sheep red blood cell rosette receptor. One interpretation of these findings is that the Tac antigen becomes associated with the virion during the viral budding process. In related studies, two monoclonal antibodies against partially-purified baboon endogenous virus were shown to react with the cellular receptor for that virus

(Cogniaux *et al.*, 1982). Furthermore, specific cell-surface binding sites for enveloped viruses, as visualized by electron microscopy, were shown to frequently occur at or near sites of virus budding (Miyamoto and Gilden, 1971). These data suggest the interesting possibility that the TCGF receptor may serve as a cellular receptor for $HTLV_I$ binding, although other mechanisms accounting for the uniform presence of TCGF receptors in $HTLV_I$-infected cells are also possible. Viral integration associated with appropriate promoter insertion could activate the gene encoding the TCGF receptor analogous to activation of *c-myc* transcription following insertion of avian leukosis viral promoter (Hayward *et al.*, 1981; Payne *et al.*, 1981). Furthermore, the presence of viral sequences actually encod- the TCGF receptor has not been excluded. Alternatively, expression of these receptors may simply reflect the state of cellular activation that follows $HTLV_I$ infection.

As noted, despite therapy, ATL often progresses with great rapidity, resulting in the early demise of these patients. A clinical trial was recently initiated to evaluate potential therapeutic effects of anti-Tac in patients with ATL. These studies involved intravenous administration of escalating amounts of unmodified anti-Tac (T. A. Waldmann, S. Broder, W. C. Greene, and associates). Should this approach prove ineffective, additional studies with anti-Tac modified with toxins or radionuclides are planned. In this regard, Fitzgerald and associates (1983) have demonstrated augmented *in vitro* killing of $HTLV_I$-infected target cells with *Pseudomonas* exotoxin covalently linked to anti-Tac. Similarly, preliminary data suggest that anti-Tac coupled to the A-chain of ricin produces greater killing of $HTLV_I$-infected leukemic cells than either anti-Tac alone or a second control murine monoclonal antibody of the same immunoglobulin subclass coupled to the ricin A-chain (M. Krönke, T. A. Waldmann, E. Vitetta, and W. C. Greene, unpublished data).

C. Expression of Receptors Recognized by Anti-Tac on Human B-Cell Malignancies

In general, most acute or chronic B-cell leukemias or lymphomas do not react with anti-Tac. Recently, Korsmeyer and colleagues (1983) studied the hairy cell leukemias (HCL, leukemic reticuloendotheliosis). Considerable controversy has existed regarding the cellular origin of this leukemia (Jansen *et al.*, 1982; Posnett *et al.*, 1982; Saxon *et al.*, 1978; Cawley *et al.*, 1978). Using DNA probes specific for heavy- and light-chain Ig genes (Ravetch *et al.*, 1981 and Hieter *et al.*, 1980), rearrangements of both heavy- and light-chain Ig genes in 14 of 14 patients with this leukemia have been detected. Furthermore, in select cases these investigators have shown that the rearranged Ig genes are transcriptionally active as evidenced by the presence of mRNA encoding the appropriate Ig. These data, coupled with expression of surface Ig and display of B_1 and HLA-Dr determinants, indicated that this leukemia represented a malignant proliferation of B cells. As expected, these cells did not react with a variety of monoclonal antibodies recognizing T-cell-associated antigens, including OKT8/Leu2, OKT4/Leu3, OKT3/Leu4, and 3A-1 (Haynes *et al.*, 1980). Unexpectedly, cells from 13 of 14 HCL patients reacted with anti-Tac. These studies were performed with enriched leukemic cell populations containing <1% T cells. Notwithstanding, these investigators confirmed by two color fluorescent-activated cell-sorting analyses that the surface Ig-positive leukemic cells were also Tac positive (Fig. 8).

Additional studies have demonstrated that the receptors displayed on HCL cells are normal in size but few in number (approximately 1000 receptors per cell) (Greene *et al.*, 1983a). Purified TCGF blocked the binding of anti-Tac to these leukemic cells (S. J. Korsmeyer, T. A. Waldmann, and W. C. Greene, unpublished data). Addition of purified TCGF to cultures of HCL cells, however, produced only a two- to three-fold increase in thymidine incorporation measured at 48 hr and did not support the long-term growth of these cells. Thus, expression of the Tac antigen in this leukemia may simply reflect transformation-associated expression of an inappropriate gene product. Alternatively, these data

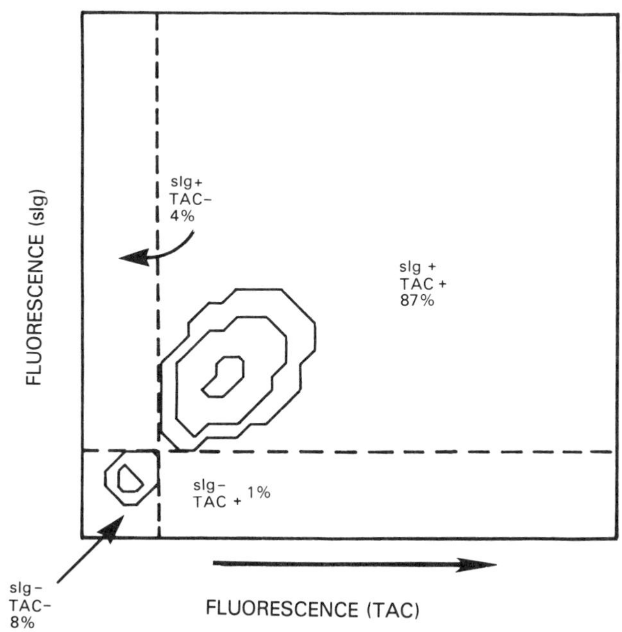

Figure 8. Linear contour plot of two-color, dual fluorescence comparison of hairy cell leukemia cells stained with FITC-anti-Tac and biotinylated anti-human λ-chain monoclonal antibody followed by avidin-linked Texas Red. Approximately 87% of the cells displayed positive fluorescence for both ligands, indicating concomitant expression of the Tac antigen and surface immunoglobulin (sIg). (Reprinted from Korsmeyer *et al.*, 1983, by permission of the *Proceedings of the National Academy of Sciences.*)

raise the probability that TCGF receptors are expressed on normal B cells, perhaps during a defined stage of differentiation or activation. In this regard, the Tac antigen has also been detected on the surface of select Burkitt's B-lymphoma cells. Receptor expression, while low, was consistently present. Additional studies are required to assess the significance of these apparent TCGF receptors on the surface of malignant B cells as well as to investigate the potential expression of these receptors on normal B cells.

VIII. CONCLUSION

The interaction of TCGF with its cellular receptor clearly forms a critical event in the evolution of the normal immune response. TCGF and its receptor represent the most completely studied of the human lymphokine–receptor systems. TCGF has now been purified and sequenced, and its posttranslational modifications have been identified. Furthermore, the gene encoding this lymphokine has been successfully isolated and expressed in both eukaryotic and bacterial cells. With the identification of anti-TCGF receptor antibodies, molecular characterization of the receptor is also proceeding at a rapid pace. The receptor has been purified, its posttranslational processing has been studied, and sensitive assays have been developed for the detection of these receptors in complex cell populations. The requirements for induction and expression of these receptors have been defined in both normal and neoplastic cells of T- and B-cell origin. Although the explanation for the uniform expression of TCGF receptors in T-leukemic cells infected with the type C retrovirus, $HTLV_I$, remains unanswered, the presence of these receptors is being actively exploited for the diagnosis and potential serotherapy of this leukemia. Future studies of the TCGF receptor will likely focus in four major areas:

1. The active site of the TCGF receptor remains to be identified; further investigation is required to define whether the receptor exists as an isolated surface glycoprotein or alternatively, as a receptor complex.
2. Little is known regarding the mechanism by which binding of TCGF to its receptor induces cellular proliferation. The potential role of second messengers and their effects on regulatory enzymatic processes remain to be identified.
3. Substantial interest will certainly focus on cloning the gene that encodes this inducible receptor.
4. With a more complete understanding of the interplay of TCGF with its receptor, coupled with the availability of large quantities of pure TCGF and/or antibodies to the TCGF receptor, *in vivo* therapeutic intervention may become possible in the pathological immune responses characteristic of various immunodeficient, autoimmune, and neoplastic diseases.

IX. REFERENCES

Abo, T., Miller, C. A., Balch, C. M., and Cooper, M. D., 1983, *J. Immunol.* **131**:1822–1826.

Altman, A., Theofilopoulos, A. N., Weiner, R., Katz, D. H., and Dixon, F. J., 1981, *J. Exp. Med.* **154**:791–808.

Andersson, J., Grönvik, K.-O., Larsson, E.-L., and Coutinho, A., 1979, *Eur. J. Immunol.* **9**: 581–587.

Andrew, M. E., Braciale, V. L., and Braciale, T. J., 1984, *J. Immunol.* **132**:839–844.

Andrus, L., Prowse, S. J., and Lafferty, K. J., 1981, *Scand. J. Immunol.* **13**:297–301.

Arya, S. K., Wong-Staal, F., and Gallo, R. C., 1984, *Science* **223**:1086–1087.

Blaney, D. W., Jaffe, E. S., Fischer, R. I., Schecter, G. P., Cossman, J., Robert-Guroff, M., Kalyanaraman, V. S., Blattner, W. A., and Gallo, R. C., 1983, *Ann. Int. Med.* **98**:144–151.

Bollum, F. J., 1979, *Blood* **54**:1203–1215.

Bonnard, G. D., Yosaka, D., and Jacobson, D., 1979, *J. Immunol.* **123**:2704–2708.

Broder, S., and Bunn, P. A. Jr., 1980, *Semin. Oncol.* **7**:310–331.

Brigham, B. A., Bunn, P. A., and Horton, J. E., 1982, *Arch. Dematol.* **118**:461–467.

Broder, S., Edelson, R., Lutzner, M., Nelson, D., MacDermott, R., Durm, M., Goldman, C., Meade, B., and Waldmann, T. A., 1976, *J. Clin. Invest.* **58**:1297–1306.

Brown, M. S., Anderson, R.G.W., and Goldstein, J. L., 1983, *Cell* **32**:663–667.

Brown, R. L., Griffith, R. L., Neubauer, R. H., and Rabin, H., 1982, *J. Immunol.* **129**:1849–1853.

Bunn, P. A. Jr., Schechter, G. P., Jaffe, E., Blayney, D., Young, R. C., Matthews, M. J., Blattner, W., Broder, S., Robert-Guroff, M., and Gallo, R. C., 1983, *N. Eng. J. Med.* **309**: 257–264.

Burnette, W. N., 1981, *Analyt. Biochem.* **112**:195–203.

Cantrell, D. A., and Smith, K. A., 1983, *J. Exp. Med.* **158**:1895–1911.

Catovsky, D., Graves, M. F., Rose, M., Galton, D. A. G., Goolden, A. W. G., McCluskey, D. R., White, J. M., Lampert, I., Bourikas, G., Ireland, R., Bridges, J. M., Blattner, W. A., and Gallo, R. C., 1982, *Lancet* **1**:639–643.

Cawley, J. C., Burns, G. F., Nash, T. A., Higgy, K. E., Child, J. A., and Roberts, B. E., 1978, *Blood* **51**:61–69.

Ceredig, R., Glasebrook, A., and MacDonald, H. R., 1982, *J. Exp. Med.* **155**:358–379.

Cheever, M. A., Greenberg, P. D., Fefer, A., and Gillis, S., 1982, *J. Exp. Med.* **155**:968–980.

Chouaib, S., and Fradelizi, D., 1982, *J. Immunol.* **129**:2463–2468.

Cogniaux, J., Otislager, R., Sprecher-Goldberger, S., and Thiry, L., 1982, *J. Virol.* **43**:664–672.

Cotner, T., Hemler, M. E., and Strominger, J. L., 1981, *Inter. J. Immunopharm.* **3**:255–268.

Cotner, T., Williams, J. M., Christenson, L., Shapiro, H. M., Strom, T. B., and Strominger, J. L., 1983, *J. Exp. Med.* **157**:461–472.

Coutinho, A., Larsson, E.-L., Grönvik, K. O., and Andersson, J., 1979, *Eur. J. Immunol.* **9**:587–592.

Dauphinée, M. J., Kipper, S. B., Wofsy, D., and Talal, N., 1981, *J. Immunol.* **127**:2483–2487.

Depper, J. M., Leonard, W. J., Robb, R. J., Waldmann, T. A., and Greene, W. C., 1983a, *J. Immunol.* **131**:690–696.

Depper, J. M., Leonard, W. J., Waldmann, T. A., and Greene, W. C., 1983b, in *Lymphokines*, Volume 9 (E. Pick, ed.), pp. 127–151, Academic Press, New York.

Depper, J. M., Leonard, W. J., Krönke, M., Noguchi, P. Cunningham, R. E. Waldmann, T. A., and Greene, W. C., 1984, *J. Immunol.* (in press).

Devos, R., Plaetinck, G., Cheroute, H., Simons, G., Degrave, W., Tavernier, J., Remout, E., and Fiers, W., 1983, *Nucleic Acid Res.* **11**:4307–4323.

Donohue, J. H., Rosenstein, M., Chang, A. E., Lotze, M. T., Robb, R. J., and Rosenberg, S. A., 1984, *J. Immunol.* **132**:2123–2128.

Eberlein, T. J., Rosenstein, M., and Rosenberg, S. A., 1982, *J. Exp. Med.* **156**:385–397.

Ek, B., Westermark, B., Wasteson, Å., and Heldin, C.-H., 1982, *Nature* **295**:419–420.

Farrar, W. L., Johnson, H. M., and Farrar, J. J., 1981, *J. Immunol.* **126**:1120–1125.

Farrar, J. J., Benjamin, W. R., Hilfiker, M. L., Howard, M., Farrar, W. L., and Fuller-Farrar, J., 1982, *Immunol. Rev.* **63**:129–166.

Fitzgerald, D., Waldmann, T. A., Pastan, I., and Willingham, M. C., 1984, *J. Clin. Invest.* (in press).

Flomenberg, N., Welte, L., Mertelsmann, R., Kernan, N., Ciobanu, N., Venuta, S., Feldman, S., Kruger, G., Kirkpatrick, D., Dupont, B., and O'Reilly, R., 1983, *J. Immunol.* **130**: 2644–2650.

Folk, J. E., 1980, *Ann. Rev. Biochem.* **49**:517–528.

Gallo, R. C. and Wong-Staal, F., 1982, *Blood* **60**:545–557.

Gallo, R. C., Mann, D., Broder, S., Ruscetti, F. W., Maeda, M., Kalyanaraman, V. S., Robert-Guroff, M., and Reitz, M. S., Jr., 1982, *Proc. Natl. Acad. Sci. USA* 79:5680–5683.

Gillis, S., and Mizel, S. B., 1981, *Proc. Natl. Acad. Sci. USA* 78:1133–1137.

Gillis, S., and Smith, K. A., 1977, *Nature* **268**:154.

Gillis, S., and Watson, J., 1980, *J. Exp. Med.* **152**:1709–1719.

Gillis, S., and Watson, J., 1981, *J. Immunol.* **126**:1245–1248.

Gillis, S., Smith, K. A., and Watson, J. D., 1980, *J. Immunol.* **124**:1954–1962.

Gillis, S., Gillis, A. E., and Henney, C. S., 1981, *J. Exp. Med.* **154**:983–997.

Glasebrook, A. L., Kelso, A., Zubler, R. H., Ely, J. M., Prystowsky, M. B., and Fitch, F. W., 1982, in: *Isolation, Characterization, and Utilization of T Lymphocyte Clones* (C. G. Fatham and F. W. Fitch, eds.), pp. 341–359, Academic Press, New York.

Gootenberg, J. E., Ruscetti, F. W., Mier, J. W., Gazdar, A., and Gallo, R. C., 1981, *J. Exp. Med.* **154**:1403–1417.

Gordon, P., Carpentier, J.-L., Cohen, S., and Orci, L., 1978, *Proc. Natl. Acad. Sci. USA* **75**: 5025–5029.

Greene, W. C., Waldmann, T. A., Cossman, J., Hsu, S.-M., Neckers, L. M., Marshall, S. L., Jensen, J. P., Bakhshi, A., Leonard, W. J., Depper, J. M., Jaffe, E. S., and Korsemeyer, S. J., 1983a, in: *Normal and Neoplastic Hematopoiesis* (P. Marx and D. Golde, eds.), pp. 501–511, Alan R. Liss, New York.

Greene, W. C., Robb, R. J., Depper, J. M., Leonard, W. J., Drogula, C., Svetlik, P., Wong-Staal, F., Gallo, R. C., and Waldmann, T. A., 1984, *J. Immunol.* **133**:1042–1047.

Grimm, E. A., Robb, R. J., Roth, J. A., Neckers, L. M., Lachman, L. B., Wilson, D. J., and Rosenberg, S. A., *J. Exp. Med.* **158**:1356–1361.

Gullberg, M., and Larsson, E.-L., 1982, *J. Immunol.* **128**:746–750.

Gullberg, M., and Larsson, E.-L., 1983, *J. Immunol.* **131**:19–22.

Gullberg, M., Ivars, F., Coutinho, A., and Larsson, E.-L., 1981, *J. Immunol.* **127**:407–413.

Haigler, H. T., Maxfield, F. R., Willingham, M. C., and Pastan, I., 1980, *J. Biol. Chem.* **255**: 1239–1241.

Hardt, C., Röllinghoff, M., Pfizenmaier, K., Mosmann, H., and Wagner, H., 1981, *J. Exp. Med.* **154**:262–274.

Harel-Bellan, A., Joskowicz, M., Fradelizi, D., and Eisen, H., 1983, *Proc. Natl. Acad. Sci. USA* 80:3466–3469.

Haynes, B. F., Mann, D. L., Hemler, M., Schroer, J. A., Shelhamer, J. H., Eisenbarth, G. S., Strominger, J. L., Thomas, C. A., Mostowski, H. S., and Fauci, A. S., 1980, *Proc. Natl. Acad. Sci. USA* 77:2914–2918.

Hayward, W. S., Neel, B. G., and Astrin, S. M., 1981, *Nature* **295**:209–215.

Hefeneider, S. H., Conlon, P. J., Henney, C. S., and Gillis, S., 1983, *J. Immunol.* **130**:222–227.

Henderson, L. E., Hewetson, J. F., Hopkins III, R. F., Sowder, R. C., Neubauer, R. H., and Rabin, H., 1983, *J. Immunol.* **131**:810–815.

Henney, C. S., Kuribayaski, K., Kern, D. E., and Gillis, S., 1981, *Nature* **291**:335–338.

Hieter, P. A., Max, E. E., Seidman, J. G., Maizel, J. F., and Leder, P., 1980, *Cell* **22**:197–207.

Hizuka, N., Gordon, P., Lesniak, M. A., Obberghen, E. V., Carpentier, J.-L., and Orci, L., 1981, *J. Biol. Chem.* **256**:4591–4597.

Howard, M., Matis, L., Malek, T. R., Shevach, E., Kell, W., Cohen, D., Nakanishi, K., and Paul, W. E., 1983, *J. Exp. Med.* **158**:2024–2039.

Inaba, K., Granelli Piperno, A., and Steinman, R. M., 1983, *J. Exp. Med.* **158**:2040–2057.

Jacobs, S., Kull, F. C., and Cuatrecasas, P., 1983, *Proc. Natl. Acad. Sci. USA* **80**:1228–1231.

Jansen, J., Schuit, H. R. E., Meijer, C. J. L. M., van Nieuwkoop, J. A., and Hijmans, W., 1982, *Blood* **59**:52–60.

Kalyanaraman, V. S., Sarngadharan, M. G., Bunn, P. A., Minna, J. D., and Gallo, R. C., 1981, *Nature* **294**:271–273.

Kasahara, T., Hooks, J. J., Dougherty, S. F., and Oppenheim, J. J., 1983, *J. Immunol.* **130**: 1784–1789.

Kawamota, T., Sato, J. D., Le, A., Polikoff, J., Sato, G. H., and Mendelsohn, J., 1983, *Proc. Natl. Acad. Sci. USA* **80**:1337–1341.

Keightly, R. G., Cooper, M. A., and Lawton, A. R., 1976, *J. Immunol.* **117**:1538–1545.

Kelso, A., and MacDonald, H. R., 1982, *J. Exp. Med.* **156**:1366–1379.

Kern, D. E., Gillis, S., Okada, M., and Henney, C. S., 1981, *J. Immunol.* **127**:1323–1328.

Kirchner, H., Tosato, G., Blaese, R. M., Broder, S., Magrath, I., 1979, *J. Immunol.* **122**: 1310–1313.

Korsmeyer, S. J., Greene, W. C., Cossman, J., Hsu, S.-M., Neckers, L. M., Marshall, S. L., Jensen, J. P., Bakhshi, A., Leonard, W. J., Depper, J. M., Jaffe, E. S., and Waldmann, T. A., 1983, *Proc. Natl. Acad. Sci. USA* **80**:4522–4526.

Kurnick, J. T., Hayward, A. R., and Altevogt, P., 1981, *J. Immunol.* **126**:1307–1311.

Lando, Z., Sarin, P., Waldmann, T. A., Gallo, R. C., and Broder, S., 1983, *Clin. Res.* **31**: 509A.

Larsson, E.-L., 1981, *J. Immunol.* **126**:1323–1328.

Larsson, E.-L., and Coutinho, A., 1979, *Nature* **280**:239–241.

Larsson, E.-L., Iscove, N. N., and Coutinho, A., 1980, *Nature* **283**:664–666.

Larsson, E.-L., Gullberg, M., and Coutinho, A., 1981, *Immunobiol.* **161**:5–20.

Leibson, H. J., Marrack, P., and Kappler, J. W., 1981, *J. Exp. Med.* **154**:1681–1693.

Leonard, W. J., Depper, J. M., Uchiyama, T., Smith, K. A., Waldmann, T. A., and Greene, W. C., 1982, *Nature* **300**:267–269.

Leonard, W. J., Depper, J. M., Robb, R. J., Waldmann, T. A., and Greene, W. C., 1983a, *Proc. Natl. Acad. Sci. USA* **80**:6957–6961.

Leonard, W. J., Depper, J. M., Waldmann, T. A., and Greene, W. C., 1983b, in: *Receptors and Recognition* (M. Greaves, ed.), Chapman and Hall Ltd., London (in press).

Linker-Israeli, M., Bakker, A. C., Kitridou, R. C., Gendler, S., Gillis, S., and Horwitz, D. A., 1983, *J. Immunol.* **130**:2651–2655.

Lotze, M. T., Line, B. R., Mathisen, D. J., and Rosenberg, S. A., 1980, *J. Immunol.* **125**: 1487–1493.

Lotze, M. T., Grimm, E. A., Mazumder, A., Strausser, J. L., and Rosenberg, S. A., 1981, *Cancer Res.* **41**:4420–4425.

Luger, T. A., Smolen, J. S., Chused, T. M., Steinberg, A. D., and Oppenheim, J. J., 1982, *J. Clin. Invest.* **70**:470–473.

Lutzner, M., Edelson, R., Sckein, P., Green, I., Kirkpatrick, C., and Akmed, A., 1975, *Ann Intern. Med.* **83**:534–552.

Maeda, S., Nishino, N., Obaru, K., Mita, S., Nomiyama, H., Shimada, K., Fujimoto, K., Teranishi, T., Hirano, T., and Onoue, K., 1983, *Biochem. Biophys. Res. Comm.* **115**: 1040–1047.

Maizel, A., Mehta, S. R., Hauft, S., Franzini, D., Lachman, L. B., and Ford, R. J., 1981, *J. Immunol.* **127**:1058–1064.

Malek, T. R., Robb, R. J., and Shevach, E. M., 1983, *Proc. Natl. Acad. Sci. USA* **80**:5694–5698.

Malkovsky, M., Asherson, G. L., Stockinger, B., and Watkins, M. C., 1982, *Nature* **300**: 652–655.

Merluzzi, V. J., Welte, K., Savage, D. M., Last-Barney, K., and Mertelsmann, R., 1983, *J. Immunol.* **131**:806–809.

Meuer, S. C., Hussey, R. E., Penta, A. C., Fitzgerald, K. A., Stadler, B. M., Schlossman, S. F., and Reinherz, E. L., 1982, *J. Immunol.* **129**:1076–1079.

Mier, J. W., and Gallo, R. C., 1980, *Proc. Natl. Acad. Sci. USA* 77:6134–6138.

Miyamoto, K., and Gilden, R. V., 1971, *J. Virol.* 7:395–406.

Miyawaki, T. A., Yachie, A., Uwandana, N., Ohzeki, S., Nagaoki, T., and Taniguchi, N., 1982, *J. Immunol.* **129**:2474–2478.

Mühlradt, P. F., and Opitz, H. G., 1982, *Eur. J. Immunol.* **12**:983–985.

Morgan, D. A., Ruscetti, F. W., and Gallo, R., 1976, *Science* **193**:1007–1008.

Nagasawa, K., and Mak, T., 1980, *Proc. Natl. Acad. Sci. USA* 77:2964–2968.

Neckers, L. M., and Cossman, J., 1983, *Proc. Natl. Acad. Sci. USA* **80**:3494–3498.

Northoff, H., Carter, C., and Oppenheim, J. J., 1980, *J. Immunol.* **125**:1823–1828.

O'Farrell, P. H., 1975, *J. Biol. Chem.* **250**:4007–4021.

Olefsky, J. M., and Kao, M., 1982, *J. Biol. Chem.* **257**:8667–8673.

Omary, M. B. and Trowbridge, I., 1981, *J. Biol. Chem.* **256**:12888–12892.

Osawa, H., and Diamantstein, T., 1983, *Immunol.* **48**:617–621.

Paetkau, V., Mills, G. B., and Bleackley, R. C., 1982, in: *The Potential Role of T Cells in Cancer Therapy* (A. Fefer and A. Goldstein, eds.), pp. 147–159, Raven Press, New York.

Palladino, M. A., Welte, K., Ciobanu, N., Mertlesmann, R., and Oettgen, H. F., 1984, in: *Thymic Hormones and Lymphokines* (A. L. Goldstein, ed.), pp. 525–529, Plenum Press, New York.

Payne, G. S., Bishop, M. J., and Varmus, M. E., 1981, *Nature* **295**:209–215.

Poiesz, B. J., Ruscetti, F. W., Mier, J. W., Woods, A. M., and Gallo, R. C., 1980a, *Proc. Natl. Acad. Sci. USA* 77:6815–6819.

Poiesz, B. J., Ruscetti, F. W., Gazdar, A. F., Bunn, P. A., Jr., Minna, J. D., and Gallo, R. C., 1980b, *Proc. Natl. Acad. Sci. USA* 77:7415–7419.

Poiesz, B. J., Ruscetti, F. W., Reitz, M. S., Kalyanaraman, V. S., and Gallo, R. C., 1981, *Nature* **294**:268–271.

Posnett, D. N., Chiorazzi, N., and Kunkel, H. G., 1982, *J. Clin. Invest.* **70**:254–261.

Ravetch, J. V., Sienbenlist, U., Korsmeyer, S. J., Waldmann, T. A., and Leder, P., 1981, *Cell* **27**:583–591.

Rey, A., Klein, B., Zagury, D., Thierry, C., and Serrou, B., 1983, *Immunol. Letters* **6**:175–178.

Robb, R. J., 1982a, *Fed. Proc.* **41**:480.

Robb, R. J., 1982b, *Lymphokine Res.* **1**:37–43.

Robb, R. J., 1984, *Immunol. Today* **5**:203–209.

Robb, R. J., and Greene, W. C., 1983, *J. Exp. Med.* **158**:1332–1337.

Robb, R. J., and Lin, Y., 1984, in: *Thymic Hormones and Lymphokines '83* (A. L. Goldstein, ed.), pp. 247–256, Plenum Press, New York.

Robb, R. J., and Smith, K. A., 1981, *Mol. Immunol.* **18**:1087–1094.

Robb, R. J., Munck, A., and Smith, K. A., 1981, *J. Exp. Med.* **154**:1455–1474.

Robb, R. J., Kutny, R. M., and Chowdhry, V., 1983a, *Proc. Natl. Acad. Sci. USA* **80**:5990–5994.

Robb, R. J., Kutny, R. M., Panico, M., Morris, H., DeGrado, W. F., and Chowdhry, V., 1983b, *Biochem. Biophys. Res. Comm.* **116**:1049–1055.

Robb, R. J., Kutny, R. M., Panico, M., Morris, H., and Chowdhry, V., 1984, *Proc. Natl. Acad. Sci. USA* (in press).

Robert-Guroff, M., Fahey, K. A., Maeda, M., Nakao, Y., Ito, Y., and Gallo, R. C., 1982, *Virology* **122**:297–305.

Rodbard, D., 1973, in: *Receptors for Reproductive Hormones* (B. W. O'Malley and A. R. Means, eds.), pp. 289–326, Plenum Press, New York.

Rosenberg, S. A., Spiess, P., Schwarz, S., 1983, *Transplantation* **35**:631–634.

Ryffel, B., Henning, C. B., and Huberman, E., 1982, *Proc. Natl. Acad. Sci. USA* **79**:7336–7340.

Saxon, A., Stevens, R. H., and Golde, D. W., 1978, *Ann. Int. Med.* **88**:323–326.

Schreier, M. H., Iscove, N. N., Tees, R., Aarden, L., and von Boehmer, H., 1980, *Immunol. Rev.* **51**:315–356.

Seigal, L. J., Harper, M. E., Wong-Staal, F., Gallo, R. C., Nash, W. G., and O'Brien, S. J., 1984, *Science* **223**:175–178.

Sekaly, R. P., MacDonald, H. R., Zalch, P., and Nabholz, M., 1982, *J. Immunol.* **129**:1407–1415.

Smith, K. A., 1980, *Immunol. Rev.* **51**:337–357.

Smith, K. A., Gillis, S., Baker, P. E., McKenzie, D., and Ruscetti, F. W., 1979, *Ann. N.Y. Acad. Sci.* **332**:423–432.

Smith, K. A., Lachman, L. B., Oppenheim, J. J., and Favata, M. F., 1980, *J. Exp. Med.* **151**: 1551–1553.

Stadler, B. M., and Oppenheim, J. J., 1982, in *Lymphokines*, Vol. 6 (S. Mizel, ed.), pp. 117–135, Academic Press, New York.

Stadler, B. M., Dougherty, S. F., Farrar, J. J., and Oppenheim, J. J., 1981, *J. Immunol.* **127**: 1936–1940.

Stadler, B. M., Berenstein, E. H., Siraganian, R. P., and Oppenheim, J. J., 1982, *J. Immunol.* **128**:1620–1624.

Steinmann, G., Conlon, P., Hefeneider, S., and Gillis, S., 1983, *Science* **220**:1188–1190.

Stötter, H., Rüde, E., and Wagner, H., 1980, *Eur. J. Immunol.* **10**:719–722.

Stickland, S., and Loeb, J. N., 1981, *Proc. Natl. Acad. Sci. USA* **78**:1366–1370.

Strous, G.J.A.M. and Lodish, H. F., 1980, *Cell* **22**:709–717.

Taniguchi, T., Matsui, H., Fujita, T., Takaoka, C., Kashima, N., Yoshimoto, R., and Hamuro, J., 1983, *Nature* **302**:305–310.

Tartakoff, A. M., Vassalli, P., and Detraz, M., 1977, *J. Exp. Med.* **146**:1332–1345.

Thoman, M. L., and Weigle, W. O., 1982, *J. Immunol.* **128**:2358–2361.

Towbin, H., Staehelin, T., and Gordon, J., 1979, *Proc. Natl. Acad. Sci. USA* **76**:4350–4354.

Tsudo, M., Uchiyama, T., Takatsuki, K., Uchino, H., and Yodoi, J., 1982, *J. Immunol.* **129**: 592–595.

Tsudo, M., Uchiyama, T., Uchino, H., and Yodoi, J., 1983, *Blood* **61**:1014–1016.

Uchiyama, T., Yodoi, J., Sagawa, K., Takatsuki, K., and Uchino, H., 1977, *Blood* **50**:481–492.

Uchiyama, T., Broder, S., and Waldmann, T. A., 1981, *J. Immunol.* **126**:1393–1397.

Ushiro, H., and Cohen, S., 1980, *J. Biol. Chem.* **255**:8363–8365.

Wagner, H., and Röllinghoff, M., 1978, *J. Exp. Med.* **148**:1523–1538.

Wagner, H., Manat, C., Heeg, K., Röllinghoff, M., and Pfizenmaier, K., 1980, *Nature* **284**: 278–280.

Waldmann, T., Greene, W., Sarin, P., Goldman, C., Frost, K., Sharrow, S., Depper, J., Leonard, W., Uchiyama, T., and Gallo, R. C., 1984, *J. Clin Invest.* **73**:1711–1718.

Walker, C., Kristensen, F., Bettans, F., and de Weck, A. L., 1983, *J. Immunol.* **130**:1770–1773.

Welte, K., Wang, C. Y., Mertelsmann, R., Venuta, S., Feldmann, S. P., and Moore, M. A. S., 1982, *J. Exp. Med.* **156**:454–464.

Yoshida, M., Miyoshi, I., and Hinuma, Y., 1982, *Proc. Natl. Acad. Sci. USA* 79:2031–2035.

Zick, Y., Whittaker, J., and Roth, J., 1983, *J. Biol. Chem.* **258**:3431–3434.

Toward the Molecular Biology of IL-2

Verner Paetkau, R. Chris Bleackley, Denis Riendeau, Delsworth G. Harnish, and Eugene W. Holowachuk

Department of Biochemistry
University of Alberta
Edmonton, Alberta
Canada T6G 2H7

I. INTRODUCTION

Reviewing the molecular biology of lymphokines in 1984 is a bit like writing a biography 10 minutes after the birth of the subject. Such a review entails both advantages and disadvantages. An advantage is that the topic is limited in content and a reasonably comprehensive review can still be attempted; this is unlikely to be the case in a few years. The major disadvantage is that some important features are still in the formative stages and likely to change soon. We have as yet only rudimentary hints about how the genetic expression of lymphokines is controlled and how they act at the molecular level. Since molecular biology is based on precise biochemical information, it may be timely to review our understanding of the molecular properties of one lymphokine, Interleukin-2 (IL-2).

This review examines some properties of primate and rodent IL-2. A comparison of purification methods is made, and the evident heterogeneity of IL-2 is considered and rationalized. Various cell lines producing high levels of IL-2 have yielded mRNA, which can be translated into biologically active IL-2 *in vitro*. Systems for mRNA translation and initial results on post-translational processing are described. An approach to the molecular biology of products of activated T lymphocytes, such as lymphokines, is illustrated. The cellular immunological context of lymphokine function is considered only in a cursory way, where necessary. Furthermore, the various lymphokines are not compared with each other in any detail. Our central purpose here is to summarize some molecular properties of IL-2 and to illustrate new directions being followed in unraveling the molecular biology of these fascinating regulatory molecules.

II. BIOLOGICAL PROPERTIES OF IL-2 AND OTHER LYMPHOKINES

A. IL-2-Dependent Responses

Various T-lymphocyte responses appear to be dependent on IL-2. When these responses are measured in mixed populations, interpretations are compromised by the possibility of secondary effects. That is, one population of cells may respond to the added lymphokine by producing another effector molecule, which in turn acts on a second population of cells. Nevertheless, responses of this type can be useful and have been important in identifying and characterizing IL-2 and other lymphokines.

One assay for IL-2 is the growth of cytotoxic T lymphocytes (CTLs) from spleen or lymph node after activation with mitogens or antigens. These cultures die out unless they are freshly stimulated with either appropriate cells or IL-2. The cultures are maintained for 1 to several weeks, and the cells are not clonally defined. However, the assay is reasonably specific for IL-2, probably because of the dominance in the cultures of the CTL generated.

Mouse thymocytes also provide a useful assay system for IL-2 (DiSabato *et al.*, 1975). They are relatively insensitive to T-cell mitogens, particularly if they are depleted of adherent cells (Mills *et al.*, 1976) or are cultured at low density (Paetkau *et al.*, 1976). Addition of IL-2 permits them to respond at much higher levels. A disadvantage of this assay is that other lymphokines, e.g., IL-1, can stimulate thymocytes as well (Mizel *et al.*, 1978).

IL-2 also restores certain kinds of T-lymphocyte responses to populations deficient in ancillary cells or stimulated with antigenic, but nonimmunogenic, target cells. Thus, it restores the CTL response of thymocytes depleted of adherent cells or stimulated by ultraviolet (UV)-irradiated tumor cells (Paetkau *et al.*, 1980). Responses of B lymphocytes to sheep erythrocytes can also be used to monitor IL-2 activity (Granelli-Piperno *et al.*, 1981; Watson *et al.*, 1979a). However, this effect is undoubtedly mediated indirectly by other cells or lymphokines (Pure *et al.*, 1982; Teranishi *et al.*, 1982; Yoshizaki *et al.*, 1982).

Given the shortcomings of the assays described, it is particularly advantageous that IL-2 activity can be defined in terms of its effects on cloned CTL. This is the T-cell growth assay (Morgan *et al.*, 1976; Gillis *et al.*, 1978). Proteins that stimulate the continuous proliferation of activated CTL (and some other kinds of T lymphocytes) and that are secreted by activated T lymphocytes are referred to as IL-2. Although other molecules may have this activity, e.g., the phorbol diester (PMA) stimulates the growth of some T-lymphocyte lines, the definition given above is probably safe if one keeps in mind the protein nature of IL-2 and its cellular source. A number of CTL lines have been cloned, and their total dependence on IL-2 for growth makes them a sensitive assay system.

B. Some Other Lymphokines

Since a number of lymphokines are mentioned in this chapter, it is worthwhile to identify and briefly describe some of these:

Interleukin-1 (IL-1): A product of macrophages (and possibly other cells) that activates lymphocytes (Mizel *et al.*, 1978), originally called lymphocyte activating factor.

Interleukin-3 (IL-3): Like IL-2, a product of T lymphocytes, that can be assayed by a number of parameters (Ihle *et al.*, 1982b); induction of the enzyme 20α-hydroxysteroid dehydrogenase (Ihle *et al.*, 1981) and the outgrowth of persistent (Clark-Lewis and Schrader, 1981), granulocytic cells from bone marrow (Ihle *et al.*, 1982b; J. Schrader, personal communication).

Colony-stimulating factor for granulocytes and macrophages (GM-CSF): Induces the outgrowth of granulocyte and macrophage colonies from bone marrow (Burgess *et al.*, 1977); is distinct from both IL-3 and CSF-1, which is selective for macrophages (Stanley and Heard, 1977).

Lymphokines acting on B lymphocytes: B-cell growth factor (BCGF) (Farrar *et al.*, 1982; Howard *et al.*, 1982) and factors that cause the differentiation of proliferating B lymphocytes to high levels of immunoglobulin (Ig) production (Isakson *et al.*, 1982). (The latter is often referred to as T-cell replacing factor (TRF), but more recently it has been termed B-cell differentiation factor, BCDF, a term that is more descriptive and that avoids certain complications attached to the earlier one. There are probably several forms of both BCDF and BCGF (Nakanishi *et al.*, 1983).

C. Specific Activity of IL-2

One problem in dealing with incompletely purified and defined biological material is establishing a generally accepted unit of activity. Until homogeneously pure material is widely available, it is necessary to resort to working definitions for a substance like IL-2. Although IL-2 activity has been quantified in various ways, it would be useful to have a means to compare the results from different sources and laboratories and to determine the relative potencies of different effector molecules. Such comparisons can be approximated by defining a unit of relative activity. In our own work, we have defined an ED_{30} unit of IL-2 activity as that amount, in a 1-ml culture, that generates 30% of the maximal response obtainable with saturating levels of IL-2 in the same assay. We use the 30% value because titration curves plotting in log–log dose-response fashion are linear in this region. By 50% of the response, the curves frequently begin to fall off the maximum linear slope. Furthermore, in the presence of inhibitors existing in crude preparations, it is difficult to obtain meaningful dose–response curves above 30%. Some workers have reported data in terms of units that stimulate 50% maximal activity. In our experience, the relative size of this unit is about 1.7 times ED_{30}. In the data discussed here, this conversion will be used in order to allow for comparisons.

As anyone who has worked with such growth factors well knows, the activities obtained in two experiments on the same cellular response can differ by severalfold even when the same preparation of factor is used. This stems from the complexity of the assay. The variation between different assays can be even larger; in our experience, the thymocyte proliferation assay requires about five times more IL-2 to produce a given fraction of the maximal response than does the CTL proliferation assay. This is partly due to the larger number of (IL-2-adsorbing) cells present in the former.

III. PURIFICATION AND BIOCHEMICAL PROPERTIES OF IL-2

A. Human IL-2

The ability to stimulate the growth of human T cells was a major starting point for IL-2 research (Morgan *et al.*, 1976; Gillis *et al.*, 1978). Several sources of human IL-2 are available, which give rise to different molecular forms of the lymphokine. Normal lymphoid cells from tonsils produced two forms of IL-2 (Welte *et al.*, 1982). Surprisingly, the form produced depended on whether the cells were stimulated with a mixture of allogeneic cells and mitogen alone or whether a lymphoblastoid line (Daudi) was also present. In the presence of Daudi cells, the apparent molecular weight (M_r) was 14,500, as estimated by polyacrylamide gel electrophoresis in sodium dodecylsulfate (SDS-PAGE). When Daudi cells were not present, similar amounts of activity of higher apparent molecular weights, 16,000 and 17,000 (two bands) were obtained.

The IL-2 produced from normal human tonsil cells was purified by a series of steps (Welte *et al.*, 1982). Both blue agarose and Procion red columns were used, as well as chromatography on DEAE and gel filtration. The final product was free of interferon (γ- and α-IFN), GM-CSF, BCDF, BCGF, and a differentiating factor for thymocytes. It can be estimated that the purified material produced a half-maximal response at a protein concentration of 0.2 ng/ml, or about 1.3×10^{-11} M (assuming an M_r of 16,000). Activity was detectable at one-tenth this concentration. The estimated potency of this material, which was probably close to 100% pure, is 8000 ED_{30} units per microgram.

Another source of human IL-2 is the Jurkat T lymphoma line. IL-2 was purified from these cells by standard gel filtration and isoelectric focusing (IEF) steps (Robb *et al.*, 1981). This material, apparently of very high purity, was used to measure receptors on responding lymphocytes. The dissociation constant estimated from Scatchard plots was in the region of 2×10^{-12} M. More recently, human IL-2 was purified from the same source with a one-step, antibody-affinity column. Monoclonal (mouse) anti-human IL-2 antibody was bound to a Sepharose column, and large volumes of crude, serum-free culture supernatant were passed through. The adsorbed material, when eluted with low pH buffer, appeared to be homogeneously pure IL-2 by two-dimensional PAGE (Robb *et al.*, 1983). It represented about two-thirds of the total IL-2 activity in the crude preparation, the other one-third having no affinity for the column. From the data given, the purified protein can be estimated to have a specific activity of about 5000 ED_{30} units/μg protein. Using an M_r of 16,000, this corresponds to a concentration of 2×10^{-11} M at 50% maximal activity. Amino acid sequence determination of this material yielded the same 36 amino terminal residues as predicted from cDNA cloning work (Section V.A), indicating that no contaminating proteins were detectable.

There is a reasonable similarity between the concentration of purified IL-2 giving half-maximal activity and the dissociation constant determined by binding, although confirmation of both numbers is required. Nevertheless, it appears that the biologically important and physically determined dissociation constants are in the range of 10^{-11}–10^{-12} M.

A new source of human IL-2 was recently described. Cell lines from a cutaneous T-cell lymphoma/leukemia (CTCL) produce IL-2 constitutively. This so-called L-TCGF is lower in pI (4.5) than the tonsil or Jurkat forms (pI 6.7–8.1). Interestingly, the difference between normal and CTCL-derived IL-2 is not altered by treatment with neuraminidase, suggesting that the basis for this difference is not sialic acid (Gootenburg *et al.*, 1982).

B. Mouse and Rat IL-2

Various standard biochemical techniques have been applied to the purification of murine IL-2. Gel filtration, anion exchange chromatography, and hydrophobic affinity chromatography (Shaw *et al.*, 1978a; Watson *et al.*, 1979a,b; Hilfiker *et al.*, 1981; Clark-Lewis and Schrader, 1982a), IEF (Shaw *et al.*, 1978a) and chromatofocusing (Pure *et al.*, 1982) have also been successfully used. When these methods were applied to IL-2 from normal mouse spleen cells stimulated with concanavalin A (Con A), material of specific activity approximately 50 ED_{30} units/μg protein was obtained, as measured in a thymocyte comitogenesis assay (Shaw *et al.*, 1978a). In terms of activity on cloned CTL, this corresponds to about 250 ED_{30} units/μg, or about 2% purity (see below, summarized in Section 3.D).

More recently, large quantities of murine IL-2 from spleen cells stimulated in serum free medium were worked up through hydroxyapatite chromatography, ion exchange, and preparative SDS-PAGE (Granelli-Piperno *et al.*, 1981). Although the purified material ran at a defined location in analytical SDS-PAGE, it was probably not homogeneously pure, as judged by the final specific activity. Activity was detectable at 4×10^{-11} M, and maximal at 10^{-9} M, suggesting that half-maximal activity occurred at about 2×10^{-10} M, or 4.6 ng/ml. The most highly purified preparations of mouse IL-2 (below) are half-maximally active around 0.2 ng/ml. The behavior on SDS-PAGE cannot be taken as evidence of purity, since this technique was used as the final purification step.

A major advantage was realized when cloned cell lines were obtained that could be induced to synthesize large quantities of IL-2. Two types of cells are in general use, T-cell lymphomas and T-cell hybridomas. T-cell lymphomas producing high levels of IL-2 when suitably stimulated were described by Farrar *et al.* (1980) and by Gillis and Watson and colleagues (Gillis *et al.*, 1980a). For example, the EL4 T-cell lymphoma variant described by Farrar *et al.* (1980) produces about 1000 times as much IL-2 per cell, under optimal conditions, as do normal spleen cells. (Since the spleen cells are normally grown at a 10-fold higher cell density, the yield per milliliter is only 100 times higher with EL4. For purposes of generating homogeneously pure material, however, it is important to realize that starting specific activities are about 1000 times higher with the EL4 line.)

We have applied several previously described purification steps in combination with reverse-phase high-performance liquid chromatography (RP-HPLC) to the isolation of IL-2 from the EL4 lymphoma line (Riendeau *et al.*, 1983). The starting material was culture supernatant from EL4 cells stimulated with PMA to produce high levels of IL-2 (Farrar *et al.*, 1980). High-producer clones of this line have been derived and preserved by freezing. This step is an important precaution, as the productivity tends to fall off after repeated passages in culture. Large volumes (5 liters or more) of culture supernatants were rapidly concentrated and dialyzed with a new ultrafiltration system (Millipore Pellicone). Sequential chromatography over Sephadex G100 (Shaw *et al.*, 1978a), phenyl Sepharose (Hilfiker *et al.*, 1981), and DEAE cellulose (Shaw *et al.*, 1978a) yielded partial purification. The G100 Sephadex and phenyl Sepharose steps separate IL-2 and IL-3 from GM-CSF and BCGF (Hilfiker *et al*, 1981; Clark-Lewis and Schrader, 1982a; Howard *et al.*, 1982). IL-3 does not bind to DEAE (Ihle *et al.*, 1982a) and is thus separated from IL-2, which is desorbed at NaCl concentrations above 0.15 M.

The greatest degree of purification occurred during subsequent separation on RP-HPLC. The hydrophobic nature of murine IL-2 caused it to be eluted at about

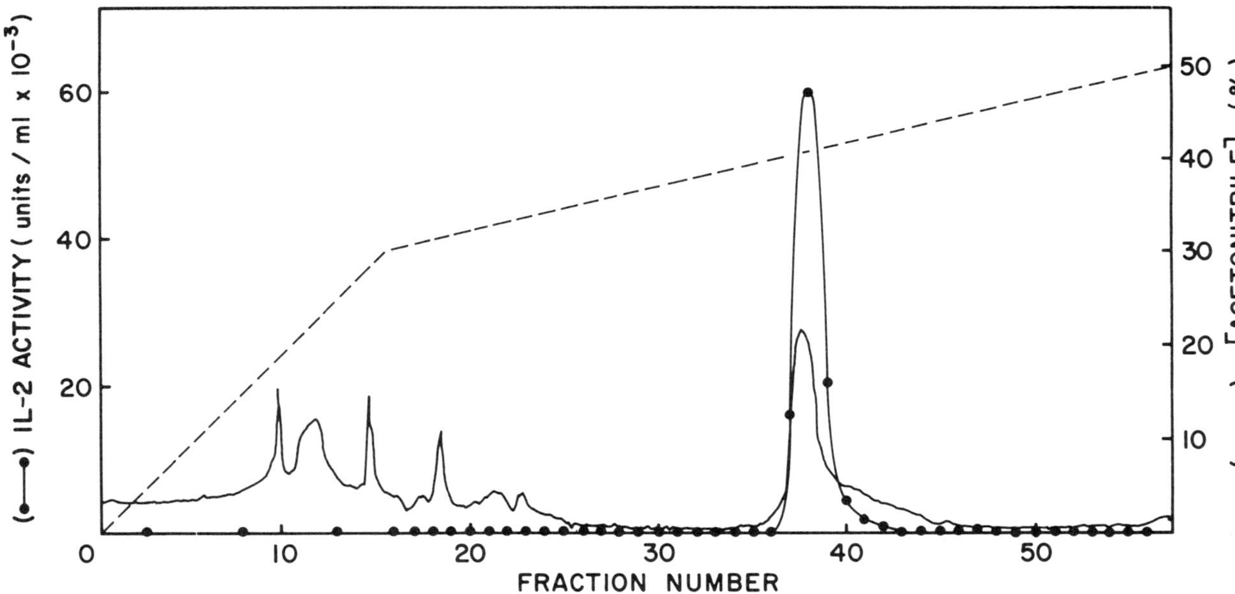

Figure 1. RP-HPLC of IL-2 derived from phorbol myristate acetate (PMA)-stimulated EL4 cells. IL-2 was partially purified by gel filtration (Sephadex G-100), hydrophobic chromatography on phenyl Sepharose, and anion-exchange chromatography on DEAE Sephacel (see text for details). The resulting sample (93,000 ED_{30} units of IL-2, volume 8 ml) was acidified with trifluoroacetic acid (TFA) to a final concentration of 0.1%; the pH was adjusted to 2 with 1 M HCl. It was then chromatographed on a Synchropak-RP C_{18} column (250 × 4.1 mm) (Linden, Ind.) using a Spectra-Physics SP8700 solvent-delivery system coupled to a Spectra-Physics SP8750 organizer pumping system. The column was washed with 0.1% TFA to obtain a stable baseline of A_{220}. Elution was effected with gradients of acetonitrile in 0.1% TFA as follows: 0–30% for 15 min, then 30–60% for 60 min, at a flow rate of 1 ml/min. IL-2 activity was assayed at a 1:10,000 final dilution. Recovery of activity was approximately 79%. Data shown represent rechromatography of the peak of activity from such a run. ED_{30}, amount of activity in 1 ml that produces 30% maximal response; IL-2, Interleukin-2; RP-HPLC, reverse-phase-high-performance liquid chromatography.

40% acetonitrile, after essentially all other proteins had been removed (Fig. 1). This feature permits even relatively crude IL-2 generated in serum-free medium, and subjected only to concentration and chromatography on G100 Sephadex, to be purified to a similar specific activity by direct application onto a C_{18} column. (A limitation is the capacity of the column, which precludes the application of this abbreviated protocol to large quantities of IL-2 with a low specific activity, such as crude preparations made from serum-containing medium.)

DEAE chromatography, although not offering a great increase in specific activity, separates IL-3 from IL-2, and is probably important since IL-3 and IL-2 emerge from C_{18} columns under almost identical conditions (comparing data of Ihle *et al.*, 1982a, with that represented in Fig. 1). Phenyl Sepharose chromatography separates GM-CSF from the T-cell-active lymphokines and facilitates its purification. This step is important if RP-HPLC is not used, since CSF-GM and IL-2 have similar pI and M_r values (Hilfiker *et al.*, 1981). Because PMA, which is used to induce IL-2 production, sticks to serum proteins and is thereby carried through purification steps (Krakauer *et al.*, 1982), it is advantageous to begin with serum-free culture supernatants. In our experience, there is little detectable PMA following the Pellicon concentration step. In a typical application of the protocol described above, the overall recovery of IL-2 after HPLC is 15-30%.

One of the features that has complicated this work is the loss of material that occurs when dilute solutions of highly purified IL-2 are handled. Procedures that are satisfactory for crude preparations, such as lyophilization, can produce enormous or even total losses when applied to IL-2, which is greater than 10% pure and less than 30 μg/ml in protein. Fortunately, several solvents overcome this problem. IL-2 is stable in the solvent used for HPLC (Fig. 1) (pH 2, 30-40% acetonitrile) and can be stored in it for long periods of time. Also, IL-2 can be recovered from SDS (Caplan *et al.*, 1981) and is stable in this detergent. At very high protein concentrations, or in the presence of added serum proteins or purified serum albumin, activity is also stable.

The usual principle in protein purification is to optimize the resolution of each step. Because of the unusual features of IL-2, i.e., its lability at low protein concentrations, the rather cumbersome time requirements for bioassay (24-hr), and its hydrophobic character, we have abandoned this principle in our present purification scheme. Instead, ion exchange and phenyl Sepharose steps are used only to remove specific components of the starting mixture. This can be realized by batch elution. Most of the BCGF is removed from crude IL-2 by gel filtration (Howard *et al.*, 1982). The IL-2 is then adsorbed onto phenyl Sepharose, and GM-CSF is eluted with starting buffer (Hilfiker *et al.*, 1981; Clark-Lewis and Schrader, 1982a), IL-2, IL-3, and any remaining BCGF (Farrar *et al.*, 1982) are stripped from the column in two steps of high ethylene glycol-low salt. No bioassay is required, and the eluate can be directly loaded onto DEAE after a brief dialysis. IL-3 washes directly off this column at low salt (Ihle *et al.*, 1982a), and IL-2 is brought off with 0.3 M NaCl. The pooled IL-2 sample is applied to the

C_{18} column for HPLC. The entire protocol can be carried out in a few days, with a reasonable recovery (15-25%) of pure material.

Material worked up through the preliminary steps indicated, and eluted from the RP-HPLC column, appeared to be homogeneous on SDS-PAGE (Fig. 2). The IL-2 activity eluted from the gel comigrated with the protein band, which had the mobility of marker proteins of M_r 22,000-23,000. The heterogeneity ob-

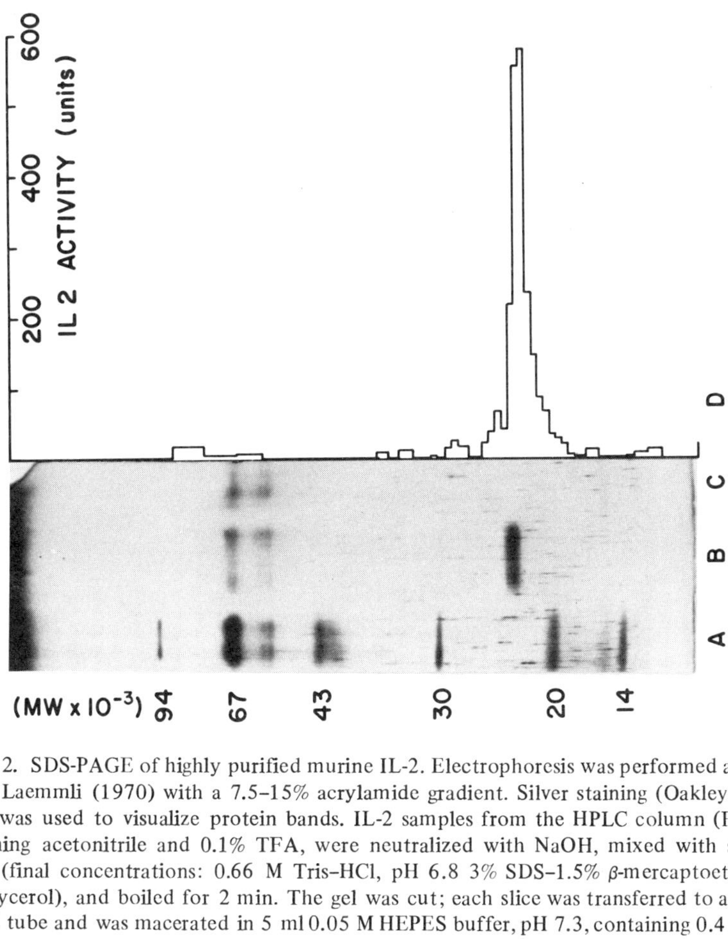

Figure 2. SDS-PAGE of highly purified murine IL-2. Electrophoresis was performed according to Laemmli (1970) with a 7.5–15% acrylamide gradient. Silver staining (Oakley *et al.*, 1980) was used to visualize protein bands. IL-2 samples from the HPLC column (Fig. 1), containing acetonitrile and 0.1% TFA, were neutralized with NaOH, mixed with sample buffer (final concentrations: 0.66 M Tris-HCl, pH 6.8 3% SDS–1.5% β-mercaptoethanol–16% glycerol), and boiled for 2 min. The gel was cut; each slice was transferred to a sterile conical tube and was macerated in 5 ml 0.05 M HEPES buffer, pH 7.3, containing 0.4 mg/ml BSA. This mixture was then incubated at 4°C for 24 hr with shaking and IL-2 activity determined at a dilution of 1:40 or more. (Lane A) Molecular weight markers (Pharmacia); (lane B) purified IL-2 (9000 ED_{30} units); (lane C) electrophoresis sample buffer (no sample); (lane D) as in B, but unstained. The slight shift between activity and stained protein seen here is an artifact arising from gel shrinkage during staining. It is impossible to align the two profiles precisely, but the average mobility of the stained band and activity in repeat experiments is the same.

served in IEF or chromatofocusing (Pure *et al.*, 1982) apparently did not lead to heterogeneity in RP-HPLC. Material eluted as a sharp peak and, when this was rerun, it again emerged as a single, well-defined peak (data not shown). This material had a specific activity of 15,000 ED_{30} units/μg protein, with a mouse CTL line as an assay. Half-maximal activity occurred at 7×10^{-12} M, assuming a M_r of 16,000. The NH_2-terminal amino acid sequence of this material is unambiguous, indicating peptide homogeneity, and corresponds through the first seven residues to that of human IL-2 (M. Bond, personal communication). Two-dimensional analysis (IEF and M_r in SDS) indicates a series of closely spaced spots by silver staining, with a similar M_r but a range of pI values, presumably due to variable content of neuraminic acid termini on carbohydrate chains (J. Ng and V. P., unpublished results).

IL-2 has been partially purified from normal rat lymphocytes by a combination of gel filtration, ion exchange, and IEF (Gillis *et al.*, 1980b). More recently, Red agarose affinity chromatography has been added (DiSabato, 1982). In the latter study, most contaminating proteins of lymphocyte origin were apparently removed, as judged from the 6000- to 8000-fold purification, but bovine serum albumin (BSA) was added to stabilize the activity, and thus the specific activity in terms of units per microgram total protein (i.e., including the added BSA) was not high. Nevertheless, on the basis of recovered, biosynthetically labeled lmphocyte proteins, it could be estimated that IL-2 activity was detectable at 10^{-11} M (DiSabato, 1982).

C. Microheterogeneity of IL-2

IL-2 derived from both normal, Con A-stimulated mouse spleen cells and from EL4 has a heterogeneous profile on IEF or chromatofocusing (Shaw *et al.*, 1978a; Gillis *et al.*, 1982; Pure *et al.*, 1982). We have repeatedly seen a range of pI from 3.9 to 5.0, with up to 10 peaks. The predominant form in IEF was at pI 3.9 in our preparations. The heterogeneity is probably due to a variable content of negatively charged carbohydrate, since either treatment with neuraminadase or blocking the addition of *N*-linked carbohydrate with tunicamycin reduces it and causes the activity to focus at the upper end of the scale (Clark-Lewis and Schrader, 1982b; Farrar *et al.*, 1982). A direct relationship between negative charge and apparent M_r on SDS-PAGE was noted by Gillis *et al.* (1982). This would be the case if a high-density negative charge reflected a higher carbohydrate content, for two reasons: (1) removal of carbohydrate chains from secreted IL-2 would reduce the M_r directly, as well as increasing the pI due to less sialic acid; and (2) high negative charge due to higher sialic acid could lead to diminished binding of SDS, and a lower mobility (higher apparent M_r) on PAGE. Results obtained with human IFN are in keeping with these predictions, i.e., removal of carbohydrate chains converted it to a form of lower apparent M_r and greater homogeneity on SDS-PAGE (Stewart *et al.*, 1977).

The behavior of murine IL-2 on gel-filtration columns suggests an M_r of 32,000 (Chen and DiSabato, 1976) or 45,000 (Shaw *et al.*, 1978a), or any value in between. The correct M_r, on the basis of combining sedimentation coefficient, Stokes radius, and partial specific volume, appears to be close to 32,000 (Shaw *et al.*, 1978a). Again, the discrepancy may be related to carbohydrate content. Material that showed a higher Stokes radius than expected on gel filtration also had a relatively low pI (predominantly 3.9) and a rather low partial specific volume, all consistent with a rather high carbohydrate content (Shaw *et al.*, 1978a). Carbohydrate would lead to greater hydration than expected for pure protein, explaining the gel-filtration data. On the other hand, other preparations from mouse spleen cells showed a less anomalous behavior on gel filtration as well as a higher overall pI, consistent with a lower carbohydrate content (Watson *et al.*, 1979a; Mochizuki *et al.*, 1980).

A range of pI values (6.7–8.1) has been seen with IL-2 from human tonsil lymphocytes (Robb and Smith, 1981); this pattern also appears to be due to sialic acid. IL-2 from the Jurkat line showed only a single band of activity, with a pI of 8.1, during IEF (Robb and Smith, 1981; Robb *et al.*, 1983). Treatment of the tonsil material with neuraminidase converted it to material with the same high pI as Jurkat IL-2 (Robb and Smith, 1981). IL-2 from tonsil lymphocytes exhibited two bands on SDS-PAGE, running with markers of 16,200 and 14,600, but the Jurkat material ran as a single band just below 15,000. Treatment with exo- plus endoglycosidases converted the higher-M_r-tonsil IL-2 to the same mobility as Jurkat. All these results can be explained by the hypothesis that greater amounts of carbohydrate result in higher M_r, lower mobility in SDS-PAGE, and a lower pI. Jurkat IL-2 would then be predicted to have the least, if any, carbohydrate. Interestingly, the Jurkat sequence deduced from cloned cDNA is predicted not to contain *N*-linked carbohydrate, although this does not rule out other polysaccharides (Taniguchi *et al.*, 1983). Indeed, the third amino acid residue from the *N*-terminus, threonine, appears to be modified in the secreted protein (Robb *et al.*, 1983) and may be a site of *O*-glycosylation.

IL-2 from human peripheral blood lymphocytes (PBL) showed a puzzling difference in pI, when generated in the presence or absence of Daudi cells (added to enhance the level of production) (Welte *et al.*, 1982). In the absence of Daudi, the pI observed was 6.7, but in their presence it was 8.1. The apparent M_r under nondenaturing conditions also differed; however, the effects were so large as to defy swift interpretation. Thus, leaving out Daudi cells produced an apparent M_r of 26,000, rather than the otherwise observed 13,000–18,000, in gel filtration—possibly the result of aggregation. In SDS-PAGE, the two preparations ran at 16,000–17,000 and 14,500, respectively, a much smaller difference (Welte *et al.*, 1982). One possible basis for the differences between the two IL-2 species could be a difference in carbohydrate content. If the presence of Daudi cells resulted in the removal of sialic acid and other carbohydrate groups by neuraminidase and glycosidases, the pI value would rise and the M_r decrease, as observed.

D. Molecular Properties of IL-2 Summarized

Much of the observed heterogeneity in IL-2 from a given species can be rationalized on the basis of variable carbohydrate content. This would explain the apparent decrease in hydrodynamic particle size and the increase in pI with removal of carbohydrate. Other aspects of heterogeneity can also be accounted for within the context of a single protein product for IL-2 in any given species. Thus, the multiple M_r forms of human IL-2 seen in nondenaturing solvents by Gillis *et al.* (1980b) appeared to consist of aggregates of a fundamental product with an M_r of about 15,000. Preliminary data (Taniguchi *et al.*, 1983) indicated that only a single gene hybridizes with Jurkat IL-2 cDNA; more recent work confirms that at least the gene coding for IL-2 produced by normal lymphocytes and Jurkat cells is present in one copy per haploid genome (Degrave *et al.*, 1983).

Human IL-2 is normally isolated as a single-chain product, with the same M_r in SDS as in nondenaturing solvents (Table I). Both methods suggest a value close to 16,000, and the cloned IL-2 cDNA predicts 15,400 as the M_r of the processed protein (Taniguchi *et al.*, 1983). By contrast, mouse IL-2 appears to

Table 1. Molecular Properties of IL-2[a, b]

	Mouse		Human		
Property	EL4, LBRM	Spleen	Normal cells	Jurkat	CTCL
Native M_r[c]	32,000	32,000	15,000–18,000	15,400	16,000
M_r of protein chain[c]	22,000–23,000	17,000	*a*	*a*	*a*
Approx. ED_{30} (pg)	75	–	135	200	–
Approximate yield (ng/nl)[d]	100–400	2	100–200	400	–
pI	3.9–5.0	3.9–4.9	6.8–8.2	8.2 (7.9)	4.5

[a] Data compiled from the following references: mouse LBRM33: Gillis *et al.*, 1982; mouse EL4: Farrar *et al.*, 1980, 1982; and our own data; mouse spleen: Shaw *et al.*, 1978a; Watson *et al.*, 1979b; human PBL: Welte *et al.*, 1982; Gillis *et al.*, 1980b, 1982; Mier and Gallo, 1980; human tonsil lymphocytes: Robb and Smith, 1981; Jurkat cells: Robb and Smith, 1981; Robb *et al.*, 1981, 1983; CTCL: Gootenberg *et al.*, 1982.

[b] CTCL, cutaneous T-cell leukemia/lymphoma; ED_{30}, amount of activity in 1 ml that produces 30% maximal response; M_r, relative molecular weight.

[c] Values are generally based on behavior displayed with gel chromatography, except for mouse spleen, which is based on sedimentation and Stokes radius (Shaw *et al.*, 1978a). Data refer to behavior on SDS-PAGE and reflect apparent M_r with reference to markers. The exception to this is the value for Jurkat, which is based on inferred protein sequence derived from cloned cDNA (Taniguchi *et al.*, 1983).

[d] Yields are estimated from the activities measured in culture supernatants on the assumption that the highest specific activity material described in the text represents essentially pure IL-2. They are not corrected for the numbers of cells, and so forth. It should be noted that typically primary leukocyte cultures (spleen, PBL) are at a higher density than are cultures of tumor cells.

exist as a dimer of two 16,000–18,000-M_r chains (Caplan *et al.*, 1981). The reason for this difference in behavior between human and mouse IL-2 is not apparent.

Thus, both human and mouse IL-2 probably consist of protein chains of M_r 15,000–18,000. Both can be isolated in various forms of glycosylation, leading to heterogeneity for each species. The two IL-2 proteins themselves are different, with mouse having an intrinsic pI near 5.0, and human near 8.2. Rat IL-2 appears to fall in between, at pI 5.4–5.6 in one report (Gillis *et al.*, 1980b) and at pI 5.5–6.3 in another (DiSabato, 1982). No extensive examination of the effects of neuraminidase treatment has been reported for rat IL-2. Both mouse and human IL-2 are extremely hydrophobic, compared with most soluble proteins. Both are relatively stable. Mouse IL-2, for example, can be denatured at 90°C in 1% SDS, with or without mercaptoethanol and the activity completely recovered (Caplan *et al.*, 1981). The specific activities of the two molecules, expressed in terms of ED_{30}, are about 10,000–15,000 and 5000–8000 units/μg protein for the purest preparations of mouse and human IL-2, respectively. Differences in the specific activity of this magnitude can easily arise from different assay conditions and are in themselves not significant. These preparations are probably near 100% in purity. The concentration of IL-2 giving 30% maximal responses in cell culture is on the order of 3 to 10×10^{-12} M. In a typical IL-2 assay, of 0.2-ml volume and sensitive to 0.05 ED_{30} units/ml, less than 1 pg of purified mouse IL-2 can be detected. The properties of human and mouse IL-2 are summarized in Table I.

IV. TRANSLATION OF LYMPHOKINE mRNA

A. mRNAs Encoding Lymphokines

With the availability of tumor cell lines producing high levels of IL-2 from several species, it has become feasible to isolate mRNA coding for this lymphokine. This approach is illustrated by results based on the mouse T-cell lymphoma EL4. In the absence of stimulation, the culture supernatants of these cells contain very little IL-2. After stimulation with the phorbol diester PMA, the IL-2 level in the medium begins to rise within 1–2 hr, reaching a maximum value at about 24 hr (Bleackley *et al.*, 1981). Since mRNA levels are probably highest at the time that the level of secreted IL-2 is rising fastest, mRNA was isolated after 12–14 hr of exposure to PMA. Total RNA was prepared by selective precipitation from guanidinium chloride-lysed cells (Przybyla *et al.*, 1979), and further purification of poly A^+ RNA was achieved by affinity chromatography on oligo-dT cellulose (Bleackley *et al.*, 1981). Typically, the yield from 10^9 cells was 200–600 μg poly A^+ RNA.

This mRNA, when injected into *Xenopus laevis* oocytes, gave biologically active IL-2, as assayed on an IL-2-dependent T-cell line, and GM-CSF, assayed by the ability to stimulate growth of granulocyte–macrophage colonies from bone marrow. However, the mRNAs for these two lymphokines were separated on a sucrose gradient (Fig. 3; Bleackley *et al.*, 1983). Thus, IL-2 and GM-CSF are encoded by different messengers with sedimentation coefficients of 11.5 and 8S, respectively. They may conceivably derive from a common, larger precursor molecule. When size-fractionated RNA was translated and assayed for IL-3 activity by stimulation of DNA synthesis in an IL-3-dependent cell line, the peak was coincident with GM-CSF mRNA (Fig. 3). The rather low sedimentation

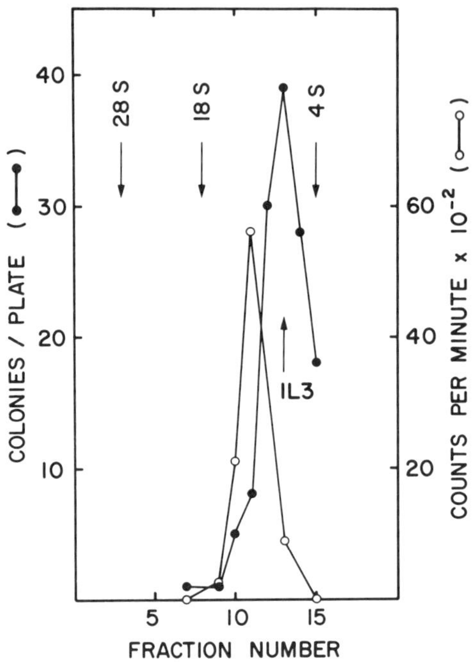

Figure 3. Sedimentation of lymphokine mRNAs. EL4 lymphoma cells were stimulated with PMA (10 ng/ml); after 14 hr in culture medium containing 4% horse serum, they were harvested and lysed with guanidinium chloride (Przybyla *et al.*, 1979), as described by Bleackley *et al.* (1981, 1983). After chromatography through oligo-dT cellulose (two cycles, with an intermediate salt wash of 0.1 M LiCl the second time), poly A^+ RNA was pooled and frozen in aliquots. Poly A^+ RNA was heated to 70°C in water just before sedimentation through 10–28% sucrose gradients in an SW 50.1 rotor (Beckman) at 48,000 rpm for 5 hr at 4°C. Gradient fractions were precipitated twice with ethanol and dissolved in water before being microinjected into *Xenopus laevis* oocytes. Oocyte supernatants were harvested; at 48 hr PMSF was added to 25 μg/ml to inhibit proteolysis; then a standard assay for IL-2 was carried out on CTL line MTL2.8 (Bleackley *et al.*, 1981, 1982). CSF-GM was also determined in the oocyte supernatant by the growth of colonies and clusters from the bone marrow of 8–12-week-old $BCDF_1$ mice (Pluznik and Sachs, 1965; Bradley and Metcalf, 1966). Material translatable into IL-2 sedimented in the region of 11.5S compared with the marker RNAs, while mRNA for CSF-GM sedimented at about 8S. In a separate experiment, oocyte translation products were also assayed for IL-3 activity by their ability to stimulate proliferation of an IL-3-dependent cell line. The mRNA for this activity (arrow) sedimented similarly to CSF-GM. Note that IL-3 and CSF-GM are not the same, as they are separated by hydrophobic affinity chromatography. BCDF, B-cell differentiating factor, CSF-GM, colony-stimulating factor for granulocytes and macrophages; CTL, cytotoxic T lymphocyte; PMSF, phenylmethylsulfuryl flouride.

coefficients of 8S for GM-CSF and IL-3 mRNAs points out the unpredictability of relating mRNA sedimentation in nondenaturing gradients to the size of the final product. IL-3 behaves like a molecule of M_r 28,000-41,000 in SDS-PAGE (Ihle *et al.*, 1982a,b), and GM-CSF as a molecule of M_r 23,000 (Burgess *et al.*, 1977) while IL-2 runs with markers of 22,000-23,000 (Fig. 2). A part of each molecule is undoubtedly carbohydrate, and it remains to be seen how much peptide is encoded by each of the respective mRNAs.

Similar IL-2 mRNAs have been isolated from a variety of other cells, including a gibbon lymphoma (Lin *et al.*, 1982), human tonsils (Efrat *et al.*, 1982), human PBL (Hinuma *et al.*, 1982), and the human Jurkat lymphoma (Taniguchi *et al.*, 1983). In each case, the mRNAs were identified by translation in *Xenopus laevis* oocytes, followed by specific bioassay for the protein. Sedimentation in sucrose gradients was used to obtain a rough idea of the size of the relevant mRNAs. Gibbon IL-2 mRNA sedimented rather broadly, and the observed sedimentation rate of 14-16S may have been partially a reflection of aggregation. IL-2 mRNA from human tonsils sedimented at 10-10.5S, with a minor component at 13-13.5S. (Evidence presented elsewhere indicates that the latter is probably an artifact of aggregation; see Taniguchi *et al.*, 1983.) The mRNA from PBL sedimented at 10-12S, while Jurkat (human) IL-2 mRNA sedimented at 11.5S. These results are consistent with the conclusion reached in Section III that the protein components of IL-2 from different species are of similar size, around 15,000 M_r. It is conceivable, but unlikely, that a single polypeptide the size of native mouse IL-2 (32,000) could be encoded by the observed mRNA.

An interesting question pertains to the induction of IL-2 activity in stimulated lymphocytes. In the EL4 lymphoma, for example, IL-2 begins to accumulate in the culture medium within 2 hr of being stimulated with PMA, and the level continues to increase for about 25 hr. Similar results are seen with normal T lymphocytes stimulated with Con A (Paetkau *et al.*, 1976) or in an MLC (Shaw *et al.*, 1978b). This induction does not appear to be due to the release of preformed IL-2 in the case of normal spleen lymphocytes, since we have been unable to find any in unstimulated cells. The question then becomes whether IL-2 is constantly being synthesized, secreted, and degraded in the absence of stimulation, or whether the increase in secreted IL-2 is a reflection of increased IL-2 mRNA. The latter is undoubtedly occurring. Unstimulated EL4 cells contained barely detectable levels of IL-2 mRNA (Bleackley *et al.*, 1981); these levels rose to their maximum value within about 12 hr of stimulation with PMA. In human lymphocytes stimulated with PHA and PMA, the level of translatable IL-2 mRNA went from undetectably low to its maximum in 16 hr, a time when IL-2 was beginning to accumulate at its maximum rate in the cell culture supernatant (Efrat *et al.*, 1982). The most likely explanation for these results is that, prior to the synthesis and secretion of high levels of IL-2, the level of IL-2 mRNA increases dramatically in the cytoplasm of the activated T lymphocytes.

B. Processing of Nascent IL-2

Mouse (Bleackley *et al.*, 1983), gibbon (Lin *et al.*, 1982), and human (Hinuma *et al.*, 1982) IL-2 translated in microinjected *Xenopus laevis* oocytes is found predominantly in the supernatants of these cultures by 40 hr. This presumably reflects the ability of oocytes to process and secrete these proteins, as is known to occur for other secretory products (Colman, 1982). To study processing of newly synthesized IL-2 we have used two cell-free translation systems, i.e., rabbit reticulocyte and wheat germ lysates.

A rabbit reticulocyte lysate system (Pelham and Jackson, 1976) is often used for cell-free translation because of its relatively high efficiency. However, we experienced only occasional success in translating IL-2 mRNA in this system. This was so, though other proteins were being translated efficiently, as measured by the incorporation of [^{35}S]methionine and PAGE analysis. By addition of authentic IL-2, we showed that the lack of success was not due to inhibition of the IL-2 assay by the lysate. We will return to the basis of this problem, which is somewhat interesting.

In contrast to the variable and generally poor translatability of IL-2 mRNA in rabbit reticulocyte lysates, wheat germ lysates (Roberts and Paterson, 1973) reproducibly synthesized biologically active IL-2 with both poly A$^+$ and gradient-purified mRNAs (Table II). When microsomes prepared from dog pancreas were added to the wheat germ translation system programmed with IL-2 mRNA, most of the IL-2 activity segregated into the microsomes (Fig. 4). These could be separated from the soluble fraction of the translation system by centrifugation through a sucrose cushion (Walter and Blobel, 1981a) and the IL-2 released with detergent. Control experiments indicated that only mRNA from PMA-stimulated EL4 cells generated significant amounts of IL-2. Furthermore, microsomes that were heat inactivated did not sequester IL-2, nor did microsomes added after translation was complete. Other control experiments showed that preformed IL-2 isolated from EL4 cells was not associated with microsomes, when added during translation of an irrelevant mRNA (placental prelactogen), which does associate with microsomes. Finally, microsome-associated IL-2 was relatively resistant to trypsin (data not shown), strong evidence that it had crossed into the luminal space (Katz *et al.*, 1977). In summary, translocation of nascent IL-2 into heterologous microsomes occurs during translation and requires functional microsomes.

Extensive studies on the processing of secreted proteins have led to a model explaining how they are marked and handled for export (Meyer *et al.*, 1982). A signal-recognition particle (SRP) (Walter and Blobel, 1981b) recognizes hydrophobic leader sequences on nascent secretory proteins and temporarily halts their translation. Docking protein (DP) (Meyer *et al.*, 1982), which is associated with rough endoplasmic reticulum, binds the SRP–nascent protein complex, releasing the inhibition and guiding the polypeptide into the microsomal lumen

Table II. Microsomes Alleviate Inhibition of IL-2 Translation Caused by Reticulocyte Lysates

Translation mix[a]	Microsomes[b]	mRNA[c]	Net IL-2 activity[d]	% [^{35}S]met incorporated[e]
Wheat germ	–	None	(0)	36
Wheat germ	–	PMA$^-$	2 ± 28	202
90% wheat germ	–	PMA$^+$	1129 ± 36	(100)
90% wheat germ 10% reticulocyte	–	PMA$^+$	51 ± 9	74
90% wheat germ	+	PMA$^+$	1398 ± 31	94
90% wheat germ 10% reticulocyte	+	PMA$^+$	256 ± 3	72

[a] Translation reactions and IL-2 assays were performed as described in Fig. 4. 90% wheat germ reactions contained 9 μl instead of 10 μl wheat germ per 30-μl incubation. Where indicated, 1 μl reticulocyte lysate (10%) was also present.
[b] Microsome samples were treated with SDS (0.5% w/v) and heated (70°C, 10 min), at the end of 60-min incubation at 25°C. SDS was removed by precipitation with 0.1 M KCl (2×) at 4°C.
[c] Poly A$^+$ RNA (mRNA) was isolated from ELY lymphoma cells either stimulated with 10 ng/ml phorbol myristate acetate (PMA$^+$) or unstimulated (PMA$^-$).
[d] Six-μl aliquots were assayed directly for IL-2 activity, given in cpm [^{125}I]dIUrd incorporated into the cloned CTL line MTL2.8 (Bleackley *et al.*, 1981, 1982). A value of 564 cpm, obtained with no mRNA, was subtracted throughout.
[e] Incorporation of [^{35}S]methionine is relative to the level observed with 90% wheat germ.

during the resumed translation. Thus, translocation through the microsomes is coupled to translation (Walter and Blobel, 1981b). Most of these features appear to apply to the coupled translation and translocations of IL-2 described here. This finding is consistent with the secretory nature of IL-2 and with its secretion from microinjected *Xenopus laevis* oocytes as well. Furthermore, it should be noted that human (Jurkat) IL-2 contains a putative 20-amino acid leader sequence with a characteristic hydrophobic nature (Taniguchi *et al.*, 1983).

The lack of translation of IL-2 in the reticulocyte lysate system is due to the action of an inhibitor, which is present to various degrees in different lysates. This was shown by adding small proportions of a reticulocyte lysate that did not translate IL-2 activity, but that was active in synthesizing other proteins (data not shown), to the wheat germ system (Table II). As little as 10% by volume of reticulocyte lysate completely inhibited translation of IL-2, in a specific way; general translation, as indicated by incorporation of [^{35}S]methionine and SDS-PAGE, was only slightly inhibited. The inhibition was probably due to the presence of SRP in the reticulocyte lysate, as reported by Meyer *et al.* (1982). Wheat germ lysates do not contain SRP. Interestingly, addition of microsomes, which contain DP and thus are able to reverse the SRP-induced inhibition by binding the SRP-nascent peptide complex, did indeed remove the inhibition to a significant degree (Table II).

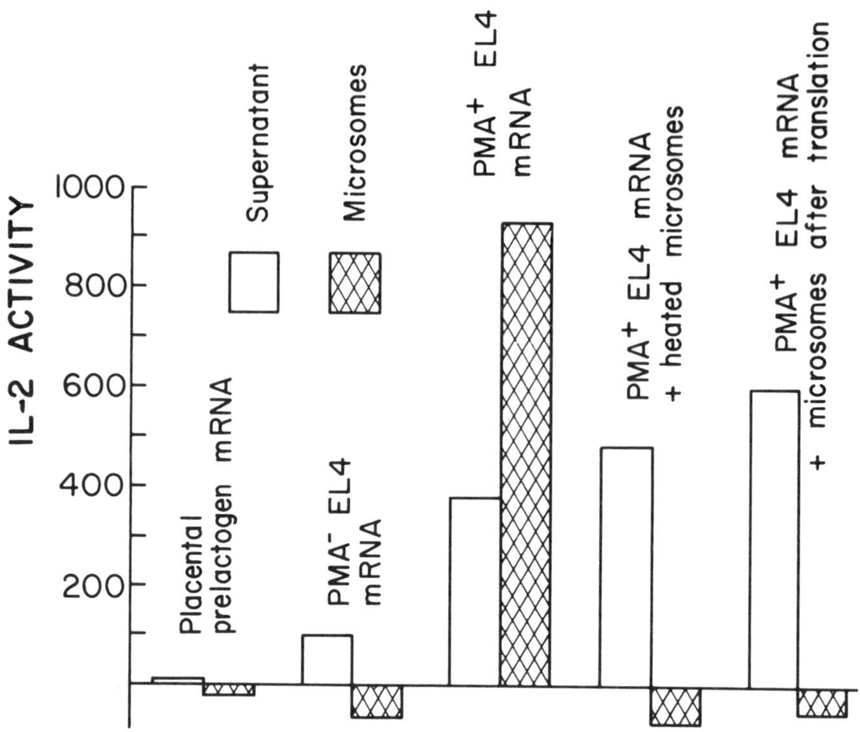

Figure 4. Effects of dog pancreatic microsomes on translation of IL-2 mRNA *in vitro*. Poly A^+ RNA (mRNA) was isolated from EL4 lymphoma cells either stimulated with 10 ng/ml phorbol myristate acetate (PMA^+) or unstimulated (PMA^-). It was translated in a wheat germ system treated with micrococcal nuclease to reduce background synthesis and purchased from Bethesda Research Laboratories. The incubation mixture contained 63.3 mM potassium acetate, 0.7 mM magnesium acetate, 1.6 μCi/μl [^{35}S]methionine (1040 Ci/mmol, NEN), 20 mM HEPES buffer (pH 7.5), 1.2 mM ATP, 0.1 mM GTP, 5.5 mM creatine phosphate, 0.2 mg/ml creatine kinase, 80 μM spermidine, 50 mM each of 19 amino acids (excluding methionine), and 30% (v/v) wheat germ extract EL4 mRNAs were added at 1-20 μg/ml. Placental prelactogen mRNA (NEN) was added to monitor the ability of added microsomes to translocate nascent protein (PAGE data not shown). Dog pancreatic microsomes (NEN) were added to 1% v/v and, at the end of incubation (60 min at 25°C), samples were layered onto a 10% (w/v) sucrose solution and the microsomes were pelleted by centrifugation in a Beckman Airfuge at 120,000 × *g* for 10 min. Microsomal pellets were washed once and then lysed in buffer containing 0.5% SDS. The detergent was removed by two precipitations with 0.1 M KCl. The material released from microsomes (clear bars) and that remaining at the top of the sucrose cushion from the centrifugation step (hatched bars) were both assayed for IL-2 using an IL-2-dependent CTL line. In one sample, microsomes were heated to 60°C for 10 min before being added. In another, no microsomes were added initially; after translation was complete at 60 min, 0.2 μg pancreatic RNase was added, and 10 min later, microsomes were added. After 30 min further incubation, the sample was processed as described above. The IL-2 assay is given as cpm [^{125}I]DIUdR incorporated 24 hr after adding test samples to the CTL line. A background value of 720 ± 40 cpm was subtracted from all data.

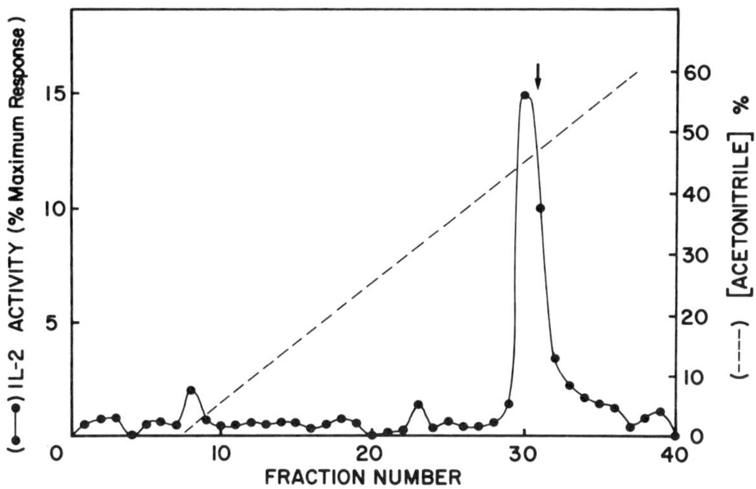

Figure 5. HPLC of IL-2 synthesized in the wheat germ translation system. RNA isolated from PMA-stimulated EL4 cells was translated in the wheat germ system as described in Fig. 4. The incubation mixture contained 100 μg/ml poly A^+ RNA. After a 1-hr incubation at 25°C, 5 ml RIPA (50 mM Tris–HCl, pH 7.2–0.15 MNaCl–0.1% SDS–1% sodium deoxycholate–1% Triton X100–1 mM PMSF), 1.5 ml of a 1:1 dilution of protein A-Sepharose CL4B (Pharmacia), and 100 μl of a rat anti-mouse IL-2 antiserum were added. The serum was obtained from rats repeatedly immunized with EL4-derived IL-2 (five to seven injections of 50,000 ED_{30} units). This antiserum inhibits IL-2 in the TCGF assay at 1:1000 dilution or less. The immunoprecipitates were incubated at 4°C for 3 hr with constant mixing. Beads were collected and washed three times with RIPA and twice with phosphate-buffered saline. Immune complexes were dissociated by incubation in 0.5 M HCl for 10 min at 4°C. The sample was then chromatographed on RP-HPLC (Varian Vista Series 5000 liquid chromatograph) using a C_{18} column, as described in Fig.1, except that a linear gradient of 0–60% acetonitrile (60 min) was used for elution. Fractions (2 ml) were lyophylized after addition of 1.6 mg bovine serum albumin (BSA) and dilution to 8 ml with distilled water. The samples were then suspended in 300 μl RHFM and assayed in triplicate (3 × 100 μl) for IL-2 activity. The arrow shows the elution position of fraction 3 IL-2 derived from PMA-induced EL4 cells and run over the same column. The difference in positions is not significant. RHFM, RPMI 1640 medium containing 5 × 10^{-5} M 2-mercaptoethanol-20 mM $NaHCO_3$-0.34 mM Na pyruvate-20 mM HEPES, pH 7.3–10% fetal bovine serum; RP-HPLC, reverse-phase-high-performance liquid chromatography.

Our results demonstrate that newly synthesized IL-2 is translocated cotranslationally into the luminal side of microsomes. Although in general the amount IL-2 synthesized was greater in the presence of microsomes than in their absence, it is clear that posttranslational processing is not essential for activity. This is most directly shown by the observation that translation in the wheat germ system in the absence of microsomes or SRP resulted in active IL-2.

We can also conclude that the hydrophobic nature of IL-2 is a property of its protein component. In Fig. 5, IL-2 synthesized in the wheat germ system was immunoprecipitated and applied to a similar HP-HPLC column as in Fig. 1. The activity emerged in essentially the same position as IL-2 secreted by EL4 cells.

V. CLONED LYMPHOKINES

A. Human IL-2

It is of paramount importance in unraveling the complex interactions between cells and molecules in the immune system to relate molecular structures to lymphokine activities. Purification of the product lymphokine is a useful approach, but it cannot, in principle, prove the relationship between a specific biological function and a given molecule. The second phase of proving such a relationship has always been the synthesis of the putative structure. For a large protein such as IL-2, organic chemical synthesis would be difficult; the modern approach is to use genetic engineering instead. In addition to providing material for biological studies and therapeutic evaluation, this method also generates the tools with which to study gene structure, regulation of expression, and evolutionary relationships between lymphokines.

In order to clone genetic elements coding for lymphokines, it is necessary to develop assays for the genes in question. This can be done by establishing efficient systems for measuring lymphokine mRNAs, as described above, or through the synthesis of oligonucleotide gene probes, deduced from amino acid sequence data. The successful cloning of a lymphokine cDNA gene was reported by Taniguchi *et al.* (1983), whose work exemplifies the approach of cloning in which the biological activity of mRNA is used as the assay and is worth summarizing.

The starting point for cloning human IL-2 was mRNA isolated from the human Jurkat cell line, which had been stimulated with Con A to produce a high level of IL-2. Poly A^+ RNA was fractionated on a sucrose gradient and assayed by injection into *Xenopus laevis* oocytes. The peak fraction of IL-2 mRNA, 11.5S, was used as a template for the synthesis of double-stranded complementary DNA (dscDNA). After selection on the basis of size, the dscDNA was inserted into the plasmid cloning vector pBR322, and the recombinant molecules were used to transfect *Escherichia coli*. Pools containing 24 recombinant plasmid DNA molecules each were bound to nitrocellulose filters and screened for IL-2 gene sequences by the ability to bind IL-2 mRNA specifically (positive RNA selection). One colony out of 432 screened was found to be positive by this assay, but displayed less coding sequence than expected for intact IL-2. The positive recombinant DNA was used to detect a second clone containing 880 base pairs of IL-2 cDNA. The frequency of IL-2 mRNA in the poly A^+ pool isolated from Con A-stimulated cells was estimated to be 0.005%. It is not surprising that the cloning of lymphokine genes has proved difficult. As further proof that the cloned sequence corresponded to IL-2, it was inserted into a Simian Virus 40 (SV40) expression vector, and the new recombinant was used to transfect monkey COS cells. Low levels of IL-2 activity were found in the cell medium 72 hr after transfection. Southern blotting indicates that there is a single gene for this sequence, which also represents the IL-2 synthesized by normal tonsil cells (Degrave *et al.*, 1983).

The amino acid sequence of human IL-2 predicted from the cloned cDNA included a 20-amino acid putative leader segment, plus coding information for a mature protein of M_r 15,400. The assignment of the cleavage point of the leader sequence is supported by amino acid sequence data of purified Jurkat IL-2 (Robb *et al.*, 1983). The mature protein was predicted to contain equal numbers of basic and acidic amino acids, consistent with the observed pI of the protein. There are no sequences typical of *N*-glycosylation sites, but other modifications cannot be ruled out. Little homology was found between IL-2 and other growth factors apart from a very limited similarity with human interferon (IFN), i.e., γ-IFN and β_1-IFN. Although the amino acid sequence contains some clusters of nonpolar amino acids, it remains to be seen whether the rather high hydrophobicity of human IL-2 can be explained by the amino acid sequence alone.

B. PMA-Inducible Expression

In addition to being a useful source of lymphokines, cell lines such as Jurkat and EL4 are interesting model systems for the induction of specific genetic readout. After stimulation with PMA, the EL4 variant secretes IL-2, IL-3, GM-CSF, BCGF, BCDFμ, and other factors that are still poorly characterized. However, overall expression of genetic functions is not greatly altered, quantitatively or qualitatively. We have observed this at both the protein and mRNA levels. In the first place, biosynthetic labeling of proteins secreted by control, or PMA-induced intact EL4 cells, followed by one- or two-dimensional PAGE analysis, has shown only a few changes out of several hundred proteins synthesized (J. Ng, manuscript in preparation). Second, cDNA probes made from mRNA generated from induced or control cells were used to analyze sequence differences by hybridization ($R_o t$ analysis) (V. Paetkau, unpublished data). The difference in bulk mRNA sequences was estimated to be less than 10% overall.

These data strongly suggest that, despite the dramatic induction of specific lymphokine expression, the overall expressed repertoire of EL4 cells is not greatly altered by stimulation with PMA. Consequently, these data can serve as a model for investigating the molecular basis of the control of expression in eukaryotic cells, perhaps even of a subset of T lymphocytes. To carry out model studies, and to confirm the hypothesis that PMA induces only a limited alteration in expression, it is necessary to derive cloned probes for the induced mRNAs. These should contain, among others, sequences for the lymphokines of interest.

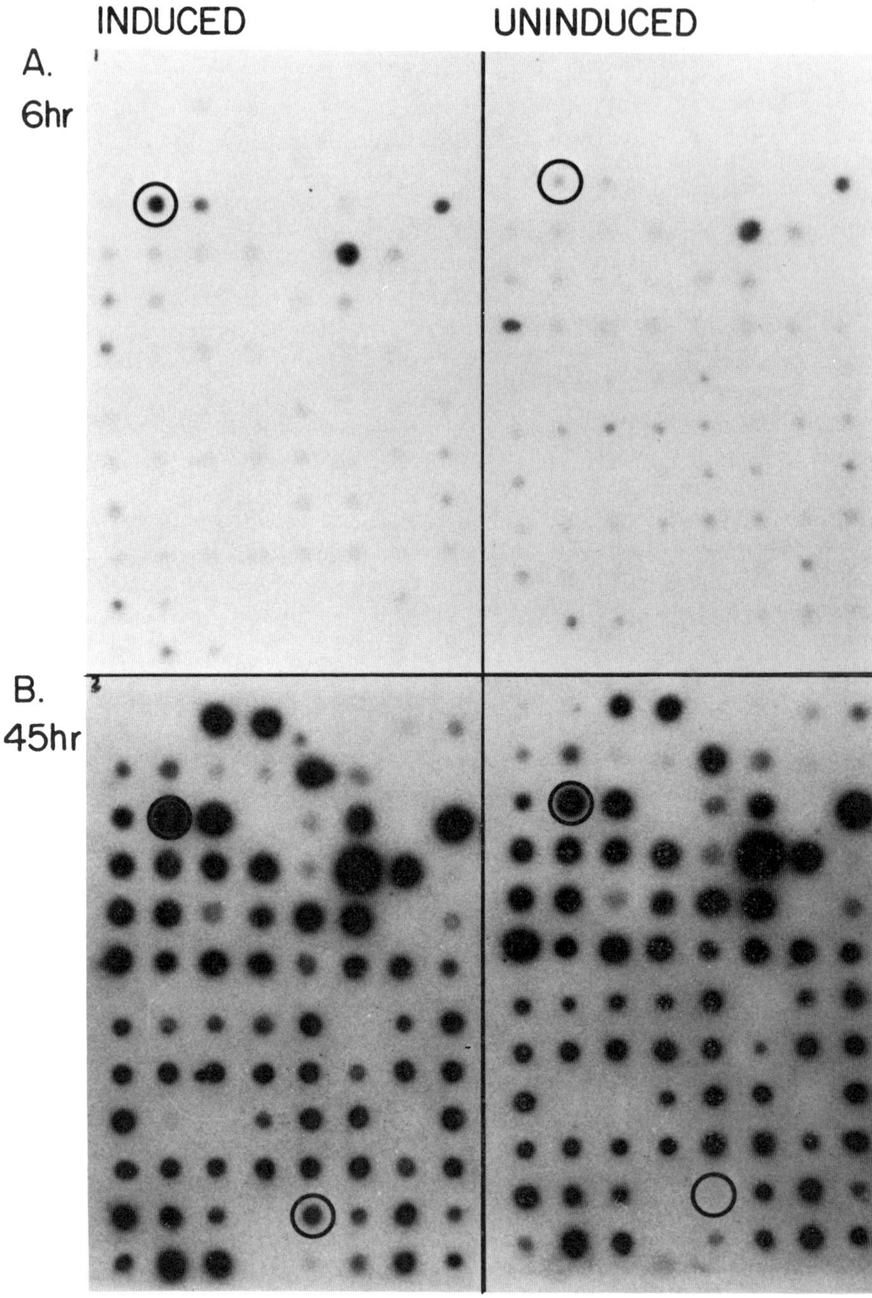

Figure 6. Screening of a cDNA library for PMA-induced sequences. Recombinant DNA was formed by linking (G-C tails) cDNA copied from poly A^+RNA purified from PMA-stimulated EL4 cells, and plasmid pBR322 DNA. This was used to transfect *Escherichia coli* cells selected for recombinant plasmids on the basis of being tetracycline resistant and ampicillin sensitive. Colonies were picked and grown to saturation in 96-well microtiter plates, replicated

Poly A^+ from PMA stimulated cells was copied into dscDNA and inserted into pBR322. The recombinant DNA was used to transfect *E. coli*, and appropriate drug-resistant transformants were selected. Recombinant clones were individually picked and put into microtiter trays. Duplicate-ordered arrays of these clones were then grown on nitrocellulose filters and screened by colony hybridization with cDNA probes copied from mRNA of either control of PMA-induced EL4 cells (Fig. 6). This method of plus-minus screening has been used to clone human γ-IFN (Gray *et al.*, 1982). Autoradiograms were scanned for colonies showing stronger hybridization with cDNA probe from PMA-induced cells than with control cDNA (Fig. 6). About 4% of the individually picked recombinants appeared to contain induced sequences by first colony hybridization but, upon rescreening by colony hybridization, only 33% of these still looked positive. Thus, the frequency of induced clones appeared to be about 1%. This result is consistent with our earlier observation that PMA stimulation results in only a limited alteration of genetic readout.

The library of sequences induced with PMA contains mRNAs of both low and moderate abundance. When colony hybridization autoradiograms were developed for 6 hr, a few sequences could already be seen to have registered as induced (Fig. 6). These presumably represent fairly abundant sequences. In contrast, some induced sequences showed up only after prolonged exposure of the autoradiogram, e.g., 48 hr, (Fig. 6B), and these probably represent low copy-number mRNAs. In addition to PMA-induced sequences, we have also observed sequences that are decreased in expression after PMA stimulation.

To confirm that at least some of cloned cDNA sequences selected by colony hybridization (Fig. 6) corresponded to PMA-induced mRNA sequences in EL4 cells, we used them as probes in the cytoplasmic dot method of analysis (White and Bancroft, 1982). Total cellular RNAs were prepared by rapid detergent lysis and fixed to nitrocellulose filters. RNA was derived from both PMA-induced and uninduced EL4, as well as from the CTL line MTL2.8 (Bleackley *et al.*, 1982). One probe corresponded to an mRNA whose level rose by about four-fold after exposure to PMA (Fig. 7). The other, as a control, hybridized equally to RNA

---

onto duplicate nitrocellulose filters, and grown to exponential phase; their plasmid DNA was amplified with chloramphenicol. The colonies were lysed and their DNA denatured and fixed onto the nitrocellulose filters (Grunstein and Hogness, 1975). The duplicate filters were hybridized with ^{32}P-labeled single-stranded cDNA synthesized with poly A^+ RNA purified from PMA-stimulated or -unstimulated EL4 cells. The specific activity of the probe was $1\text{–}2 \times 10^8$ cpm/μg, and hybridization conditions were based on the work of Thomas (1980), as described by Bleackley *et al.* (1982). The filters were washed and exposed to X-ray film. (A, B) are Autoradiograms of 6-hr and 45-hr exposure, respectively. Two colonies that show greater hybridization with ^{32}P-probe from PMA-induced cells than with probe from unstimulated cells are circled. Short exposure times were necessary to identify recombinants harboring highly abundant sequences (A) because the intensity differential was not as obvious after long exposures. (B) Recombinants carrying sequences of moderate to low abundance required long exposures.

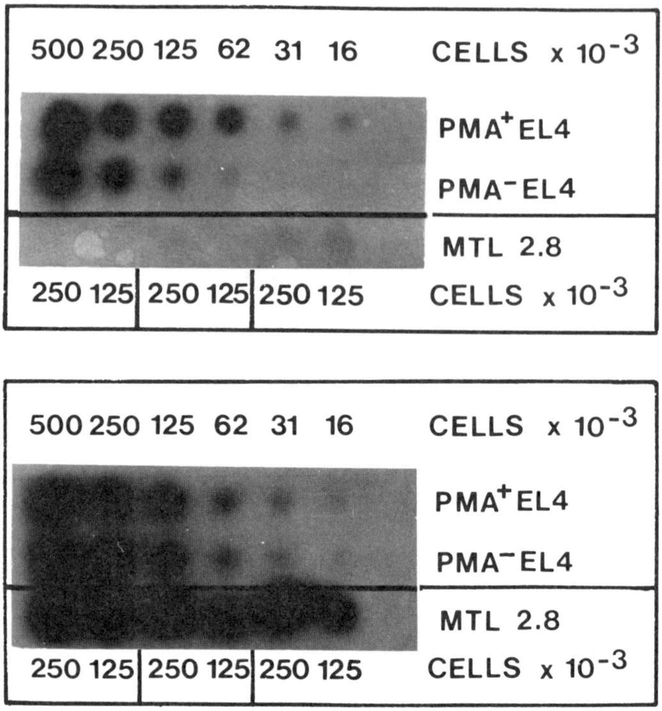

Figure 7. Analysis of mRNA levels in (PMA)-induced EL4 cells. EL4 cells stimulated with 10 ng/ml PMA for 24 hr (PMA^+) and control cells (PMA^-) were harvested. Total cytoplasmic RNA samples were prepared essentially as described by White and Bancroft (1982). Cells were lysed with the nonionic detergent NP-40 and nuclei removed by centrifugation. The supernatant samples were subjected to denaturation in formaldehyde and various proportions were bound to nitrocellulose. Serial two-fold dilutions of the cytoplasmic samples were used. As a control, cytoplasmic RNA from three subclones of the CTL line MTL2.8 (Bleackley *et al.*, 1982) was hybridized to the same probes. These samples represented 250,000 and 125,000 cells each, as indicated. Hybridization to the nick-translated cloned cDNA probes was performed according to Thomas (1980). Probe 7 (A) is a relatively high-abundance cDNA encoding a putative PMA-induced sequence in EL4 cells. It corresponds to the circled recombinant in Fig. 6A. Probe 10 is a cDNA of similar abundance, but its level is apparently not increased after exposure to PMA. Probe 7 had a specific activity of 5.8×10^7 cpm/μg, and probe 10 contained 7.3×10^7 cpm/μg. Probe 7 (B) evidently represents an EL4 sequence enhanced about four-fold after PMA induction and present at an undetectably low concentration in MTL2.8 cells. In contrast, probe 10 corresponds to a sequence that is not enhanced after PMA and that is much more common (at least 10-fold) in MTL2.8 than in EL4.

from both EL4 cell preparations. Both are fairly high-abundance sequences. Interestingly, the induced sequence (probe 7, Fig. 7) was undetectable in MTL2.8 cells, but the unchanging sequence (probe 10) was more abundant in MTL2.8 than in either EL4 preparation.

We have not yet identified the protein product represented by probe 7. However, by building up a library of such induced sequences, representing the enhanced readout of less than 1% of the mRNA sequences synthesized in EL4 cells, we expect to produce clones corresponding to both the identified and unidentified lymphokines secreted by this line after PMA stimulation. A valuable adjunct in this work is the sequestering of secretory proteins translated *in vitro* into microsomes when these are present during translation.

The library of induced sequences from this cellular source can be used to probe various parameters of T-lymphocyte function. Both T-lymphoma cells of the EL4 type, normal T lymphocytes selected on the basis of surface markers, and cloned, functional T lymphocytes could be profitably examined. In this way, the study of lymphokines will be brought into the context of cellular and molecular biology. In addition, models will be created for genetic regulation of the highly differentiated cells represented by T lymphocytes.

ACKNOWLEDGMENTS

The work supported in this review was supported by the Alberta Heritage Foundation, Medical Research Council of Canada, and the NCIC through its Terry Fox Special Initiatives Program.

VI. REFERENCES

Bleackley, R. C., Caplan, B., Havele, C., Ritzel, R. G., Mosmann, T. R., Farrar, J. F., and Paetkau, V., 1981, *J. Immunol.* **127**:2432–2435.
Bleackley, R. C., Havele, C., and Paetkau, V., 1982, *J. Immunol.* **128**:758–767.
Bleackley, R. C., Horak, H., McElhaney, J., Havele, C., Shaw, A. R. E., Turner, A. R., and Paetkau, V. H., 1983, *Nucleic Acids Res.* **11**:3027–3035.
Bradley, T. R., and Metcalf, D., 1966, *Aust. J. Exp. Biol. Med. Sci.* **44**:287–300.
Burgess, A. W., Camakaris, J., and Metcalf, D., 1977, *J. Biol. Chem.* **252**:1998–2003.
Caplan, B., Gibbs, C., and Paetkau, V., 1981, *J. Immunol.* **126**:1351–1354.
Chen, D.-M., and DiSabato, G., 1976, *Cell. Immunol.* **22**:211–224.
Clark-Lewis, I., and Schrader, J. W., 1981, *J. Immunol.* **127**:1931–1947.
Clark-Lewis, I., and Schrader, J. W., 1982a, *J. Immunol.* **128**:168–174.
Clark-Lewis, I., and Schrader, J. W., 1982b, *J. Immunol.* **128**:175–180.
Colman, A., 1982, *Trends Biochem. Sci.* **7**:435–437.
Degrave, W., Tavernier, J., Duerinck, F., Plaetinck, G., Devos, R., and Fiers, W., 1983, *EMBO J.* **2**:2349–2353.
DiSabato, G., 1982, *Proc. Natl. Acad. Sci. USA* **79**:3020–3023.

DiSabato, G., Chen, D.-M., and Erickson, J. W., 1975, *Cell. Immunol.* **17**:495–504.
Efrat, S., Pilo, S., and Kaempfer, R., 1982, *Nature* **297**:236–239.
Farrar, J. J., Fuller-Farrar, J., Simon, P. L., Hilfiker, M. L., Stadler, B. M., and Farrar, W. L., 1980, *J. Immunol.* **125**:2555–2558.
Farrar, J. J., Benjamin, W. R., Hilfiker, M. L., Howard, M., Farrar, W. L., and Fuller-Farrar, J., 1982, *Immunol. Rev.* **63**:129–166.
Gillis, S., Ferm, M. M., Ou, W., and Smith, K., 1978, *J. Immunol.* **120**:2027–2032.
Gillis, S., Scheid, M., and Watson, J., 1980a, *J. Immunol.* **125**:2570–2578.
Gillis, S., Smith, K. A., and Watson, J., 1980b, *J. Immunol.* **124**:1954–1962.
Gillis, S., Mochizuki, D. Y., Conlon, P. J., Hefeneder, S. H., Ramthun, C. A., Gillis, A. E., Frank, M. B., Henney, C. S., and Watson, J. D., 1982, *Immunol. Rev.* **63**:167–209.
Gootenberg, J. E., Ruscetti, F. W., and Gallo, R. C., 1982, *J. Immunol.* **129**:1499–1505.
Granelli-Piperno, A., Vassalli, J., and Reich, E., 1981, *J. Exp. Med.* **154**:422–430.
Gray, P. W., Leung, D. W., Pennica, D., Yelverton, E., Najarian, R., Simonsen, C. C., Derynck, R., Sherwood, P. J., Wallace, D. M., Berger, S. L., Levinson, A. D., and Goeddel, D. V., 1982, *Nature* **295**:503–508.
Grunstein, M., and Hogness, D. S., 1975, *Proc. Natl. Acad. Sci. USA* **72**:3961–3965.
Hilfiker, M. L., Moore, R. N., and Farrar, J. J., 1981, *J. Immunol.* **127**:1983–1987.
Hinuma, S., Onda, H., Naruo, K., Ichimori, Y., Koyama, M., and Tsukamoto, K., 1982, *Biochem. Biophys. Res. Commun.* **109**:363–369.
Howard, M., Farrar, J., Hilfiker, M., Johnson, B., Takatsu, K., Hamaoka, T., and Paul, W. E., 1982, *J. Exp. Med.* **155**:914–923.
Ihle, J. N., Pepersack, L., and Rebar, L., 1981, *J. Immunol.* **126**:2184–2189.
Ihle, J. N., Keller, J., Henderson, L., Klein, F., and Palaszynski, E., 1982a, *J. Immunol.* **129**:2431–2436.
Ihle, J. N., Rebar, L., Keller, J., Lee, J. C., and Hapel, A., 1982b, *Immunol. Rev.* **63**:5–32.
Isakson, P. C., Pure, E., Vitetta, E. S., and Krammer, P. H., 1982, *J. Exp. Med.* **155**:734–748.
Katz, F. N., Rothman, J. E., Lingappa, V. R., Blobel, G., and Lodish, H. F., 1977, *Proc. Natl. Acad. Sci. USA* **74**:3278–3282.
Krakauer, T., Mizel, D., and Oppenheim, J. J., 1982, *J. Immunol.* **129**:939–941.
Laemmli, U. K., 1970, *Nature* **227**:680–685.
Lin, Y., Stadler, B. M., and Rabin, H., 1982, *J. Biol. Chem.* **257**:1587–1590.
Meyer, D. I., Krause, E., and Dobberstein, B., 1982, *Nature* **297**:647–650.
Mier, J. W., and Gallo, R. C., 1980, *Proc. Natl. Acad. Sci. USA* **77**:6134–6138.
Mills, G., Monticone, V., and Paetkau, V., 1976, *J. Immunol.* **117**:1325–1330.
Mizel, S. B., Oppenheim, J. J., and Rosenstreich, D. L., 1978, *J. Immunol.* **120**:1497–1503.
Mochizuki, D., Watson, J., and Gillis, S., 1980, *J. Immunol.* **125**:2579–2583.
Morgan, D. A., Ruscetti, F. W., and Gallo, R., 1976, *Science* **193**:1007–1008.
Nakanishi, K., Howard, M., Moraguchi, A., Farrar, J., Takatsu, K., Hamaoka, T., and Paul, W. E., 1983, *J. Immunol.* **130**:2219–2224.
Oakley, B. R., Kirsch, D. R., and Morris, N. R., 1980, *Anal. Biochem.* **105**:361–363.
Paetkau, V., Mills, G., Gerhart, S., and Monticone, V., 1976, *J. Immunol.* **117**:1320–1324.
Paetkau, V., Shaw, J., Caplan, B., Mills, G. B., and Lee, K.-C., 1980, *J. Supramol. Struct.* **13**:271–280.
Pelham, H. R. B., and Jackson, R. J., 1976, *Eur. J. Biochem.* **67**:247–256.
Pluznik, D. M., and Sachs, L., 1965, *J. Cell. Physiol.* **66**:319–324.
Przybyla, A. E., MacDonald, R. J., Harding, J. D., Pictet, R. L., and Rutter, W. J., 1979, *J. Biol. Chem.* **254**:2154–2159.
Pure, E., Isakson, P. C., Paetkau, V., Caplan, B., Vitetta, E. S., and Krammer, P. H., 1982, *J. Immunol.* **129**:2420–2425.

Riendeau, D., Harnish, D. G., Bleackley, R. C., and Paetkau, V., 1983, *J. Biol. Chem.* **258**:12114–12117.

Robb, R. J., and Smith, K. A., 1981, *Mol. Immunol.* **18**:1087–1094.

Robb, R. J., Munck, A., and Smith, K. A., 1981, *J. Exp. Med.* **154**:1455–1474.

Robb, R. J., Kutny, R. M., and Chowdhry, V., 1983, *Proc. Natl. Acad. Sci. USA* **80**:5990–5994.

Roberts, B., and Paterson, B. M., 1973, *Proc. Natl. Acad. Sci. USA* **70**:2330–2334.

Shaw, J., Monticone, V., and Paetkau, V., 1978a, *J. Immunol.* **120**:1967–1973.

Shaw, J., Monticone, V., Mills, G., and Paetkau, V., 1978b, *J. Immunol.* **120**:1974–1980.

Stanley, E. R., and Heard, P. M., 1977, *J. Biol. Chem.* **252**:4305–4312.

Stewart, E. W., Lin, L. S., Wiranowska-Stewart, M., and Cantell, K., 1977, *Proc. Natl. Acad. Sci. USA* **74**:4200–4204.

Taniguchi, T., Matsui, H., Fujita, T., Takaoka, C., Kashima, N., Yoshimoto, R., and Hamuro, J., 1983, *Nature* **302**:305–310.

Teranishi, T., Hirano, T., Arina, N., and Onoue, K., 1982, *J. Immunol.* **128**:1903–1908.

Thomas, P. S., 1980, *Proc. Natl. Acad. Sci. USA* **77**:5201–5205.

Walter, P., and Blobel, G., 1981a, *J. Cell Biol.* **91**:551–556.

Walter, P., and Blobel, G., 1981b, *J. Cell Biol.* **91**:557–561.

Watson, J., Aarden, L. A., Shaw, J., and Paetkau, V., 1979a, *J. Immunol.* **122**:1633–1638.

Watson, J., Gillis, S., Marbrook, J., Mochizuki, D., and Smith, K. A., 1979b, *J. Exp. Med.* **150**:849–861.

Welte, K., Wang, C. Y., Mertelsmann, R., Venuta, S., Feldman, S. P., and Moore, M. A. S., 1982, *J. Exp. Med.* **156**:454–464.

White, B. A., and Bancroft, F. C., 1982, *J. Biol. Chem.* **257**:8569–8572.

Yoshizaki, K., Nakagawa, T., Kaieda, T., Muraguchi, A., Yamamura, Y., and T. Kishimoto, 1982, *J. Immunol.* **128**:1296–1301.

Interleukin-2 and the Regulation of Natural Killer Activity in Cultured Cell Populations

Colin G. Brooks

Program in Basic Immunology
Fred Hutchinson Cancer Research Center
Seattle, Washington 98104

and

Christopher S. Henney

Immunex Corporation
Seattle, Washington 98101

I. INTRODUCTION

The recent immunology literature is replete with examples of effector T-cell populations, the proliferation and function of which are potentiated by culture medium containing Interleukin-2 (IL-2), formerly T-cell growth for factor (TCGF). Indeed, it is often taken as axiomatic that all T cells can respond to IL-2, in conjunction with other signals, and, conversely, that all cells that respond to IL-2 are T cells. An apparent exception to this general rule was provided by the observation that IL-2 could enhance natural killer (NK) activity and that medium containing this lymphokine could support the continuous growth of cell lines with NK-like activity. This chapter reviews the now extensive literature pertaining to these phenomena and describes some newer data that demonstrate some interesting and previously undocumented interrelationships between cytotoxic T cells (CTL) and NK cells.

NK cells themselves are an ill-defined and poorly understood component of the immune system. These cells have, however, attracted considerable attention because of their ability to lyse spontaneously a large variety of malignant cells, virus-infected cells, and even some uninfected normal cell types. These observations have raised the possibility that NK cells may be the principal component of an immunosurveillance system against neoplasia and/or may play a role in antiviral defenses or in normal immune regulation. Therapeutic regulation of their activity could therefore be of benefit in a variety of disease situations. Although direct experimental evidence delineating the true function of NK cells is still lacking, a multitude of studies in laboratory animals have strongly implicated NK cells in the destruction of tumor cells *in vivo* (Kiessling *et al.*, 1975; Talmadge *et al.*, 1980; Brooks *et al.*, 1981; Gorelik and Herberman, 1981; Kawase *et al.*, 1982; Pollack and Hallenbeck, 1982).

The mechanism by which NK cells exert their antitumor effects either *in vivo* or *in vitro* is still unclear. Indeed, the mechanism by which NK cells recognize their targets, the nature of the structures on the target cells to which NK cells bind, and even the hematopoietic lineage to which NK cells belong are still controversial issues. Given all these uncertainties, it is difficult to formulate a coherent and comprehensive definition of an NK cell. For the purposes of this discussion, we shall consider an NK cell to be any cell present in lymphoid tissues or established *in vitro* from such sources, which is capable of lysing, in the absence of exogenous stimuli, prototypical NK-cell targets (YAC-1 in the mouse, K562 in humans) in an antigen-nonspecific manner.

One aspect of the biology of NK cells that is now comparatively well understood is the regulation of NK activity. Early in the study of NK cells it was observed that *in vivo* administration of a variety of substances, such as Bacillus Calmette–Guérin (BCG) (Wolfe *et al.*, 1976), *Corynebacterium parvum* (Ojo *et al.*, 1978), viruses (Herberman *et al.*, 1977; Welsh and Zinkernagel, 1977), polynucleotides (Oehler *et al.*, 1978), and even tumor cells themselves (Herberman *et al.*, 1977) caused boosting of NK activity. The observation that NK-cell boosting by tumor cells was mediated via the induction of interferon (IFN) provided a breakthrough in NK-cell research (Trinchieri *et al.*, 1978; Trinchieri and Santoli, 1978). That IFN is a major regulator of NK activity was rapidly confirmed in other laboratories (Gidlund *et al.*, 1978; Welsh, 1978; Djeu *et al.*, 1979a); this finding provided a satisfying explanation of how the diverse substances described above could augment NK activity, for all are known as potent IFN inducers. All three major species of IFN (α, β, and γ) have the ability to boost NK activity. This field was recently comprehensively reviewed by Welsh (1983).

More recently it was observed that IL-2 could also augment NK activity (Henney *et al.*, 1981). Whereas IFN apparently potentiates NK activity principally by enhancing the cytolytic activity of NK cells directly, the mechanism of action of IL-2 appears to be more complex. At least two distinct pathways have been described. First, IL-2 can, via a complex series of cell–cell interactions, induce the production of γ-IFN, which itself enhances cytolysis by NK cells. Second, it appears that IL-2 can induce the expression of NK-like function in cells belonging to the CTL lineage by a process more akin to differentiation than to activation.

Before discussing the results that support these conclusions, an important cautionary note must be made. It is still relatively common to find the term T-cell growth factor (TCGF), or IL-2, being used in the literature to describe crude unfractionated, or minimally fractionated, supernatants obtained from cultures of mitogen-stimulated spleen cells or peripheral blood lymphocytes. Such supernatants obviously contain a multitude of biologically active molecules. Given the ample descriptions of methods for obtaining highly purified IL-2 (Gillis *et al.*, 1982; Granelli-Piperno *et al.*, 1981; Acuto *et al.*, 1982; Stadler *et al.*, 1982), it is a pity that so much work on this important lymphokine has been performed with such impure material that meaningful analysis of the data generated is often not possible.

The two most important contaminants in IL-2 preparations, whose removal is a *sine qua non* for studying NK cell boosting, are residual mitogen (or, in some cases, phorbol myristate acetate, PMA) and IFN. Many workers attempt to remove mitogen by a simple one-step process such as absorption by Sephadex or red blood cells. Rarely have unambiguous checks on the efficiency of the procedure, such as using radiolabeled mitogen tracers, been performed. Separation of IL-2 and IFN occurs readily during the early stages of conventional protein-purification procedures (by ion-exchange chromatography, for example). Treatment of partially purified IL-2 preparations at pH 2.0 for 24 hr may also be advantageous, as IL-2 is stable under these conditions, whereas γ-IFN (the species of IFN that normally contaminates IL-2) is destroyed. Clearly, supernatants obtained from IL-2-secreting tumor cells (Gillis *et al.*, 1980), which contain a more limited number of lymphokines than do cultures of mitogen-stimulated peripheral blood cells, represent a more suitable starting material. Jurkat tumor cells, for example, produce copious amounts of IL-2, but no demonstrable IFN.

II. BOOSTING OF MURINE NK ACTIVITY BY IL-2 IN SHORT-TERM CULTURES

The first evidence demonstrating that IL-2 could enhance NK activity was obtained in murine systems (Henney *et al.*, 1981; Kuribayashi *et al.*, 1981). Spleen-cell mitogen-induced murine IL-2, purified by sequential ammonium sulfate precipitation, gel exclusion, ion-exchange chromatography, and flatbed isoelectric focusing, induced profound activation of NK activity during a 24-hr culture period (Fig. 1). Both the kinetics and magnitude of the activation induced by IL-2 were comparable to those achieved with the synthetic polynucleotide, polyinosinic-polycytidylic acid (poly I:C), a potent inducer of α- and β-IFN (Kuribayashi *et al.*, 1981). High NK activity persisted for greater than 5 days in cultures treated with a single pulse of either poly I:C or IL-2. More detailed kinetic analysis of NK potentiation by both IL-2 and mouse β-IFN were subsequently performed. These studies showed that, whereas β-IFN was able to induce significant boosting of NK activity within 2 hr, IL-2-induced boosting of NK activity was not significant before 8 hr (Kuribayashi, unpublished data). This difference in kinetics suggested that IL-2 might be acting indirectly, perhaps through the participation of non-NK cells and/or via the induction of other soluble mediators. These suppositions were subsequently confirmed by cell-separation procedures (Kawase *et al.*, 1983a).

An interesting observation made during these early studies was that admixture of poly I:C and IL-2 or of β-IFN and IL-2 (Fig. 1) led to a synergistic effect on NK-cell potentiation. Similar effects were noted when spleen cells were pretreated with poly I:C for 24 hr, then washed prior to exposure to IL-2. The ability of poly I:C pretreatment to enhance the subsequent response to IL-2 could have been due to promotion of the expression of IL-2 receptors on either NK cells themselves or on some other cell involved in the boosting mechanism. Direct evidence supporting this hypothesis was obtained from absorption experiments (Table I). Thus, whereas fresh CBA spleen cells, or spleen cells cultured for 24 hr without stimulation, were unable to absorb IL-2, spleen cells cultured with poly I:C had considerable absorptive capacity. This was true even if the spleen cells had been depleted of T cells by treatment with anti-Thy-1 and complement, indicating that poly I:C could induce the appearance of IL-2 receptors on Thy-1$^-$ (non-T) cells.

It was presumed that the appearance of IL-2 receptors on spleen cells following culture with poly I:C was mediated by IFN produced in the cultures. Evidence supporting this hypothesis has been obtained by Riccardi *et al.* (1983) using a limiting dilution method of analysis. Pretreatment of BALB/c spleen cells with IFN increased the frequency of microwell cultures containing either proliferating colonies or cytotoxic (putative NK) colonies after 7 days' incubation with partially purified rat IL-2. Similar results were obtained with both human cells (Vose *et al.*, 1983) and with BALB/c-*nu*/*nu* spleen cells, although in the latter case the frequency of both types of colony was much lower (Riccardi *et al.*, 1983). More recently, an analogous phenomenon has been observed with cloned mouse cell lines (Brooks, 1983). Some NK activity could be induced in such cells by either IFN or IL-2, but very strong NK activity was induced by an admixture of the two mediators (for further discussion, see Section VI).

The issue of whether human NK cells express IL-2 receptors has recently been directly addressed by Abo *et al.* (1983). These workers have made use of two monoclonal antibodies: one directed against the HNK-1 antigen, which is present on virtually all NK cells (Abo and Balch, 1981), and one directed against the Tac-1 antigen, which is probably a determinant on the IL-2 receptor (Leonard *et al.*, 1982). Freshly isolated blood mononuclear cells were found to con-

Figure 1. Potentiation of NK activity of CBA/J spleen cells following incubation for 24 hr with partially purified mouse fibroblast IFN and partially purified IL-2. The IL-2 was purified from the supernatants of mitogen-stimulated spleen cells by ammonium sulfate precipitation, gel filtration, ion-exchange chromatography, and flatbed isoelectric focusing. In those experiments in which IFN was added to a constant amount of IL-2, the IL-2 dilution was 1:20. Lysis was measured on YAC-1 targets in a 4-hr chromium release assay at an effector: target ratio of 25:1. (Adapted from Kuribayashi *et al.*, 1981, with permission.) IFN, interferon; IL-2, Interleukin-2.

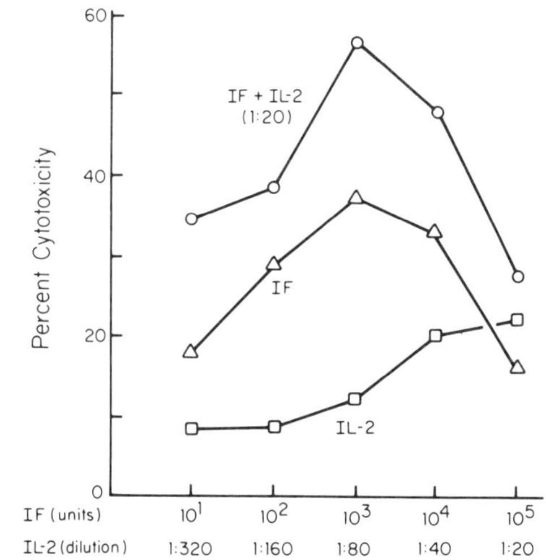

tain no detectable Tac-1⁺ cells. Within a few hours of culture with phytohemagglutin (PHA), the Tac-1 antigen appeared on 25% of HNK-1⁺ cells. The Tac-1⁺ HNK-1⁺ cells belonged to the subset of HNK-1⁺ cells that express T-cell markers, e.g., E receptor, Leu 4, and OKT3, and that exhibit low but significant NK activity (Abo *et al.*, 1982a). The HNK-1⁺ subclass that represents the bulk of the blood NK activity and which expresses OKM1 but lacks T-cell markers, did not acquire

Table I. Capacity of Cell Populations to Absorb IL-2 Activity[a, b]

Cell population used for adsorption[c]	IL-2 remaining (U/ml)	%absorption
None	3.00	0
Fresh CBA spleen	3.17	0
Fresh, Thy-1-depleted CBA spleen	2.94	6
24-hr-cultured CBA spleen	3.06	0
24-hr Poly I:C-stimulated CBA spleen	1.23	59
24-hr Poly I:C-stimulated Thy-1 depleted CBA spleen	1.01	66
48-hr LPS-stimulated C57BL/6 spleen	3.10	0
48-hr Con A-stimulated C57BL/6 spleen	0.74	76
120-hr MLC-stimulated C57BL/6 spleen[d]	0.90	70
Long-term-cultured IL-2-dependent CTLL 2-Clone 8[e]	0.06	98

[a](Adapted from Kuribayashi *et al.* (1981), with permission.

[b]Con A, Concanavalin A; LPS, lipopolysaccharide; MLC, mixed lymphocyte culture; poly I:C, polyinosinic–polycytidylic acid.

[c]Four-hr absorption 3.00 U/ml IL-2, 4°C. Dose-response curve for each absorbing cell population was employed. Data shown are for cell concentration of 10^8 cells/ml.

[d]C57BL/6 spleen versus X-irradiated (1500 R) BALB/c spleen.

[e]C57BL/6 anti-H-2^d killer T-cell line.

the Tac-1 antigen. These studies indicate that most freshly isolated blood NK cells do not express IL-2 receptors, but after being cultured with mitogens, the NK subpopulation most similar phenotypically to T cells will express IL-2 receptors. Interestingly, these cells proliferate only slowly in response to mitogen, compared with HNK-1⁻ T cells (Abo and Balch, 1982), unless an excess of a crude IL-2 preparation is added to the cells (Abo and Balch, 1983). It will be important to determine the role played by IFN in the induction of IL-2 receptors on HNK-1⁺ cells and whether those cells displaying IL-2 receptors show enhanced NK activity when challenged with IL-2.

Although the genetics of IL-2-induced NK-cell boosting have not yet been systematically investigated, our preliminary studies indicate that good boosting is obtained with most mouse strains, e.g., CBA, C57BL/6, BALB/c, and DBA/2. However, spleen cells from C57BL/6-*bg/bg* mutant mice, which have deficient intrinsic NK activity and which are poorly boosted by IFN (Roder, 1979), fail to develop augmented NK activity when cultured for 24 hr with IL-2 (Kawase *et al.*, 1983a). Strong boosting of NK activity is observed with BALB/c-*nu/nu* mice, comparable to that observed in euthymic strains, indicating that mature T cells are not an absolute requirement for NK-cell boosting (Kawase *et al.*, 1983a). In the limiting dilution system of Riccardi *et al.* (1983), BALB/c-*nu/nu* spleen cells gave 10- to 100-fold lower frequencies of IL-2-dependent cytotoxic colonies than did BALB/c-*nu/+* spleens. The discrepant results obtained in the short-term bulk cultures and in the long-term limiting dilution cultures most likely reflect the existence of two different mechanisms by which IL-2 can induce NK-like reactivities. In the former system, the predominant mechanism is probably of NK-cell activation via IL-2-induced γ-IFN; in the latter system, the predominant mechanism appears to involve differentiation of CTL or CTL precursors into promiscuously cytotoxic cells. A full discussion of these mechanisms is presented in Section IV.

A major issue in the early studies of NK boosting by IL-2 preparations was the unambiguous definition of the material responsible for the biological activity. Simply put, was NK boosting actually caused by IL-2, or by a contaminating lymphokine? At the simple phenomenological level, a strong correlation was observed between the IL-2 concentration in various lymphokine-containing supernatants and their ability to augment NK-cell activity (Kuribayashi *et al.*, 1981). More persuasively, the purest preparations of murine IL-2 available at that time, obtained by sequential ammonium sulfate precipitation, gel-exclusion and ion-exchange chromatography, isoelectric focusing (IEF), and sodium dodecylsulfatepolyacrylamide gel electrophoresis (SDS-PAGE), were as active on a unit-for-unit basis as were crude IL-2 preparations (Henney *et al.*, 1981). Such preparations contained no detectable IFN. More recently, IL-2 purified to homogeneity by high-performance liquid chromatography (HPLC) has been shown to retain NK-potentiation activity (Urdal *et al.*, unpublished data). In addition, depletion of IL-2 from concanavalin A (Con A)-induced spleen-cell supernatants by immunoabsorption with a monoclonal antibody to IL-2 (Henney *et al.*, 1981) concomitantly removed NK-potentiating activity. Taken together, these results provided compelling evidence that IL-2 is indeed a regulator of NK function. As emphasized in Section I, however, it does not follow that boosting of NK activity by IL-2-containing preparations is necessarily due solely to the presence of IL-2.

The specificity of the cytotoxicity induced by IL-2 during short-term (24-hr) culture of murine spleen cells is essentially identical to that of uncultured normal spleen cells or of spleen cells from poly I:C-treated mice (Henney *et al.*, 1981). Particularly useful in analysis of NK specificity have been two clones of the L5178Y murine lymphoma. One of these, clone 27v, is NK sensitive, while the other, clone 27av, is NK resistant, yet both clones are equally susceptible to alloimmune cytotoxic T lymphocytes (CTL) (Durdik *et al.*, 1980). IL-2-boosted spleen cells show augmented lysis of YAC-1 and clone 27v targets but give little or no lysis of clone 27av cells or of other NK-resistant targets.

The observation that IL-2 can augment murine NK-cell activity has now been confirmed in several laboratories. Minato *et al.* (1981) observed activation of NK-cell activity following culture of mouse spleen cells with partially purified IL-2 obtained from the supernatants of mixed lymphocyte cultures. Because of the extended culture period used by these investigators (4–5 days), activation of CTL-like cells also occurred. Saxena *et al.* (1983) reported that the YAC-1 killer cells activated by IL-2 in short-term cultures bore asialo-GM_1 (a marker selectively expressed by NK cells, but not by CTL) and lacked Lyt-2 (a marker selectively expressed by CTL, but not by NK cells). Lattime *et al.* (1983), who studied NK cell augmentation by partially purified rat IL-2 in 24-hr cultures, also found no evidence of CTL-like (Qa-5^-) killer cells capable of lysing YAC-1. These workers went on to compare the requirements for activation of both NK cells (Qa-5^+ cells, which lyse YAC-1) and NC cells (Qa-5^- cells, which lyse Meth A tumor cells). They found that poly I:C, presumably acting via IFN production, and IL-2, but not IL-3, could boost NK activity, whereas IL-2 and IL-3, but not poly I:C, boosted NC activity. [IL-3 is a lymphokine currently defined by its ability to induce expression of 20α-hydroxysteroid dehydrogenase in lymphoid cells and to promote the growth of certain lymphoid cell lines (Ihle *et al.*, 1983).] These studies collectively support the hypothesis that, in short-term cultures, IL-2 activates predominantly classical NK cells and NC cells.

As is clear from the work of Lattime *et al.* (1983) and from our own unpublished observations, rat IL-2 will activate mouse NK cells. Human IL-2, purified by ammonium sulfate precipitation and CM-Sepharose chromatography from the supernatants of Jurkat-JA1 lymphoma cells stimulated with PHA and PMA, was also found to be highly stimulatory to murine NK cells in 24-hr cultures (Kawase *et al.*, 1983a). By contrast, Merluzzi *et al.* (1983) reported an inability to boost murine NK activity by human IL-2 in short-term cultures, but did find promiscuous cytotoxicity to develop in 72-hr cultures. The reasons for these discrepancies are unclear.

Given the potential therapeutic importance of IL-2-induced NK-cell potentiation, it was important to determine whether NK boosting could be demonstrated *in vivo*. Hefeneider *et al.* (1983) treated CBA/J mice with a single intraperitoneal injection of IL-2, purified from the supernatant of PHA-stimulated LBRM-33 cells by sequential ammonium sulfate precipitation, gel-exclusion and ion-exchange chromatography, hydrophobic affinity chromatography, and isoelectric focusing. Such IL-2 preparations lacked detectable IL-1, IFN, and colony-stimulating factor (CSF). Two days after injection of an Interleukin-2-bovine serum albumin (IL-2–BSA) mixture, anti-YAC-1 cytotoxic activity was markedly enhanced in both peritoneal exudate cells and in spleen cells, compared with that observed in control mice treated with saline–BSA. Further testing showed that the induced cytotoxic activity had the same specificity displayed by normal spleen cells. Thus, it appears that IL-2 can potentiate NK-cell activity *in vivo* as well as *in vitro*.

III. BOOSTING OF HUMAN NK ACTIVITY BY IL-2 IN SHORT-TERM CULTURES

There appears to have been relatively little investigation in this area, with only one detailed report published to date. Domzig *et al.* (1983) found that human IL-2 purified by successive phenyl-Sepharose chromatography, DEAE chromatography, gel filtration, and isoelectric focusing was a potent activator of human NK-like activity. Activation was measured in blood mononuclear preparations enriched for NK activity by density-gradient fractionation.* Activation was extremely rapid, and up to 20-fold boosting was observed when these IL-2-containing preparations were added directly to 4-hr NK assays. Most intriguingly, Domzig and co-workers reported that a monoclonal antibody prepared against human IL-2 would inhibit the intrinsic NK activity of human NK cells, implying that IL-2 was required for the normal expression of NK function. Unfortunately, no data demonstrating that the antibody would inhibit NK potentiation by exogenous IL-2 were presented. These studies are reminiscent of earlier ones in which antisera to IFN were found to inhibit intrinsic NK activity (Herberman *et al.*, 1979). Collectively, these findings imply that expression of NK function may be dependent on IL-2-mediated IFN production. However, more detailed examination of the specificity of the various antibodies and exclusion of indirect effects (such as induction of suppressor cells by these antibodies) would be required before such a conclusion could be rigorously established.

Two other preliminary reports have been published in this area. Ramsey *et al.* (1983) reported the ability of highly purified IL-2 to enhance NK activity

*Such preparations are generally termed large granular lymphocytes (LGL) because of their large cells containing azurophilic granules that do not show a monocytic staining pattern with reagents that detect nonspecific esterases (Saksela *et al.*, 1980a).

during short-term incubation with density-gradient-purified human NK cells, and Weigent *et al.* (1983) had observed IL-2 to enhance human NK activity via γ-IFN induction (for details, see Section IV). The extent to which the specificity and phenotype of the cells displaying IL-2-induced cytotoxicity was examined was not clear, and therefore whether the induced cytotoxicity resides in NK cells or in CTL-like killers is unknown. However, given the speed of activation by IL-2 in human systems and the evidence for the IFN-based mechanism (Weigent *et al.*, 1983), it seems very likely that classical NK-cell activation is predominant. It appears from these limited reports that activation of human NK cells by IL-2 is much more rapid and/or more potent than is activation of murine cells by IL-2, but parallel studies need to be performed to evaluate this possibility.

IV. MECHANISM OF NK POTENTIATION BY IL-2

It is now clear that two different classes of cytolytic activity involving two different, but possibly related, cell types can be induced by IL-2-containing preparations. The induction of promiscuous cytotoxicity in CTL-like killers has already been alluded to and is discussed in detail in Section V. In this section we confine our attention to the mechanism by which IL-2 activates classical NK activity in short-term cultures.

Given the prominent role of IFN in mediating NK-cell potentiation, our first experiments were designed to investigate whether IL-2 could induce IFN production in spleen cells (Kawase *et al.*, 1983a). We found that partially purified preparations of both LBRM-33-derived murine IL-2 and Jurkat-derived human IL-2 induced significant amounts of IFN during 24-hr incubation with CBA/J spleen cells; both IL-2 preparations induced strong NK activation (Table II). The species of IFN generated was apparently of the γ class, as it was destroyed by dialysis against pH 2.0 buffer and was not neutralized by an antiserum that reacted with both α- and β-IFN. While these studies were in progress, Yamamoto *et al.* (1982) published results showing that highly purified IL-2 obtained from EL4 tumor cells could induce IFN from murine spleen cells, but not from thymocytes (even cortisone-resistant thymocytes). These workers also showed that the IFN was of the γ class, as it was neutralized by antiserum to γ-IFN but not by antiserum to α- or β-IFN.

Somewhat surprisingly, in view of the general belief that IL-2 interacts solely with T cells, equally good titers of IFN were obtained when spleen cells from *nu/nu* mice were incubated with IL-2 (Table II). In addition, when spleen cells from euthymic mice were treated with monoclonal anti-Thy 1 and complement, under conditions in which all cytotoxic T-cell activity and responsiveness to Con A were eliminated, IL-2-induced γ-IFN production (and NK potentiation) remained similar to that observed with untreated spleen cells. These results,

Table II. Induction of IFN and Boosting of NK Activity by IL-2[a]

Responder spleen cells	Source of IL-2[c]	Dose of IL-2 (U/ml)	NK activity[d] (% Lysis)	IFN titer (U/ml)
Experiment I				
CBA		0	2	<25
	Mouse	0.37	15	<25
	Mouse	0.75	23	<25
	Mouse	1.5	51	100
	Mouse	3.0	64	150
BALB/c *nu/nu*		0	5	<25
	Mouse	0.37	30	100
	Mouse	0.75	58	100
	Mouse	1.5	72	150
	Mouse	3.0	72	250
Experiment II				
CBA		0	3	<6[e]
	Mouse	3.0	45	>400[e]
	Human	1.0	15	400[e]
	Human	4.0	32	>400[e]

[a]Adapted from Kawase *et al.* (1983a) with permission.
[b]IFN, interferon; NK, natural killer; PHA, phytohemagglutinin; PMA, phorbol myristate acetate.
[c]Mouse IL-2 was obtained from PHA-stimulated LBRM-33 cells and was purified by ammonium sulfate precipitation. Sephadex G100 chromatography, and flatbed isoelectric focusing. Human IL-2 was prepared from Jurkat JAI lymphoma cells stimulated with PHA and PMA; it was purified by ammonium sulfate precipitation and CM-sepharose chromatography.
[d]NK activity was measured in a 4-hr chromium release assay with YAC-1 targets and an effector: target cell ratio of 50:1.
[e]The supernatants were concentrated four fold before IFN assay.

together with the finding that cortisone-resistant thymocytes do not secrete IFN in response to IL-2 (Yamamoto *et al.*, 1982), provide convincing evidence that the IFN produced by normal lymphoid cells treated with IL-2 does not originate from mature T cells, nor are mature T cells required.

Further experiments were performed to identify the source of IFN (Kawase *et al.*, 1983a). Spleen cells were treated with anti-asialo-GM_1 serum and complement or with anti-NK-2.1 serum and complement under conditions that eliminated >90% of NK activity but that had no effect on either CTL activity or Con A or Lipopolysaccharide (LPS) responsiveness. Both types of treatment strongly inhibited IL-2-induced IFN production but had no effect on poly I:C-induced IFN production. It has been known for some time that poly I:C-induced splenic IFN probably originates in macrophages (Djeu *et al.*, 1979b). The new data obtained in these experiments strongly suggested that NK cells themselves played a crucial role in IFN secretion in response to IL-2. A simple, attractive model might be that IL-2 bound to mature NK cells induced the release of γ-IFN, which then activated NK cytolytic activity in immature NK cells. The prediction on the basis of this model would be that IL-2 should induce IFN-mediated NK potentiation in purified NK populations. This prediction was not fulfilled.

Rigorous depletion of adherent cells, by passing spleen cells over two successive nylon–wool columns, abrogated IL-2-induced IFN production and NK-cell boosting. Full responsiveness could be restored by the addition of small numbers of splenic adherent cells. As expected, the NK-2.1$^+$ cell required in this system resided in the nonadherent compartment. Further valuable information on the nature of the cellular interactions involved in this pathway was provided by the discovery that supernatant obtained by incubating splenic adherent cells with IL-2 for 24 hr could induce nylon–wool-nonadherent spleen cells to secrete IFN. Supernatant obtained from splenic adherent cells incubated without IL-2 was unable to induce IFN in nonadherent cells, even when such cultures were supplemented with IL-2. It therefore appears that treatment of splenic adherent cells with IL-2-containing preparations causes release of a soluble factor which, either acting alone or in conjunction with IL-2, can induce γ-IFN production from a nonadherent non-T spleen cell.

These experiments demonstrated that short-term, IL-2-mediated, NK-cell potentiation is a much more complex process than anticipated. Perhaps the most intriguing of the many new issues raised by these experiments was the suggestion that IL-2 could interact directly with macrophages and, by implication, that macrophages have IL-2 receptors. Given the general dogma that IL-2 is a lymphokine restricted to the T-cell (and perhaps NK-cell) compartments, alternative explanations for these data were considered. For example, the macrophage monolayers may have been contaminated with T cells but, because T cells apparently play no role in IL-2-mediated NK potentiation, such contamination would be irrelevant. It was also possible that the IL-2 preparations used in this study contained a contaminant. Yet, given the compelling evidence that IL-2 is indeed an activator of NK cells (see Sections II and III), there remains the problem of explaining the macrophage requirement.

Another issue that is not yet fully resolved is the nature of the cell that secretes IFN. It is established that an NK alloantigen-bearing cell is involved in this process, but formal proof that the IFN is derived from NK cells is currently lacking. Handa *et al.* (1983) showed that cloned murine NK-like cells secrete γ-IFN in response to IL-2. However, the nature of the relationship between such killer cell clones and splenic NK cells is not clear (see Section VI). Nonetheless, there is increasing evidence implicating NK cells as major IFN producers in various systems. There are several reports that NK cells are required for IFN production in mixed-lymphocyte–tumor-cell cultures (MLTC) (Trinchieri *et al.*, 1978; Minato *et al.*, 1980; Shellam *et al.*, 1980; Saksela *et al.*, 1980b). Recent work by Kawase *et al.* (1983b) has shown remarkable parallels between the mechanism of IFN production in MLTC and in response to IL-2: splenic adherent cells mixed with tumor cells secrete a soluble mediator that can induce

IFN production from nonadherent, thymus-independent cells bearing NK alloantigens. Curiously, in these MLTC NK-dependent systems, the species of IFN varies, being alternatively α, β, or γ, or a mixture of components. It should be noted that in none of these systems was there direct evidence that NK cells were the IFN producers. However, Saksela *et al.* (1980b) showed that some tumor-cell-binding cells (putative NK cells) could be stained with antiserum to IFN. In a different system, Djeu *et al.* (1982) reported that a fraction of human blood mononuclear cells, highly enriched for NK cells was the predominant source of IFN following infection with influenza or herpes viruses. It has also been reported that the cell in human mononuclear cell preparations responsible for γ-IFN production in response to PHA has the NK-like phenotype OKM1$^+$, FcR$^+$, OKT11A$^+$ (O'Malley *et al.*, 1983).

The ability of IL-2 to induce γ-IFN has been verified in a human system. Kasahara *et al.* (1983) showed that IL-2 prepared from mitogen-stimulated human mononuclear cells by successive phenyl-Sepharose chromatography and DEAE-Sephacel chromatography would induce IFN in a process dependent on nonadherent E-rosette-forming cells. Removal of OKT4$^+$ or OKT8$^+$ cells by treatment with antibody and complement did not affect IL-2-induced IFN production. It was concluded that both T4$^+$ and T8$^+$ T cell subsets made IFN in response to IL-2. An alternative explanation would be that a T4$^-$, T8$^-$, E$^+$ NK cell was required. In support of this possibility, treatment with OKM1 antibody together with complement reduced IFN titers, but whether this was caused by removal of NK cells or monocytes or both was not clear. Weigent *et al.* (1983) have also reported, in a preliminary communication, that IL-2 induces γ-IFN in both murine and human systems. Antibodies to γ-IFN blocked IL-2-induced NK boosting, but did not block IL-2-induced cell proliferation. Assuming that the antibodies were truly IFN specific, these experiments provide direct confirmation that IL-2-induced NK potentiation in short-term cultures occurs principally via the induction of γ-IFN. The synergism between IL-2 and β-IFN reported in the early studies of this phenomenon (Henney *et al.*, 1981; Kuribayashi *et al.*, 1981) might be explained in one of the following ways: (1) γ-IFN and β-IFN act synergistically on NK cells; (2) β-IFN enhances the expression of IL-2 receptors; or (3) β-IFN activates some other component in the complex pathway by which IL-2 induces γ-IFN production. It is interesting to note that an apparent synergism between different classes of IFN has been observed in the activation of macrophage cytotoxicity (Schultz, 1982; Schultz and Kleinschmidt, 1983); such synergism has been known for some time in regard to the antiviral effects of IFN (Fleischmann *et al.*, 1979).

IL-2 not only induces γ-IFN directly, but can also promote γ-IFN production in response to mitogens or antigens. For example, γ-IFN production by mouse spleen cells cultured with staphylococcal enterotoxin A was greatly enhanced in cultures supplemented with exogenous IL-2 (Yamamoto *et al.*, 1982). During mixed-lymphocyte reactions, IL-2 production was found to be a prerequisite for the generation of γ-IFN from Thy-1$^+$ Lyt-2$^+$ T cells (Farrar *et al.*, 1981). In this type of system, IL-2 presumably acts, at least in part, by promoting more vigorous and prolonged proliferation of those T cells that respond to mitogen or antigen and secrete γ-IFN.

V. INDUCTION OF CTL-LIKE REACTIVITIES BY IL-2 IN LONG-TERM CULTURES OF NK CELLS

The first indication that IL-2 might activate or induce cytolytic activities other than those attributable to classical NK cells arose from the studies of Minato *et al.* (1981). These workers used IL-2 and IFN preparations separated on Biogel columns from the supernatants of mixed lymphocyte cultures. When normal murine spleen cells were cultured without lymphokine supplementation, three classes of cytotoxic cells could be discerned: (1) NK_I cells, which were Thy-1^-, Qa5^+; (2)NK_T cells, which were Thy-1^+, Qa-5^+ (both classes lysed only NK targets); and (3) CTL-like killers, TK, which were Thy-1^+, Qa-5^- and lysed an NK-resistant target. Addition of IFN to cultures caused rapid activation of both NK_I and NK_T cells in a process not requiring Thy-1^+ cells. In contrast, IL-2 caused a slower (4–5-day) activation of NK_T and TK, but not NK_I, cells in a process absolutely dependent on Thy-1^+ cells. The requirement for Thy-1^+ cells distinguishes this protracted IL-2-dependent activation process, which leads to the generation of a mixture of NK and CTL-like effectors, from the short-term (24-hr) activation of NK cells discussed above. It is worth noting that these studies, in which the IL-2 was prepared from supernatants of mixed-lymphocyte cultures, provide definitive proof that traces of lectin, which may exist in most preparations of IL-2, are not required for either NK-cell activation or for the development of CTL-like killers.

At about the same time, a number of laboratories began examining whether placement of blood mononuclear cells from cancer patients into supernatants containing high concentrations of IL-2 would promote the growth of CTL specifically reactive against autologous tumor cells. Hersey *et al.* (1981) cultured blood mononuclear cells from melanoma patients for 6 days with a mitogen-depleted crude supernatant from PHA-stimulated lymphocytes. These investigators found that the cultured cells displayed potent cytolytic activity not only toward autologous tumor cells, but also against allogeneic tumor cells and K562 targets. Furthermore, identical reactivities developed in cultures of mononuclear cells from healthy patients. No cytotoxicity appeared in control cultures lacking PHA-induced supernatant. Cold target competition assays indicated that with some cancer patients specific reactivities to autologous tumor cells did develop but were superimposed on a high background of nonspecific killing. Essentially similar observations were made by Lotze *et al.* (1981) and Grimm *et al.* (1982). These workers showed that partially purified IL-2 preparations depleted of IFN by pH 2 treatment were effective at inducing promiscuous cytotoxicity in normal blood mononuclear cells. Cytotoxic activity first appeared on day 2 of culture and rose progressively over a 5–7-day culture period. The fresh tumor target cells used in these studies were completely resistant to lysis by NK cells in normal peripheral blood. Analysis of effector cells (Grimm *et al.*, 1983) with monoclonal antibodies and complement confirmed that they were not classical NK cells. Their phenotype was $OKT3^+$, $OKT4^-$, $OKT8^+$, Leu-1^+, $OKM1^-$—that of a CTL (as opposed to the phenotype of NK cells, which is $OKT3^-$, $OKT4^-$, $OKT8^-$, Leu-1^-, $OKM1^+$). Further analysis showed that the precursor cells did not form E rosettes and, in fact, lacked all surface markers tested, i.e., OKT3, OKT8, OKT11, OKM1, Leu-1, and HNK-1. (Because surface markers were evaluated using complement-dependent lysis, it is conceivable that the precursor cells were simply resistant to complement.) They were also found to be low-density cells; they were widely distributed, being present in thymus, spleen, lymph node, and thoracic duct, as well as in blood.

It thus appears that long-term culture of blood mononuclear cells with IL-2-containing supernatants can induce the appearance of cells with CTL phenotype (perhaps arising by differentiation of primitive precursor cells), which display potent promiscuous lytic activity against transformed cells. These general observations have been confirmed in other laboratories. For example, Gray *et al.* (1983) observed that IL-2-containing supernatant, obtained from the monkey cell line MLA-144, induced the development of cytotoxic cells capable of lysing both NK-sensitive and NK-resistant targets in blood mononuclear cell cultures. Such effectors could still arise if the mononuclear cells were depleted of NK cells before being cultured, or if thymocytes or lymph node cells, which lack NK activity, were used. Both Gray *et al.* (1983) and Torten *et al.* (1982) reported that the development of these cellular reactivities was facilitated if irradiated allogeneic blood mononuclear cells or allogeneic lymphoblastoid cells were added to the cultures. Whether such cells act simply as feeders or as providers of an antigenic stimulus is not clear. An apparently similar cellular reactivity can be induced in blood mononuclear cells after 2 days' incubation with Con A or PHA (Strausser *et al.*, 1981) or after 7 days of culture with pooled allogeneic stimulator cells (Mazumder *et al.*, 1983). The effector cells were $OKT3^+$ $OKM1^-$ cells, and their generation in these two systems required $OKT3^+$ $OKM1^-$ cells. By contrast, in cultures stimulated with IL-2 alone (see above), $OKT3^+$ cells were not required. It seems likely that the difference between these two systems is explainable in terms of the requirement for IL-2 production from $OKT3^+$ cells in the mitogen- and alloantigen-stimulated cultures. The same phenomenon has also been observed in a murine system. Killer cells capable of lysing freshly explanted syngeneic tumors, but not syngeneic blast cells, were generated by culturing murine spleen cells for 1–3 days with PHA, Con A, or crude supernatants containing IL-2 (Gonzales *et al.*, 1983).

The type of broad cytolytic reactivity developing in these culture systems is reminiscent of the "anomalous killer" (AK) cell activities which develop when human or mouse lymphoid cells are incubated in medium containing fetal bovine serum (Zielske and Golub, 1976; Ortaldo *et al.*, 1977; Golub *et al.*, 1979), in mixed cultures of lymphoid cells and lymphoblastoid or other tumor cell lines (Poros and Klein, 1978; Koide and Takasugi, 1978; Jondal and Targan, 1978; Zarling *et al.*, 1981b; Biron *et al.*, 1981), and in mixed-lymphocyte cultures (MLC) with stimulator cells derived from single (Callewaert *et al.*, 1978; Seeley *et al.*, 1979; Karre and Seeley, 1979; Paciucci *et al.*, 1980a, b; Karre *et al.*, 1983; Hurrel and Zarling, 1983) or multiple (Zarling and Bach, 1978; Zarling and Kung, 1980; Zarling *et al.*, 1981a; Paciucci *et al.*, 1980a, b; Strassmann *et al.*, 1983) donors. Studies of the AK phenomenon have been fragmentary, and the wide variety of systems evaluated has indicated a degree of complexity that may be more apparent than real. The unifying notion that lymphokines, particularly IL-2, may play a dominant role in the evolution of AK activity provides a basis for an analysis of current knowledge in this area and for further experimentation.

What is clear is that the effectors of AK activity are neither specific CTL (directed against the immunizing antigen) nor, in most cases, classical NK cells. Three lines of evidence distinguish AK cells from immunogen-specific CTL. First, AK activity usually peaks 1-2 days before the peak of specific CTL activity (Karre and Seeley, 1979; Seeley and Golub, 1978; Callewaert *et al.*, 1978). Second, generation of AK activity, but not immunogen-specific CTL, is often resistant to treatments (exposure to BUdR and light or to irradiation) that inhibit cell division (Callewaert *et al.*, 1978; Paciucci *et al.*, 1980a; Zarling *et al.*, 1981a). Under some conditions, however, these procedures do inhibit the development of AK cells (Zarling *et al.*, 1981a; Karre *et al.*, 1983). Third, no cross-competition between AK and immunogen-specific CTL occurs (Zarling and Bach, 1978; Karre and Seeley, 1979; Seeley *et al.*, 1979; Karre *et al.*, 1983). For example, in an early study of the development of AK activity in murine MLC, Karre and Seeley (1979) showed that AK-mediated lysis of YAC-1 cells was not inhibited by stimulator strain target cells and conversely that lysis of these specific target cells by the immunogen-specific CTL arising in MLC was not inhibited by YAC-1.

Somewhat surprisingly, especially as prototype NK targets are frequently employed to monitor AK activity, no convincing evidence that classical NK cells participate as mediators of AK function has been presented. For example, in human MLC (using pooled stimulator cells), the AK effectors that lysed K562 targets were $OKT3^-$ and $OKT8^-$, as are normal NK cells. However, the AK cells were also $OKM1^-$, whereas most blood NK cells are $OKM1^+$ (Zarling and Kung, 1980). Biron *et al.* (1981) reported that the anti-K562 killer cells generated after stimulation with autologous lymphoblastoid cell lines were heterogeneous in size, but generally much larger than normal or IFN-activated NK cells. Similarly, in mouse MLC, the AK effectors that kill YAC-1 cannot be removed by treatment with anti-NK alloantisera and complement under conditions that eliminate all splenic NK activity (Karre *et al.*, 1983). Somewhat tantalizingly, there is compelling evidence in both sytems that NK cells participate in the generation of AK activity. Strassmann *et al.* (1983) reported that prior removal of B73.1$^+$ cells (or OKM1$^+$ cells) abolished the development of K562 killers in human MLC. Among blood mononuclear cells, expression of B73.1 antigen is restricted to NK cells and indeed appears to be a determinant on the Fc receptor of NK cells (Perussia *et al.*, 1983). Karre *et al.* (1983) found that pretreatment of mouse spleen cells with anti-NK alloantisera and complement prevented the appearance of YAC-1 killer cells in mouse MLC. One interpretation of these results would be that NK cells can differentiate into AK cells in a process involving loss of the OKM1 antigen or of sensitivity to NK alloantisera and complement. Alternatively, NK cells may participate as regulatory cells, promoting the evolution of a distinct cellular reactivity. Such a hypothesis is supported by the growing evidence (see Section IV) that NK cells are intimately involved in the production of at least one lymphokine, i.e., IFN. It should be noted, however, that in two other AK systems in which K562 cells were used as targets, removal of Fc receptor-bearing cells (including NK cells) prior to culture had no noticeable effect (Ortaldo *et al.*, 1977; Seeley *et al.*, 1979). In addition, Abo and Balch (1982) found that when purified HNK-1$^-$ cells (i.e., the NK$^-$ fraction of blood mononuclear cells) were cultured in MLC, neither HNK-1$^+$ cells nor LGL developed, yet potent AK activity against K562 and other NK-sensitive and NK-resistant targets developed.

The most common finding is that AK cells have close phenotypic resemblance to CTL but lack specific cytolytic activity against the immunizing antigens. This is particularly true for those AK cells that lyse NK-resistant targets. Human AK cells arising in MLC and that can kill autologous lymphoblastoid cell line (LCL) targets were OKT3$^+$ and OKT8$^+$ (Zarling *et al.*, 1981a). Similar OKT8$^+$ AK cells were found in cultures in which autologous LCL were used as the stimulators in the MLC (Zarling *et al.*, 1981b). In contrast to the class of AK cells active against K562 cells, the OKT8$^+$ AK required neither OKM1$^+$ nor B73.1$^+$ cells for development (Strassmann *et al.*, 1983) and were sensitive to BUdR and light treatment (Zarling *et al.*, 1981a). In mouse MLC, AK cells active against a variety of syngeneic tumors were found to be Ly 2$^+$ (Hurrell and Zarling, 1983), a marker for cytotoxic/suppressor T lymphocytes and absent from NK cells.

Taken together, the studies of AK activity indicate that there are probably two distinct classes of effector cells: CTL-like (but not immunogen-specific) killers capable of lysing a wide variety of NK-resistant targets, and non-CTL killers, possibly derived from NK cells, which lyse prototype NK targets. This situation is reminiscent of that described by Minato *et al.* (1981), in which prolonged culture of lymphoid cells with IL-2 led to activation of both classical NK cells and of CTL-like killers. The implication is that IL-2 and IFN, generated in the culture systems in which AK arises, may be responsible for the development of these effectors. Such a hypothesis is supported by the kinetics of AK development, which often follow the kinetics expected for IL-2 production. However, few studies have addressed this issue directly. Trinchieri *et al.* (1978), and later Koide and Takasugi (1978), showed that human blood mononuclear cells cultured with certain tumor cells released mediators, in particular IFN, which could boost NK activity. More recently, Hurrell and Zarling (1983) found that the induction of Ly 2^+ AK cells in mouse MLC could be mimicked by treating spleen cells with MLC-derived culture supernatants. It is also interesting to note that the presence of small numbers of T cells appears to be an essential requirement for generation of AK activity. Thus, although AK effectors can still develop in MLC in which the responder cells have been treated with anti-Thy 1 and complement or are derived from *nu/nu* mice, they fail to develop if the irradiated stimulator cells are also lacking in T cells (Paciucci *et al.*, 1980b; Karre *et al.*, 1983). It is well documented that irradiation of T cells does not abrogate their ability to secrete lymphokines.

An interesting study that provides some insight into the complexity of AK systems and the possible role of IL-2 is that of Lopez-Botet *et al.* (1982). When human MLC-derived cells, after 5–7 days of culture, were separated by density-gradient fractionation, all specific alloreactive CTL were found to be low-density cells, whereas AK activity toward K562 was found in both low-density and high-density fractions. The AK activity in the high-density cells was dependent on the presence of FcγR-bearing cells in the starting population, could not be boosted by IL-2, and showed true NK specificity. The activity in the low-density cells was independent of FcγR cells, was boosted by IL-2, and had a broad specificity, lysing both NK-sensitive and NK-resistant targets. Although these AK cells had the same density found in the specific CTL cold target competition assays, monolayer absorptions and surface-marker studies confirmed that these populations were different.

Much more work needs to be performed in AK systems before a full description of this phenomenon becomes available. Current indications are that such studies might provide insight into some previously unrecognized, but potentially important, aspects of the cellular immune system. In particular, the ability of lymphokines, secreted in antigen-specific immune responses, to induce the development of a variety of antigen-nonspecific cytotoxic reactivities may have important implications for our understanding of autoimmune diseases, resistance to infections, inflammatory responses, and graft rejection. Furthermore, the preliminary indication from these systems that cells in the NK and CTL lineages may exist in multiple differentiation states associated with distinct marker profiles and cellular reactivities merits extensive study. There is already convincing evidence that antigen-specific CTL can undergo a lymphokine-driven differentiation into cells displaying NK reactivity and, subsequently, into cells exhibiting promiscuous lytic activity (see Section VI).

Although the precise nature of AK cells and the role of IL-2 in their generation remain to be determined, there is no doubt that partially purified IL-2 preparations can promote the long-term growth of cells with NK-like activity. In the mouse, Kuribayashi *et al.* (1981) showed that spleen cells pretreated with poly I:C and then incubated in IL-2-containing medium for 24 hr displayed a specificity identical to that of fresh splenic NK cells. In some cases, especially where the spleen cells were depleted of Thy-1^+ cells prior to culture, this NK specificity could persist for several days, and sometimes weeks. Generally, however, when incubation with IL-2 was prolonged beyond 24 hr, marked alterations in specificity occurred, with a progressive increase over a period of days in lytic activity against NK-resistant targets. Particularly striking was the loss of discrimination between the NK-sensitive (cl 27v) and NK-resistant (cl 27av) clones of L5178Y (K. Kuribayashi and C. G. Brooks, unpublished data). Such broad cytolytic reactivities are often called NK-like but are more appropriately termed promiscuous. Although detailed comparisons have not been reported, the specificity of these long-term IL-2 cultures is clearly reminiscent of that seen in some AK systems. There seems to be some selectivity toward lysis of transformed target cells, and at least with murine clones (Brooks *et al.*, 1982) some restriction for lysis of lymphoma cells of the same species. In this context, it is interesting to note that normal thymocytes or neuraminidase-treated T cells display an innate binding preference for cells of the same species (Galili *et al.*, 1978).

At least in the early stages of IL-2-stimulated cultures, the predominant cellular phenotype was asialo-GM_1^+, Thy-1^+, Lyt-2^- (Kuribayashi *et al.*, 1981). However, when cloned cell lines were developed from these cultures (Brooks *et al.*, 1982), using IL-2-containing medium, two types of cytotoxic cells were identified; a Thy-1^+, Ig^-, Lyt-1^-, Lyt-2^-, Ly-5^+, asialo-GM_1^+, Qa-5^+, Mac-1^-, $Fc\gamma R^-$, NK-alloantigen$^+$ cell, and a cell with identical surface markers except for the presence of Lyt-2. In all other respects, the two types of cloned lines were identical. They were extremely cytolytic for YAC-1 targets, often giving 50% lysis in a 4-hr chromium release assay at effector: target ratios lower than 1:1. They had the same specificity, lysing a variety of NK-sensitive and some NK-resistant murine lymphomas, but with much lower activity against NK-sensitive murine solid tumor-derived targets or against xenogeneic targets. All were large cells, with prominent granules (Brooks *et al.*, 1982) that ultrastructurally resembled the granules of basophilic leukocytes (Galli *et al.*, 1982; S. Galli and A. M. Dvorak, personal communication). Similar lines, with NK-like activity and showing heterogeneity of Lyt-2 expression, were described by Kedar *et al.* (1982).

Whether the Lyt-2^- lines arise from Lyt-2^+ lines by simple antigen loss, as has been observed with conventional CTL clones (Dialynas *et al.*, 1981; Giorgi *et al.*, 1982) or whether Lyt-2^- and Lyt-2^+ lines arise from separate precursors is not clear. Recent work by Suzuki *et al.* (1983) favors the latter hypothesis. These investigators observed that low-density murine spleen cells, which contain most of the intrinsic splenic NK activity, could be propagated indefinitely by partially purified IL-2. Pretreatment of these low-density spleen cells with anti-asialo-GM_1 and complement abolished NK activity and severely reduced proliferative potential. The proliferating cells were large and granular and had the predominant phenotype Thy-1$^-$, Lyt-1$^-$, Lyt-2$^-$, Ly-5$^+$, asialo-GM$_1^+$, FcγR$^-$—the same as splenic NK cells. Clones derived from these cultures retained this phenotype and displayed high cytolytic activity against prototype NK targets and also against some NK-resistant targets. Given the apparent absence of Lyt-2 during the development of these clones, it seems likely that they arose from Lyt-2$^-$ precursors, perhaps NK cells themselves. Suzuki *et al.* (1983) also observed that high-density spleen cells, which contain small T cells but few NK cells, could not be induced to proliferate unless IL-2, mitogen, and either macrophages or IL-1 were present in the cultures. Cell lines developing from such cultures contained cytolytic activity (but less than in the former cultures), as well as Lyt-2$^+$ cells. In the studies of Brooks *et al.* (1982) and Kedar *et al.* (1982), which used unfractionated spleen cells and/or preparations containing residual mitogen, development of both Lyt-2$^-$ and Lyt-2$^+$ lines would be expected.

Studies similar to those of Suzuki *et al.* (1983) have been performed in human subjects by Timonen *et al.* (1982) and Ortaldo *et al.* (1982). Highly purified NK cells (the E receptor negative fraction of low-density nylon–wool nonadherent mononuclear cells) and small T cells (high-density nylon–wool nonadherent cells) were both found to proliferate rapidly in medium supplemented with crude IL-2. Ten- to 20-day cultures established from the NK cell fraction were composed of large granular cells and had high cytolytic activity with a specificity similar to that of fresh NK cells. Cultures established from the small T-cell fraction were composed mainly of large agranular cells and displayed little cytolytic activity. An important observation was that within the first 10 days of culture of the NK-cell fraction, a remarkable shift in surface-marker phenotype occurred from predominantly OKT3$^-$ Ia$^-$, OKT10$^+$, OKM1$^+$, FcγR$^+$ (typical of blood NK cells) to OKT3$^+$, Ia$^+$, OKT10$^-$, OKM1$^-$, FcγR$^-$ (the same phenotype as the CTL-like killer cells observed in the systems studied by Rosenberg and associates (Mazumder *et al.*, 1983)). The cultures with this phenotype retained the NK-like cytolytic activity. Whether the change in phenotype occurred as a consequence of differentiation of the classical NK cells that constituted the majority of the cells at the initiation of culture or was due to selective proliferation of a contaminating low-density (activated?) T cell or pre-T cell was unclear.

A large number of reports have now been published describing similar experiments in which continuous cell lines and clones displaying NK-like reactivities were generated from both mouse and human lymphoid cells using medium containing crude preparations of IL-2. Space limitations do not permit a detailed analysis of these investigations here, but a comprehensive review appears elsewhere (Brooks, 1984). In general, such cell lines and clones display strong cytolytic activity not only against NK-sensitive target cells, but against certain NK-resistant targets as well. Their surface-marker profile tends to be somewhat variable, especially among the human clones, but in general is more similar to that of CTL than NK cells.

Of particular relevance to the present review is the nature of the factors that support the growth and activity of these cells. The general assumption that IL-2 was necessary for the growth of these cell lines was recently confirmed using cloned lines of mouse NK-like cells (Olabuenaga *et al.*, 1983). Thus, both crude and partially purified mouse and rat IL-2 preparations were able to stimulate thymidine uptake in a 24-hr assay in both cloned NK-like cells and CTLL-2 cells, a cloned CTL line widely used for the assay of IL-2 (Gillis *et al.*, 1978). Similar findings with other NK-like cell lines have been reported (Flomenberg *et al.*, 1983; Ortaldo *et al.*, 1982; Suzuki *et al.*, 1983). Indeed, when NK-like cells themselves were used to quantitate IL-2 in a miscellaneous set of lymphokine preparations, the results were identical to those obtained with the standard CTLL-2 cell line. In addition, cloned NK-like cells could readily absorb IL-2; on a cell-for-cell basis, they had somewhat greater absorptive capacity than did CTLL-2 cells. It was repeatedly observed, however, that, although purified IL-2 was capable of supporting the indefinite growth of CTLL-2 cells, it would not support the long-term growth of cloned NK-like cells. This was true even if the IL-2 was supplemented with Con A or IFN. The nature of the putative auxiliary growth factors required by these cells has not yet been established. Interestingly, Grimm and Rosenberg (1982) reported that the ability of lymphokine-containing supernatants to support the long-term growth of human CTL cell lines did not correlate with their IL-2 content.

The results discussed in the preceding paragraphs indicate that cells present in the low-density fractions of spleen or blood mononuclear cells can be induced by crude lymphokine or partially purified lymphokine preparations (containing IL-2 and probably auxiliary growth factors) to enter continuous growth. Although these fractions are highly enriched in NK cells, the nature of the cell that is the progenitor of these cell lines has not been clearly established. The remarkable changes of phenotype that can occur within the first few days of culture suggest either that a major differentiation of NK cells is taking place or that the progeny of a minor progenitor cell population becomes predominant within the culture. In some cases, traces of mitogen and IL-1 in the medium may permit activation of small T cells, which could then proliferate rapidly in the presence of IL-2. These speculations raise the important question of whether the progenitor cell expresses IL-2 receptors before initiation of culture. As already indicated in Sections II and IV, although NK cells can be activated in cultures containing IL-2, it is unclear whether NK cells themselves express IL-2 receptors. Perhaps the progenitor cell is an activated T cell that acquired IL-2 receptors *in vivo*. Clearly, identification of the progenitor cell would provide insight into the true nature of the cell lines displaying NK-like activity. It would also be important to know what relationship these cell lines bear to the CTL-like and AK cells activated by IL-2 and in MLC, respectively. Some of the most recent experimentation addressing these issues is discussed in the next section.

VI. INTERRELATIONSHIPS BETWEEN NK AND CTL POPULATIONS: INFLUENCE OF IL-2

One approach to the complex issues of whether classical NK cells can proliferate in response to IL-2 is limiting dilution analysis (LDA). Riccardi *et al.* (1983) studied the development of colonies with anti-YAC-1 activity following limiting dilution in the presence of partially purified IL-2. Since the frequency of such colonies was increased by IFN pretreatment, this may imply that the majority of potential proliferating cells in such cultures do not display IL-2 receptors prior to culture. Even after treatment with IFN, only about 1:6000 BALB/c spleen cells gave colonies with NK activity. This is well below the frequency of NK cells in mouse spleen (of the order of 1:100). Thus, under the culture conditions used, either partially purified IL-2 induced the proliferation of only a small proportion of NK cells or, alternatively, the progenitor cell was not an NK cell. In support of the latter conclusion, spleen cells from BALB/c *nu/nu* mice, which contain a higher proportion of NK cells than do spleen cells from euthymic mice, gave very low frequencies of cytotoxic colonies, of the order of 1 per 10^6 spleen cells without IFN pretreatment and 1 per 10^5 spleen cells with IFN pretreatment. These results in fact suggest that a thymus-dependent cell is the progenitor of the vast majority of colonies with anti-YAC-1 activity.

Similar studies were performed in the human by Vose and Bonnard (1983) and Vose *et al.* (1983). NK cells were highly purified by successive incubation on plastic, passage through nylon-wool columns, density-gradient centrifugation, and depletion of E rosette-forming cells. When such cells were studied in LDA, using crude or partially purified IL-2, an average 1:200 cells was capable of cytotoxic colony formation. Pretreatment with IFN increased this figure slightly, but it was clear that the vast majority of cells in these highly purified NK cell fractions were unable to form cytotoxic colonies. Pretreatment with OKT3 plus complement had no effect on cytotoxic colony frequency, but treatment with OKM1 plus complement enhanced slightly the frequency of such colonies (Vose and Bonnard, 1983). Because most blood NK cells are OKM1$^+$ (Zarling and Kung, 1980), this provides direct evidence that NK cells in general are unable to cause formation of cytotoxic colonies. This conclusion is consistent with the observation that most NK cells do not acquire IL-2 receptors when placed in culture (Abo *et al.*, 1983) and that purified HNK-1$^+$ cells, which comprise the bulk of blood NK activity, do not proliferate in medium containing IL-2 without lectin. If PHA is added, the minor subpopulation of HNK-1$^+$ cells bearing T-cell markers proliferates and acquires promiscuous cytotoxicity (Abo and Balch, 1983).

A complication in the limiting dilution analyses is that the cultures contained irradiated lymphoid feeder cells. The possibility exists that, in at least some cases, the growing colonies were themselves not cytotoxic, but rather secreted factors that promoted cytotoxic activity in some cell in the feeder population. However, such indirect cytotoxic activities would lead to an overestimation, rather than to an underestimation, of the frequency of progenitors of cytotoxic colonies.

Moretta *et al.* (1983) investigated a limiting dilution system in which PHA and IL-2 were added. Under the conditions used, they found that virtually every human peripheral blood T cell could form a colony and that about 30% of these colonies displayed mitogen-dependent cytotoxic activity, and were therefore presumably of the CTL lineage. Of these colonies, about one-half displayed lytic activity toward K562, implying that a large proportion of CTL colonies possessed NK-like activity. Unfortunately, the possibility that residual mitogen in the cultures promoted mitogen-dependent lysis of K562 was not investigated.

A more detailed study in a murine system was described by Shortman *et al.* (1983). In limiting dilution cultures of murine spleen cells, containing Con A and IL-2, promiscuously cytotoxic colonies arose with very high frequency; indeed, virtually every Lyt-2^+ spleen cell could generate such a colony. The cytotoxicity was apparently not lectin-dependent, because it was still observable when 100 mM α-methylmannoside, a potent inhibitor of Con A binding, was added to the assay system. Shortman and co-workers also showed that the cytotoxic cells were derived from the input population and not from the feeder cells. These studies demonstrate that, under appropriate conditions, a high proportion of murine Lyt-2^+ T cells can, after a period of culture, display promiscuous cytolytic activity. A further implication from these studies is that estimates of the frequency of specific CTL precursors by LDA may not always be accurate. Depending on the susceptibility of the test target cell to promiscuous cytotoxicity, varying degrees of overestimation of the specific precursor frequency will be made. Such problems were noticed during studies of precursor CTL frequencies to minor (Von Boehmer *et al.*, 1982) and major (Teh *et al.*, 1982) histocompatibility antigens.

With regard to the nature of the cytotoxic cells developing in long-term cultures containing IL-2, considerable progress has recently been made. The important clue came from the observation that the cells of certain murine NK-like clones simultaneously displayed a marker highly specific for cells of the CTL (and suppressor T cell) lineage, Lyt-2, and a marker highly specific for NK cells, NK-alloantigen (Brooks *et al.*, 1982). This finding suggested that there may be a close relationship between cells of the CTL and NK lineages. In order to explore this relationship further, experiments were initiated to determine whether antigen-specific CTL might, under certain conditions, be induced to express NK activity. Monoclonal CTL lines were prepared by culturing mouse spleen cells through three successive cycles of MLR, then cloning by limiting dilution in medium containing low concentrations of IL-2-containing supernatant. Many of the lines obtained were recloned to ensure monoclonality. The lines were clearly CTL by the following criteria: (1) they expressed Thy-1 and Lyt-2 antigens; (2) their proliferation was antigen-dependent and specific for the immunizing haplotype; and (3) they displayed exquisite antigen-specific cytolytic activity toward normal lymphoblast targets.

It was readily determined that these antigen-specific CTL lines expressed low quantities of NK-alloantigens (Brooks *et al.*, 1983a). CTL clones derived from C57BL/6 mice expressed both NK-1.1 and NK-2.1 antigens and CTL clones derived from CBA mice expressed NK-2.1, but not NK-1.1 antigens, as expected from the genetics of NK-alloantigens. Furthermore, cloned CTL lines were able to absorb antibodies from NK-alloantisera, which caused complement-dependent lysis of fresh splenic NK cells. These observations confirmed directly that cells in the CTL lineage could express membrane molecules previously identified as specific markers of NK cells.

Most importantly, it was observed that about one-half of the antigen-specific CTL clones displayed cytolytic activity against YAC-1 cells (Brooks *et al.*, 1983b). In some cases, the specificity of this cytolytic activity was similar to the promiscuous cytotoxicity of the NK-like clones studied earlier. However, in most cases, examination of the specificity on a panel of NK-sensitive and NK-resistant lines showed it to be identical to that of splenic NK cells. Daughter clones obtained by recloning of such CTL clones also possessed both antigen-specific and NK functions. Furthermore, cold target competition assays using unlabeled YAC-1 cells established that the antigen-specific cytolytic activity of CTL clones having NK activity, but not those lacking NK activity, could be inhibited by YAC-1. These studies demonstrated that a cell could simultaneously express both antigen-specific CTL function as well as NK activity.

When CTL clones were transferred into medium containing higher concentrations of crude IL-2-containing supernatant, a series of remarkable changes occurred (Brooks *et al.*, 1983b; Brooks, 1983). First, the cells went through a phase of rapid proliferation and became somewhat enlarged and more rounded. During this period, there was a slight increase in antigen-specific cytolytic activity, but a spectacular increase in NK activity. Indeed, even CTL clones that were initially devoid of NK function acquired it (Fig. 2). The induced NK activity was initially identical in specificity to that of splenic NK cells. However, after a certain period of time (which varied from a few days to a few weeks, depending on the particular clone), the specificity degenerated toward promiscuous cytotoxicity, as manifested by the acquisition of lytic activity against NK-resistant targets. At least over the period during which the CTL expressed true NK specificity, the changes were reversible; after transfer back to medium containing low concentrations of IL-2-containing supernatant, the cells ceased to divide, gradually (over a period of several days) lost NK activity, and reverted back to small spindle-shaped cells. By contrast, in cells kept in high concentrations of IL-2-containing supernatant, the rate of division slowed, and sometimes the cells went through a crisis period, but no loss of cytolytic activity occurred.

Eventually, the cultures became overgrown with large, highly granular cells

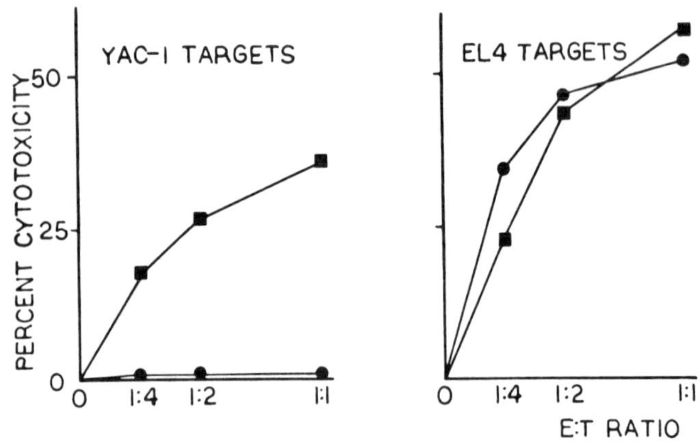

Figure 2. Induction of NK activity in a CBA/J anti-C57BL/6 (k anti-b) CTL clone (A1G7). The clone was generated using procedures similar to those described by Glasebrook and Fitch (1980). Cloning was by limiting dilution at 1 cell/well, followed by two successive reclonings at 1 cell/well, and was maintained in Click's medium containing 10% FBS and 2–4% supernatant from Con A-stimulated rat spleen cells, with periodic stimulation with antigen (irradiated C57BL/6 spleen cells). Two weeks after the last stimulation with antigen, CTL were purified on Ficoll-Hypaque and aliquots of 1×10^5 cells incubated in 1 ml regular growth medium (•) or in the same medium supplemented with 30% supernatant from Con A-stimulated mouse spleen cells (▪). Two days later, cells were washed and tested for cytotoxicity on YAC-1 (H-2^a) and EL4 (H-2^b) targets in a 4-hr chromium release assay using the effector : target (E : T) ratios shown.

that were able to proliferate indefinitely in the absence of antigen, lacked antigen-specific cytolytic activity, had a potent promiscuous cytotoxic actitity and, indeed, were identical on the basis of morphology, surface markers, and function to the NK-like clones studied previously. During the latter stages of the lymphokine-induced differentiation of CTL, profound changes in cell-surface glycolipids and glycoproteins were observed. A time-dependent loss of specific cytotoxic activity, leaving only nonspecific lytic activity, has also been noted in antigen-independent CTL clones studied by Acha-Orbea *et al.*, (1983).

All attempts to induce these cells to revert to antigen-specific CTL have failed, and it appears that the NK-like clones described by ourselves and others (for review, see Brooks, 1984) are, at least in some cases, derived by an irreversible differentiation process from cells in the CTL lineage. The observation that NK-like cells of this type often lack the Lyt-2 marker suggests that this marker may be readily lost during differentiation, or that some of these cells arise from Lyt-2^- precursors. In the latter case, an intriguing possibility is that pre-T cells or immature T cells, perhaps already programmed as CTL precursors, can differentiate into NK-like cells. At any rate, the studies described above have established several observations:

1. NK activity can reside in cells of indisputable T-cell lineage.

2. CTL are not, as was previously assumed, restricted to antigen-specific cytotoxic activity. [By antigen-specific is meant cytolytic activity involving participation of the antigen-specific receptor on these cells. It is clear from the recently published elegant experiments of Binz *et al.* (1983) that the NK function of CTL does not require the participation of these receptors.]

3. CTL are not necessarily end cells and can be induced, by factors in Con A-induced spleen cell supernatant, to differentiate further.

In sum, it is noted that these studies provide direct confirmation, at the clonal level, of the hypothesis proposed by Klein (see Klein, 1980; Vanky and Klein, 1983) that NK activity can be mediated by activated CTL.

Preliminary studies indicate that both IL-2 and IFN participate in the induction of NK activity in CTL (Brooks, 1983). Treatment of cloned CTL, lacking NK activity, for 2–3 days with IL-2 obtained from LBRM-33 cell supernatant by sequential ammonium sulfate precipitation, Sephadex G100 chromatography, and isoelectric focusing, led to induction of some NK activity (Fig. 3). The level of NK activity induced in repeat experiments using the same IL-2 preparation was surprisingly variable, ranging from almost undetectable levels to levels comparable to those induced by crude Con A-induced spleen-cell supernatants. Addition of Con A usually inhibited, and never augmented, induction of NK activity by partially purified IL-2. It would appear that the responsiveness of a given CTL clone to the induction of NK function by IL-2 varies, but what controls this responsiveness is currently unknown. Partially purified mouse fibroblast (β) IFN consistently induced some NK activity in CTL clones, and this induction was completely inhibited by antibodies to β-IFN. However, by far the most ef-

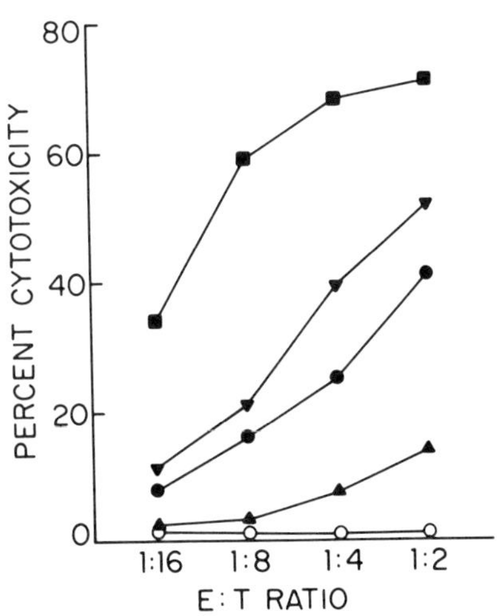

Figure 3. Induction of NK activity in a B6-C-H-2^{bm1} ByJ anti-C57BL/6 (bm1 anti-b) CTL clone (F3). This clone was prepared and maintained as described in Fig. 2. Aliquots of 1×10^5 CTL were incubated for 3 days in Click's/10% FBS containing 2% rat Con A spleen-cell supernatant (○), 30% mouse Con A spleen-cell supernatant (●), 10 U/ml partially purified mouse IL-2 (▲), 10^4 U/ml mouse β-IFN + 2% rat Con A spleen-cell supernatant (▼), or 10 U/ml IL-2 + 10^4 U/ml β-IFN (■). Cytotoxicity was measured on YAC-1 targets in a 4-hr chromium release assay at the E:T ratios shown.

fective protocol, producing levels of NK activity that exceeded those induced by crude spleen-cell supernatant, was incubation of CTL with both β-IFN and IL-2 (Fig. 3). These results are of interest not only because of the light they shed on NK function, but because they provide model systems in which to study the biochemistry through which two well-defined lymphokines, both available in highly purified form, can induce functional differentiation in a cloned T-cell line.

The synergy observed between IFN and IL-2 is itself interesting, because the first studies of IL-2-induced NK activation in murine spleen cells uncovered the same phenomenon of cooperativity between the two ligands (see Section II). It would be relatively simple to determine whether IFN acts by enhancing expression of IL-2 receptors. As with the short-term boosting of NK activity, discussed extensively in Section V, it is possible that IL-2 may act in some cases by inducing IFN from CTL clones, which could then cooperate with IL-2 in the induction of NK activity. It has indeed been shown that at least some CTL clones secrete IFN in response to antigens and mitogens (Klein *et al.*, 1982; McKimm-Berschkin *et al.*, 1982) and that some NK-like clones also secrete IFN (Kedar *et al.*, 1982; Matsuyama *et al.*, 1982; Handa *et al.*, 1983).

VII. CONCLUDING REMARKS

It is now clear that IL-2 plays a central role in the immunobiology of cytotoxic cells. In this review we have not dealt with the well-documented participation of IL-2 in the development and clonal expansion of antigen-specific CTL during immune responses. This area has been reviewed previously (see Moller, 1982) and elsewhere in this volume. Rather, we have concentrated on delineating the pathways by which IL-2 can promote the expression of NK and NK-like activities. Many of the studies in this area are incomplete, and our aim has been to assimilate a coherent viewpoint, even though at times this has required a certain degree of license with data at hand.

What appears compelling from the evidence available at this time is that there exist at least two distinct pathways through which IL-2 can potentiate NK activity. First, it can act as an inducer of γ-IFN, which can then activate NK cells (or pre-NK cells) directly (see Welsh, 1983). Because of the complexity of the pathway by which IL-2 induces IFN, many basic questions remain to be answered, not the least important being whether NK cells themselves interact with IL-2, and which cell produces the γ-IFN.

Second, IL-2 alone, but more often in concert with IFN, can induce cells of apparent CTL lineage, including conventional antigen-specific CTL, to express NK activity.

In short-term (≤ 24-hr) cultures of fresh spleen or blood cells, the former pathway, i.e., activation via IFN production, is predominant. When incubations are continued for longer than 24 hr, increasingly greater contributions are made by the second pathway. In some experiments, relatively immature cells may acquire a CTL-like phenotype and potent cytolytic activity. In other cases, more mature CTL, perhaps triggered to express IL-2 receptors by recent exposure to antigen, to serum protein in the culture medium, or to traces of lectin or other lymphokines in the IL-2 preparations, can acquire NK-like activity. Prolonged exposure of CTL to IL-2 (and perhaps other factors present in crude IL-2 preparations) causes the NK specificity to degenerate into a more promiscuous cytolytic activity and can induce profound and irreversible changes in morphology, biochemistry, and growth characteristics.

It is clear from these studies that the mature CTL can no longer be considered an end cell and that a careful delineation of the differentiation pathways and signals that regulate the interrelationships between the CTL and NK compartments poses an exciting challenge to cellular immunologists and molecular biologists. At the same time, with increasing access to lymphokines obtained by recombinant DNA technology, future studies on the mechanism of action of these important immunoregulatory molecules should be more definitive. Both the IL-2 and various interferon genes have recently been cloned and expressed in *E. coli*; studies on the mechanism of action of these gene products should now proceed quickly, concomitant with an assessment of their clinical potential.

VIII. REFERENCES

Abo, T., and Balch, C. M., 1981, *J. Immunol.* **127**:1024.

Abo, T., and Balch, C. M., 1982, *J. Immunol.* **129**:1758.

Abo, T., and Balch, C. M., 1983, *Eur. J. Immunol.* **13**:383.

Abo, T., Miller, C. A., Cooper, M. D., and Balch, C. M., 1983, *J. Immunol.* **131**:1822.

Acha-Orbea, H., Groscurth, P., Lang, R., Stitz, L., and Hengartner, H., 1983, *J. Immunol.* **130**:2952.

Acuto, O., Cianfriglia, M., Columbatti, B., Chapius, B., and Nabholz, M., 1982, *J. Immunol. Methods* **53**:15.

Binz, H., Fenner, M., Frei, D., and Wigzell, H., 1983, *J. Exp. Med.* **157**:1252.

Biron, C. A., Hult-Fletcher, L. M., Wentz, G. T., and Pagano, J. S., 1981, *Int. J. Cancer* **27**:185.

Brooks, C. G., 1983, *Nature* **305**:155.

Brooks, C. G., Flannery, G. R., Willmott, N., Austin, E. B., Kenwrick, S., and Baldwin, R. W., 1981, *Int. J. Cancer* **28**:191.

Brooks, C. G., Kuribayashi, K., Sale, G., and Henney, C. S., 1982, *J. Immunol.* **128**:2326.

Brooks, C. G., Burton, R. C., Pollack, S. B., and Henney, C. S., 1983a, *J. Immunol.* **131**:1391.

Brooks, C. G., Urdal, D., and Henney, C. S., 1983b, *Immunol. Rev.* **72**:43.

Brooks, C. G., 1984, in: *Immunobiology of Natural Killer Cells* (E. Lotzova, ed.), CRC Press, Boca Raton, Florida (in press).

Callewaert, D. M., Lightbody, J. J., Kaplan, J., Jaroszewski, J., Peterson, W. D., and Rosenberg, J. C., 1978, *J. Immunol.* **121**:81.

Dialynas, D. P., Loken, M. R., Glasebrook, A. L., and Fitch, F. W., 1981, *J. Exp. Med.* **153**:595.
Djeu, J. Y., Heinbaugh, J. A., Holden, H. T., and Herberman, R. B., 1979a, *J. Immunol.* **122**:175.
Djeu, J. Y., Heinbaugh, J. A., Holden, H. T., and Herberman, R. B., 1979b, *J. Immunol.* **122**:182.
Djeu, J. Y., Stocks, N., Zoon, K., Stanton, G. J., Timonen, T., and Herberman, R. B., 1982, *J. Exp. Med.* **156**:1222.
Domzig, W., Stadler, B. M., and Herberman, R. B., 1983, *J. Immunol.* **130**:1970.
Durdik, J. M., Beck, B. N., Clark, E. A., and Henney, C. S., 1980, *J. Immunol.* **125**:683.
Farrar, W. L., Johnson, H. M., and Farrar, J. J., 1981, *J. Immunol.* **126**:1120.
Fleischmann, W. R., Georgiades, J. A., Osborne, L. C., and Johnson, H. M., 1979, *Infect. Immun.* **25**:248.
Flomenberg, N., Welte, K., Mertelsmann, R., O'Reilly, R., and Dupont, B., 1983, *J. Immunol.* **130**:2635.
Galili, V., Galili, N., Vanky, F., and Klein, E., 1978, *Proc. Natl. Acad. Sci. USA* **75**:2396.
Galli, S., Dvorak, A. M., Ishizaka, T., Nabel, G., Der Simonian, M., Cantor, H., and Dvorak, H. F., 1982, *Nature* **298**:288.
Gidlund, M. Orn, A., Wigzell, H., Senik, A., and Gresser I., 1978, *Nature* **273**:759.
Gillis, S., Ferm, M. M., Ou, W., and Smith, K. A., 1978, *J. Immunol.* **120**:2027.
Gillis, S., Scheid, M., and Watson, J., 1980, *J. Immunol.* **125**:2570.
Gillis, S., Mochizuki, D. Y., Conlon, P. J., Hefeneider, S. H., Ramthun, C. A., Gillis, A. E., Frank, M. B., Henney, C. S., and Watson, J. D., 1982, *Immunol. Rev.* **63**:167.
Giorgi, J. V., Zawadoski, J. A., and Warner, N. L., 1982, *Eur. J. Immunol.* **12**:831.
Glasebrook, A. L., and Fitch, F. W., 1980, *J. Exp. Med.* **151**:876.
Golub, S. H., Golightly, M. G., and Zielske, J. V., 1979, *Int. J. Cancer* **24**:273.
Gonzales, H., Kariger, K., Sharma, B., and Vaziri, N., 1983, *Fed. Proc.* **42**:1195.
Gorelik, E., and Herberman, R. B., 1981, *Int. J. Cancer* **27**:709.
Granelli-Piperno, A., Vassalli, J. D., and Reich, E., 1981, *J. Exp. Med.* **154**:422.
Gray, J. D., Torten, M., and Golub, S. H., 1983, *Fed. Proc.* **42**:680.
Grimm, E. A., and Rosenberg, S. A., 1982, in: *Isolation, Characterization, and Utilization of T Lymphocyte Clones* (C. G. Fathman and F. W. Fitch, eds.), pp. 57–82, Academic Press, New York.
Grimm, E. A., Mazumder, A., Strausser, J. L., and Rosenberg, S. A., 1982, *J. Exp. Med.* **155**:1823.
Grimm, E. A., Ramsey, K. M., Mazumder, A., Wilson, D. J., Djeu, J. Y., and Rosenberg, S. A. 1983, *J. Exp. Med.* **157**:884.
Handa, K., Suzuki, R., Matsui, H., Shimizu, Y., and Kumagai, K., 1983, *J. Immunol.* **130**:988.
Hefeneider, S. H., Conlon, P. J., Henney, C. S., and Gillis, S., 1983, *J. Immunol.* **130**:222.
Henney, C. S., Kuribayashi, K., Kern, D. E., and Gillis, S., 1981, *Nature* **291**:335.
Herberman, R. B., Nunn, M. E., Holden, H. T., Staal, S., and Djeu, J. Y., 1977, *Int. J. Cancer* **19**:555.
Herberman, R. B., Ortaldo, J. R., and Bonnard, G. D., 1979, *Nature* **277**:221.
Hersey, P., Bindon, C., Edwards, A., Murray, E., Phillips, G., and McCarthy, W. H., 1981, *Int. J. Cancer* **28**:695.
Hurrell, S. M., and Zarling, J. M., 1983, *J. Immunol.* **131**:1017.
Ihle, J. N., Keller, J., Oroszlan, S., Henderson, L. E., Copeland, T. D., Fitch, F., Prystowsky, M. B., Goldwasser, E., Schrader, J. W., Palaszniski, E., Dy, M., and Lebel, B., 1983, *J. Immunol.* **131**:282.
Jondal, M., and Targan, S., 1978, *J. Exp. Med.* **147**:1621.
Karre, K., and Seeley, J. K., 1979, *J. Immunol.* **123**:1511.
Karre, K., Seeley, J. K., Eriksson, E., Burton, R. C., and Kiessling, R., 1983, *J. Exp. Med.* **157**:385.
Kasahara, T., Hooks, J. J., Dougherty, S. F., and Oppenheim, J. J., 1983. *J. Immunol.* **130**:1784.

Kawase, I., Urdal, D., Brooks, C. G., and Henney, C. S., 1982, *Int. J. Cancer* **29**:567.
Kawase, I., Brooks, C. G., Kuribayashi, K., Olabuenaga, S., Newman, W., Gillis, S., and Henney, C. S., 1983a, *J. Immunol.* **131**:288.
Kawase, I., Urdal, D., Newman, W., and Henney, C. S., 1983b, *Int. J. Cancer* **31**:365.
Kedar, E., Ibejim, B. L., Strendi, B., Bonavida, B., and Herberman, R. B., 1982, *Cell Immunol.* **69**:305.
Kiessling, R., Petranyi, G., Klein, G., and Wigzell, H., 1975, *Int. J. Cancer* 15:933.
Klein, E., 1980, *Immunol. Today* **I**:iv.
Klein, J. R., Raulet, D. M., Pasternak, M. S., and Bevan, J. J., 1982, *J. Exp. Med.* **155**:1198.
Koide, Y., and Takasugi, M., 1978, *J. Immunol.* **121**:872.
Kuribayashi, K., Gillis, S., Kern, D. E., and Henney, C. S., 1981, *J. Immunol.* **126**:2321.
Lattime, F., Pecoraro, G. A., and Stutman, O., 1983, *J. Exp. Med.* **157**:1070.
Leonard, W. J., Depper, J. M., Uchiyama, T., Smith, K. A., Waldmann, T. A., and Greene, W. C., 1982, *Nature* **300**:207.
Lopez-Botet, M., Silva, A., Rodriguez, J., and de Landazuri, M. O., 1982, *J. Immunol.* **129**:1109.
Lotze, M. T., Grimm, E. A., Mazumder, A., Strausser, J. L.,, and Rosenberg, S. A., 1981, *Cancer Res.* **41**:4420.
Matsuyama, M., Sugamara, K., Kawade, Y., and Hinuma, Y., 1982, *J. Immunol.* **129**:450.
Mazumder, A., Grimm, E. A., and Rosenberg, S. A., 1983, *J. Immunol.* **130**:958.
Merluzzi, V. J., Welte, K., and Mertelsmann, R., 1983, *Fed. Proc.* **42**:440.
Minato, N., Reid, L., Cantor, H., Lengyel, P., and Bloom, B. R., 1980, *J. Exp. Med.* **152**:124.
Minato, N., Reid, L., and Bloom, B. R., 1981, *J. Exp. Med.* **154**:750.
Moller, G. (ed.), 1982, *Immunol. Rev.* **63**.
Moretta, A., Pantaleo, G., Moretta, L., Cerottini, J.-C., and Mingari, M. C., 1983, *J. Exp. Med.* **157**:743.
McKimm-Breschkin, J. L., Mottram, P. L., Thomas, W. R., and Miller, J. F. A. P., 1982, *J. Exp. Med.* **155**:1204.
Oehler, J. R., Lindsay, L. R., Nunn, M. E., and Herberman, R. B., 1978, *Int. J. Cancer* **21**:210.
Ojo, E., Haller, O., Kimura, A., and Wigzell, H., 1978, *Int. J. Cancer* **21**:444.
Olabuenaga, S., Brooks, C. G., Gillis, S., and Henney, C. S., 1983, *J. Immunol.* **131**:
O'Malley, J. A., Nursbaum-Blumenson, A., Sheedy, D., Grossmeyer, B. J., and Ozer, M., 1983, *J. Immunol.* **128**:2522.
Ortaldo, J. R., Bonnard, G. D., and Herberman, R. B., 1977, *J. Immunol.* **119**:1351.
Ortaldo, J. R., Timonen, T. T., Vose, B. M., and Alvarez, J. A., 1982, in: *The Potential Role of T Cells in Cancer Therapy* (A. Ferfer and A. Goldstein, eds.), pp. 191–205, Raven Press, New York.
Paciucci, P. A., Macphail, S., Zarling, J. M., and Bach, F. H., 1980a, *J. Immunol.* **124**:370.
Paciucci, P. A., Macphail, S. S., Bach, F. H., and Zarling, J. M., 1980b, *J. Immunol.* **125**:36.
Perussia, B., Starr, S., Abraham, S., Fanning, V., and Trinchieri, G., 1983, *J. Immunol.* **130**:2133.
Pollack, S. B., and Hallenbeck, L. A., 1982, *Int. J. Cancer* **29**:203.
Poros, A., and Klein, E., 1978, *Cell Immunol.* **41**:240.
Rabin, H., Ortaldo, J. R., Henderson, L. E., and Neubauer, R. H., 1983, *Fed. Proc.* **42**:1239.
Ramsey, K. M., Stocks, N., Kasahara, T., and Djeu, J. Y., 1983, *Fed. Proc.* **42**:1379.
Riccardi, C., Vose, B. M., and Herberman, R. B., 1983, *J. Immunol.* **130**:228.
Roder, J. C., 1979, *J. Immunol.* **123**:2168.
Saksela, E., Timonen, T., Ranki, A., and Hayry, P., 1980a, *Immunol. Rev.* **44**: 71.
Saksela, E., Timonen, T., and Cantell, K., 1980b, *Ann. N.Y. Acad. Sci.* **350**:102.
Saxena, Q. B., Saxena, R. K., and Adler, W. H., 1983, *Fed. Proc.* **42**:450.
Schultz, R. M., 1982, *J. Interferon Res.* **2**:459.
Schultz, R. M., and Kleinschmidt, W. J., 1983, *Nature* **305**:239.
Seeley, J. K., and Golub, S. H., 1978, *J. Immunol.* **120**:1415.
Seeley, J. K., Masucci, G., Poros, E., Klein, E., and Golub, S. H., 1979, *J. Immunol.* **123**:1303.

Shellam, G. R., Winterbourn, V., and Dawkins, H. J. S., 1980, *Int. J. Cancer* **25**:331.
Shortman, K., Wilson, A., Scollay, R., and Chen, W-F., 1983, *Proc. Natl. Acad. Sci. USA* **80**:2728.
Stadler, B. M., Bernstein, E. H., Siraganian, R. P., and Oppenheim, J. J., 1982, *J. Immunol.* **128**:1620.
Strassmann, G., Bach, F. H., and Zarling, J. M., 1983, *J. Immunol.* **130**:1556.
Strausser, J. L., Mazumder, A., Grimm, E. A., Lotze, M. T., and Rosenberg, S. A., 1981, *J. Immunol.* **127**:266.
Suzuki, R., Handa, K., Itoh, K., and Kumagai, K., 1983, *J. Immunol.* **130**:981.
Talmadge, J. E., Meyers, K. M., Prieur, D. J., and Starkey, J. R., 1980, *Nature* **284**:622.
Teh, H.-S., Bennink, J., and Von Boehmer, H., 1982, *Eur. J. Immunol.* **12**:887.
Timonen, T. T., Ortaldo, J. R., Stadler, B. M., Bonnard, G. D., Sharrow, S. O., and Herberman, R. B., 1982, *Cell. Immunol.* **72**:178.
Torten, M., Sidell, N., and Golub, S. H., 1982, *J. Exp. Med.* **156**:1545.
Trinchieri, G., and Santoli, D., 1978, *J. Exp. Med.* **147**:1314.
Trinchieri, G., Santoli, D., Dee, R. R., and Knowles, B. B., 1978, *J. Exp. Med.* **147**:1299.
Vanky, F., and Klein, E., 1982, *Immunogenetics* **15**:31.
Von Boehmer, H., Bennink, J., and Langhorne, J., 1982, *Eur. J. Immunol.* **12**:892.
Vose, B. M., and Bonnard, G. D., 1983, *J. Immunol.* **130**:687.
Vose, B. M., Riccardi, R. C., Bonnard, G. D., and Herberman, R. B., 1983, *J. Immunol.* **130**:768.
Weigent, D. A., Stanton, G. J., and Johnson, H. M., 1983, *Fed. Proc.* **42**:1072.
Welsh, R. M., 1978, *J. Exp. Med.* **148**:163.
Welsh, R. M., 1983, *CRC Crit. Rev. Immunol.* **1** (in press).
Welsh, R. M., and Zinkernagel, R. M., 1977, *Nature* **268**:584.
Wolfe, S. A., Tracey, D. E., and Henney, C. S., 1976, *Nature* **262**:584.
Yamamoto, J. K., Farrar, W. L., and Johnson, H. M., 1982, *Cell. Immunol.* **66**:333.
Zarling, J. M., and Bach, F. M., 1978, *J. Exp. Med.* **147**:1334.
Zarling, J. M., and Bach, F. M., 1979, *Nature* **280**:685.
Zarling, J. M., and Kung, P. C., 1980, *Nature* **288**:394.
Zarling, J. M., Dierckins, M. S., Sevenich, E. A., and Clouse, K. A., 1981a, *J. Immunol.* **127**:2118.
Zarling, J. M., Bach, F. H., and Kung, P. C., 1981b, *J. Immunol.* **126**:375.
Zielske, J. V., and Golub, S. M., 1976, *Cancer Res.* **36**:3842.

Biochemical and Biological Properties of Interleukin-3: A Lymphokine Mediating the Differentiation of a Lineage of Cells That Includes Prothymocytes and Mastlike Cells

James N. Ihle

Basic Research Program-LBI
NCI-Frederick Cancer Research Facility
Frederick, Maryland 21701

I. INTRODUCTION

The initial characterization of Interleukin-3 (IL-3) came from a series of studies designed to identify the factors regulating early T-cell differentiation. The approach used took advantage of a series of observations demonstrating that the enzyme 20 α-hydroxysteroid dehydrogenase (20 αSDH) was uniquely associated with the T-cell lineage (Weinstein, 1977; Weinstein *et al.*, 1977; Pepersack *et al.*, 1980). The enzyme is readily detectable in lymphoid tissues of normal mice, in which it is predominantly associated with Thy-1$^+$ cells. The enzyme is either not detectable or occurs at low levels in fetal liver or spleen cells and is absent in spleen cells from genetically athymic or neonatally thymectomized mice. These results demonstrated that 20 αSDH expression is not associated with either B-cell differentiation or the majority of differentiation of myeloid, erythroid, or monocytelike lineages. The *in vivo* distribution of 20 αSDH was thus most consistent with a unique T-cell lineage expression, which was further supported by examining a variety of tissue-culture cell lines. In particular, 20 αSDH was not detectable in B-cell lines, macrophage/monocyte lines, or erythroid cell lines. In contrast, T-cell lines with a helper phenotype had low levels of 20 αSDH.

Cytotoxic IL-2-dependent, T-cell lines were found to have high levels of 20 αSDH. Of particular interest was the observation that terminal transferase (TdT)-positive T-cell lymphomas had no detectable 20 αSDH, consistent with the *in vivo* data demonstrating that 20 αSDH occurs uniquely in the medullary, hydrocortisone-resistant thymic population. In addition to these data, it has been suggested that 20 αSDH expression is associated with granulopoiesis (Garland and Dexter, 1982, 1983) based on the presence of 20 αSDH in a series of factor-dependent cell lines established from long-term bone marrow cultures. As will be seen, however, the characteristics of these cell lines (i.e., the expression of Thy 1) make it difficult to determine how the lines are related to normal myeloid differentiation. Nevertheless, the available evidence supports the hypothesis that 20 αSDH expression is characteristic of a lineage of cells that includes functional T cells.

The observation that splenic lymphocytes from neonatally thymectomized mice or genetically athymic mice lack a 20 αSDH^+ population of lymphocytes prompted experiments to determine whether a factor exists that is capable of inducing the differentiation *in vitro* of 20 αSDH^+ cells. This approach was of particular interest in that a number of studies had demonstrated that, under appropriate conditions, a precursor for functional, IL-2-responsive cytolytic T cells could be demonstrated in *nu/nu* spleens (Gillis *et al.*, 1979). In examining a variety of sources of potential factors, it was found that conditioned medium from activated T cells had a readily detected factor that, in cultures of *nu/nu* splenic lymphocytes, induced 20 αSDH activity (Ihle *et al.*, 1981). Increases in 20 αSDH occurred after a lag of approximately 6 hr and subsequently increased linearly over the next 36 hr. This rapid rise in 20 αSDH activity suggested a direct interaction of a factor with a precursor cell, resulting in its differentiation. On the basis of this assay as a measure of early T-cell differentiation, the T-cell origin of the factor involved, and its biochemical uniqueness, the term Interleukin-3 (IL-3) was proposed to distinguish this lymphokine from other T-cell-derived factors affecting lymphocyte differentiation.

A number of the parameters of the induction of 20 αSDH in *nu/nu* splenic lymphocyte cultures have been examined. Induction is rapid, and the increases observed are consistent with the *de novo* induction of 20 αSDH rather than the expansion of a 20 αSDH^+-population. The precursor population is hydrocortisone sensitive, whereas the induced population is hydrocortisone resistant. Both the precursor population and the initially induced populations are Thy 1^-, consistent with a possible early T-cell stage of differentiation. Induction of differentiation was inhibited by inhibitors of DNA synthesis, suggesting that cell division is required for differentiation. From this initial assay it has been possible to purify IL-3 to homogeneity and to begin to define the events mediated by this lymphokine. These studies have revealed a dramatic role in promoting differentiation of an early stem cell that may differentiate along multiple pathways (see Section IV). This review attempts to summarize the immunological phenomena that can currently be ascribed to IL-3 but, more importantly, attempts to present a potential lineage scheme for differentiation that is most consistent with the available data.

II. PURIFICATION AND BIOCHEMICAL PROPERTIES OF IL-3

In the initial approaches to purifying IL-3 from conditioned media of mitogen-activated lymphocytes, it was observed that the induction of 20 αSDH was associated with a unique biochemical entity that could be resolved from a number of other lymphokines. The assay therefore appeared specific for a single factor, in contrast to many assays, such as colony formation or lymphocyte proliferation, which can detect a variety of biochemically unique factors. Whether the induction of 20 αSDH with all lymphoid tissues *in vitro* can be uniquely related to IL-3 is less clear. In particular, Garland and Dexter (1982) detected 20 αSDH induction in long-term bone marrow cultures that does not appear to be due to IL-3. This induction, however, is at levels 10- to 20-fold lower than that observed in cultures of *nu/nu* splenic lymphocytes. The low levels of activity detected have not permitted a systematic study of this phenomenon. Nevertheless, the assay using *nu/nu* splenic lymphocytes has been sufficiently specific and rapid to provide an assay that can be used for the purification of IL-3.

IL-3 is predominantly, if not exclusively, a product of activated T cells. In particular, T-cell mitogens, but not B-cell mitogens, induce normal splenic lymphocytes to produce IL-3. Among normal splenic lymphocytes, limiting cell-dilution analysis has demonstrated that IL-2 and IL-3 are produced by the same lymphocyte (Miller and Stutman, 1983). In addition, cloned antigen-specific T cells have been shown to produce IL-3 after antigen or mitogen stimulation (Prystowsky *et al.*, 1982). Finally, the inability of *nu/nu* splenic lymphocytes to produce IL-3 after mitogen stimulation supports the exclusive T-cell origin of IL-3 and is consistent with the apparent lack of IL-3 promoted differentiation in *nu/nu* spleen. From a practical standpoint the most important source of IL-3 is conditioned medium from the WEHI-3 cell line (Lee *et al.*, 1982). This line constitutively produced IL-3, and conditioned medium contains 50- to 100-fold more IL-3 than conditioned medium from mitogen-stimulated splenic lymphocytes. The observation that WEHI-3 produced IL-3 was unexpected, since this line has been classified as a myelomonocytic leukemia. However, the production of IL-3 clearly distinguishes the WEHI-3 cell line from other myelomonocytic leukemias, such as the P388D1 cell line. In addition, the WEHI-3 cell line can be distinguished from other myelomonocytic cells by the expression of the Thy-1 marker. Nevertheless, the WEHI-3 cell line has proved of immense value in the purification of IL-3 by providing a constant source of IL-3 under conditions of large-scale cell cultures.

Using large volumes of WEHI-3 conditioned medium, a purification scheme has been developed that permits purification of IL-3 to homogeneity. The details of this procedure have been published and will not be considered in detail here (Ihle *et al.*, 1982b). It is important to note that this purification scheme has been used on muliple purifications and in most cases has resulted in a final preparation of homogeneous IL-3. This observation is in contrast to other procedures employing blue-Sepharose chromatography, which isolated a minor molecular form of IL-3 (Ihle *et al.*, 1982c), and as noted, gave only poor yields of purified material. The large-scale purification of IL-3 employs a variety of chromatographic procedures. One of the initial purification steps employs DEAE-cellulose. At a neutral pH, IL-3 does not bind to DEAE and therefore can be separated rapidly from the bulk of the protein. This chromatographic step is also important in resolving IL-3 from a variety of lymphokines found in conditioned medium from mitogen-stimulated lymphocytes, including the major colony-stimulating factor (CSF) activity and IL-2.

In addition to DEAE-cellulose columns, hydroxylapatite column chromatography is used. This step in purification is interesting in resolving several species of IL-3. Generally, a single major species is observed that on further purification has been characterized as a 28,000-dalton protein. Other forms of IL-3 are minor forms that appear to differ in carbohydrate content. In particular, Fig. 1 illustrates the differences observed. In this case, the IL-3 peak in the runthrough fractions from hydroxylapatite was purified to homogeneity and compared with the major IL-3 peak. The purified proteins were iodinated and subjected to either acid or acid with cyanogen bromide cleavage to compare the peptide patterns. Both fractions gave a comparable acid-generated cleavage pattern. As illustrated, in acid the major IL-3 species migrated on sodium dodecylsulfate (SDS) gels as a tight protein band with an apparent molecular weight of 28,000. By contrast, the runthrough fraction migrated in a more diffuse band with a higher apparent M_r of approximately 32,500. Both forms, however, gave comparable cyanogen bromide cleavage patterns, with the exception that the 32,500-M_r component was more diffuse. These results are most consistent with the interpretation that the protein moieties are the same and that the heterogeneity is not associated with the presence or absence of a specific peptide or glycosylation of a specific peptide, but rather with a more general extent of carbohydrate substitution. This is consistent with the observation that multiple forms of IL-3 are detectable in isoelectric focusing (IEF) and that neuraminidase can minimize this heterogeneity. In support of these results, *N*-terminal sequence analysis of the two preparations produced identical sequences. In spite of these differences, the specific activities and range of biological activities are identical, suggesting that heterogeneity of carbohydrate substitution has no effect on the biological activity. The heterogeneity of the size of IL-3 and of charge, due to the state of glycosylation, is a biochemical property similar to that observed with the colony stimulating factor, CSF-1 (Stanley and Guilbert, 1981).

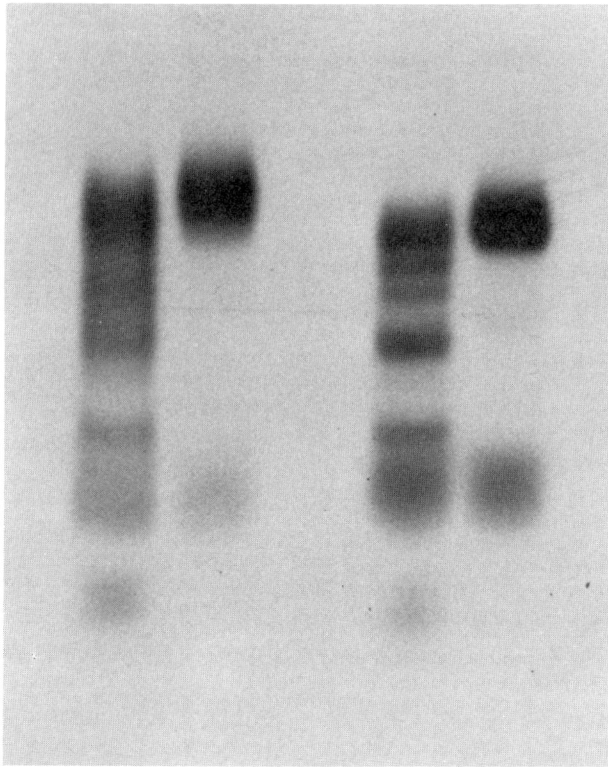

Figure 1. SDS-PAGE analysis of two forms of IL-3. The major peak of IL-3 from hydroxylapatite and a minor peak, eluting in the runthough fractions, were purified to homogeneity and iodinated with ^{125}I. The samples were subsequently treated with cyanogen bromide in formic acid (lanes 1 and 3 from left) or acid alone (lanes 2 and 4). The major IL-3 species migrated in acid with apparent molecular weights of 28,000 and 32,500.

The final step in the large-scale purification of IL-3 involves chromatography on C18 hydrophobic supports in reverse-phase high-performance liquid chromatography (RP-HPLC). IL-3 readily binds to such columns under acid conditions and can be eluted in a linear gradient of acetonitrile. In spite of the acid conditions and organic acid conditions and organic solvents, the biological activity is completely retained during purification and IL-3 is quite stable for long periods of time at -20°C in the eluting buffer. Similar to the results with hydroxylapatite, the multiple forms of IL-3, when not resolved by hydroxylapatite, can be resolved on HPLC, although not as readily.

The protein sequence of IL-3 has been established biochemically (Ihle *et al.*, 1983) and more recently from the sequence of cDNA clones for the IL-3 gene (Fung *et al.*, 1984; Yokota *et al.*, 1984). The complete amino acid sequence for

IL-3 deduced from a cDNA clone is shown in Figure 2. The sequence indicates the presence of a hydrophobic leader sequence which constitutes residues 1–32. From the protein sequence analysis of purified IL-3, the NH_2-terminal of the mature protein corresponds to the Asp in position 33. Based on a comparison of leader sequences of other proteins it has been speculated that the actual leader sequence may extend only to residue 27 and that a second cleavage may be involved in removing a small NH_2-terminal pentapeptide (Fung *et al.*, 1984). From residues 33–61 there is a complete agreement between the sequence obtained from the cDNA clones and the sequence that could be established from protein sequencing (Ihle *et al.*, 1983; J. N. Ihle, Oroszlan and Copeland, unpublished data).

As illustrated in Table I there is also agreement between the amino acid composition of purified IL-3 and that predicted from the sequence of the cDNA clones. On the basis of the cDNA sequence a molecular weight of approximately 15,000 daltons is predicted for the protein, whereas homogeneous IL-3 has an apparent molecular weight of 28,000 based on SDS-PAGE analysis. This discrepancy is due to the presence of carbohydrate on the mature protein. On analysis of homogeneous IL-3, 12 μg of glucosamine was found per 100 μg of IL-3 protein suggesting a considerable carbohydrate moiety. Assuming that an average complex moiety contains $\frac{1}{3}$ glucosamine, IL-3 could contain about 36% carbohydrate by weight. This would account for the difference in the predicted and observed molecular weights. From the cDNA sequence potential glycosylation sites are evident at residues 42, 70, 77, and 112. From the protein sequencing data no Asn residue was detectable at the position corresponding to residue 42, which strongly suggests that in the mature protein this site is glycosylated. Whether all of the potential sites are glycosylated is not known.

Whether the carbohydrate is required for the biological activity of IL-3 is not known. We have attempted to assess this possibility by using trifluoromethanesulphonate to remove the carbohydrate moiety. Unfortunately, under relatively mild conditions that do not remove the carbohydrate (as determined by SDS-PAGE), the biological activity is rapidly lost. Therefore, the acid is sufficiently strong to destroy biological activity prior to the conditions required to remove carbohydrate, thus this approach cannot be used to assess the role of the carbohydrate moiety. This conclusion is in contrast to the results of Bazill *et al.* (1983), who concluded that carbohydrate is necessary for one of the activities of IL-3 based on the loss of activity in trifluoromethanesulfonate. However, these workers provided no evidence for a direct correlation between removal of carbohydrate and loss of biological activity.

Purified IL-3 has been examined by several parameters to establish that the IL-3 activity is due to the major protein purified. Several aspects of these studies should be noted because of the spectrum of biological activities demonstrated

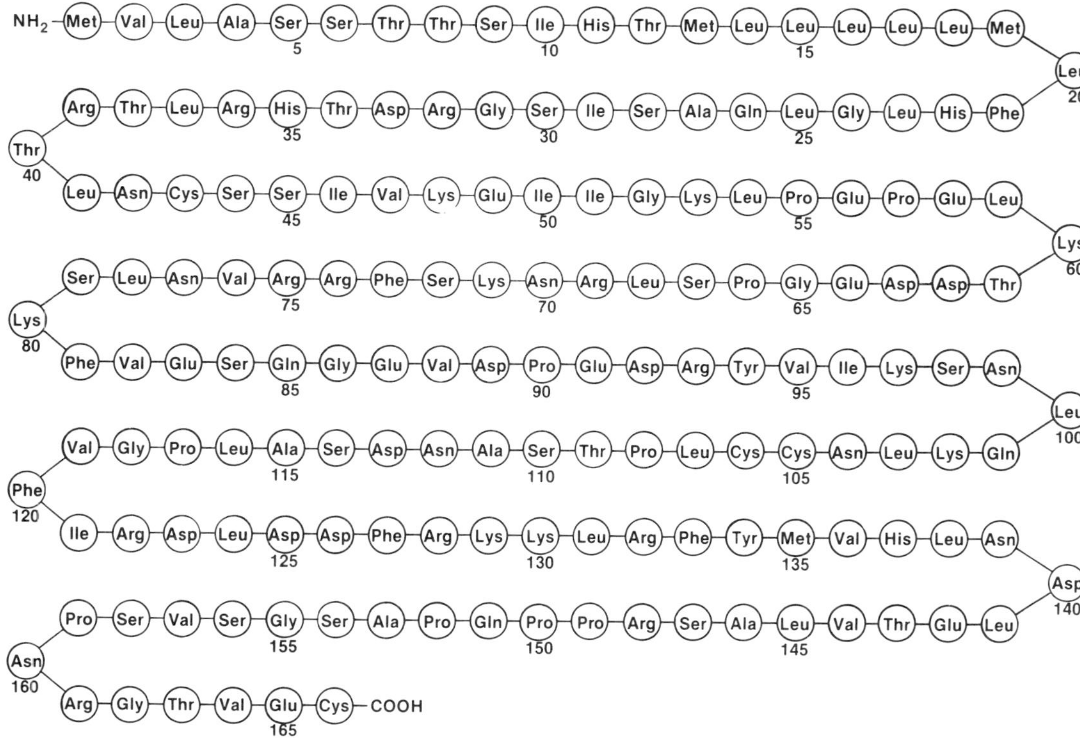

Figure 2. Amino acid sequence of IL-3. The sequence was deduced from the nucleotide sequence of a cDNA clone for IL-3 (Yokota *et al.*, 1984). As noted in the text, NH_2-terminal sequence analysis of purified IL-3 has demonstrated that the mature protein begins at residue 33. The deduced sequence from positions 33–61 is in complete agreement with the protein sequence that can be definitely identified in this region.

Table I. Amino Acid Composition of Murine IL-3[a]

	Predicted from cDNA sequence	Determined
Phe	5	4.2
Leu	15	16.7
Ile	5	4.8
Met	1	1.2
Val	10	8.3
Ser	13	11.3
Pro	10	7.1
Thr	8	7.1
Ala	3	4.2
Tyr	2	1.8
His	2	2.4
Glu, Gln	12	13.7
Asp, Asn	18	16.1
Lys	9	9.5
Cys	4	ND
Trp	0	ND
Arg	11	9.5
Gly	6	8.3

[a]The amino acid composition data was normalized to the size of mature IL-3 predicted from the cDNA sequence (Fung *et al.*, 1984). The normalization was done using the values for Glu and Asp. ND, not determined.

for IL-3. First, the published purification procedure has been used to purify numerous preparations of IL-3, which in all cases yielded a major IL-3 activity species of 28,000 daltons that, on cyanogen bromide cleavage, gave a peptide pattern identical to that in Fig. 1. In addition, when capable of being examined, the same *N*-terminal sequence has been obtained. The specific activity of these IL-3 preparations has been approximately 0.05–0.2 ng/ml for 50% maximal biological activity, corresponding to approximately 10^{-12} M. This value is within the range expected of a homogeneous growth factor, strongly suggesting that the major protein has the biological activity. In addition, an antiserum against IL-3 concomitantly immunoprecipitates the iodinated protein and inhibits its biological activity. Perhaps the most important observation, however, is that the iodinated 28,000-dalton protein shows specific binding to cell lines that are IL-3 dependent for growth but not to cell lines that do not require IL-3 for growth. Taken together with the sequence information obtained from the cDNA clones, these data provide substantial evidence supporting the contention that the major protein is homogeneous IL-3.

III. MULTIPLE BIOLOGICAL ACTIVITIES ASSOCIATED WITH IL-3

Early in the biochemical and biological studies of IL-3 it became apparent that the factor capable of inducing 20 αSDH might be capable of mediating a number of additional biological effects. The observation that IL-3 was constitutively produced by the WEHI-3 cell line prompted experiments to determine whether IL-3 was equivalent to a growth factor required for cell lines derived from long-term bone marrow cultures (Greenberger *et al.*, 1979; Dexter *et al.*, 1980). Moreover, the observation that long-term cultures of *nu/nu* splenic lymphocytes yield homogeneous populations of mastlike cells suggested a possible relationship of IL-3 to the mast cell growth factor described by several groups (Yung *et al.*, 1981; Nagao *et al.*, 1981; Razin *et al.*, 1981; Nabel *et al.*, 1981). To explore these possibilities, homogeneous IL-3 has been subjected to a variety of assays, the characteristics of which are shown in Table II. The activity of homogeneous IL-3 in several of these assays is shown in Fig. 3. As illustrated, the dose–response curves for IL-3 in all the assays in which it is active have been identical, demonstrating the equivalence of the biological activity. In addition, the ability of an antiserum against IL-3 to block activity in a variety of the assays has been examined and has been found to block the activities comparable to the inhibition of 20 αSDH induction. Since the characteristics of most of the activities listed in Table II have been reported elsewhere (references cited in Table II), only summary statements concerning the various assays are given here.

Regarding the differentiation mediated by IL-3, one of the most interesting activities is the WEHI-3 growth factor activity. This activity involves the ability of IL-3 to sustain the long-term tissue culture growth of a series of factor-dependent cell lines derived from bone marrow cultures. All the lines examined are characterized by an absolute dependence on IL-3 for growth, the presence of readily detectable high-affinity receptors for IL-3, and expression of the enzyme 20 αSDH. From a practical standpoint, these lines have been extremely important in providing a rapid, sensitive assay for IL-3, obviating the more cumbersome induction of 20 αSDH in *nu/nu* splenic lymphocyte cultures (Ihle *et al.*, 1982c). In addition, they have provided homogeneous populations of IL-3-responsive populations, permitting a detailed characterization of the IL-3 receptors (Palaszynski and Ihle, 1984). All the cell lines we have examined are nongranulated, lymphoblastic cells, which are relatively easy to maintain over long periods of time in the presence of a source of IL-3. During the period in which we have worked with these cell lines, they have maintained an absolute factor dependence. Using several of these lines, the specificity of the response to IL-3 has been examined. In either WEHI-3 conditioned media or conditioned media from mitogen-activated lymphocytes, the major proliferation-inducing activity is associated

TABLE II. Biological Activities of Homogeneous IL-3[a]

Factor/activity	Description	Uniqueness to IL-3	Reference
20 αSDH-inducing activity	Induction of 20αSDH	Unique	Ihle *et al.* (1981)
WEHI-3 hematopoietic growth factor	Growth factor for cell lines established from long-term bone marrow cultures	Unique	Dexter *et al.* (1980)
WEHI-3 growth factor	Growth factor for cell lines established from long-term bone marrow cultures	Unique	Greenberger *et al.* (1979)
Mast cell growth factor	Stimulates proliferation of mastlike cells grown from cultures of normal lymphoid tissues in CM from mitogen-stimulated lymphocytes	Major if not exclusive factor involved	Yung *et al.* (1981) Nagao *et al.* (1981) Razin *et al.* (1981) Nabel *et al.* (1981)
P-cell stimulating factor	Stimulates proliferation of a P cell grown in cultures of normal lymphoid tissues in CM from mitogen-stimulated lymphocytes	Major if not exclusive factor involved	Schrader *et al.* (1981)
Histamine-producing cell-stimulating factor	Increases histamine synthesis in cultures of normal spleen or bone marrow cells	Major if not exclusive factor involved	Dy *et al.* (1981)
Colony-stimulating factor	Induces colonies in soft agar cultures of normal bone marrow cells	Constitutes <5% of the total CSF activity	Ihle *et al.* (1983)
Burst-promoting activity	Stimulates the production of erythropoietin inducible erythroid colonies	Not unique	Goldwasser *et al.* (1983)
Hemopoietin-2	Stimulates the differentiation of lymphoid cells having receptors for CSF-1	Not known	Bartelmez *et al.* (1984)
NK cell growth factor	Causes the proliferation in tissue culture of splenic lymphocytes	Not known	Lattime *et al.* (1983); Djeu *et al.* (1982)

TABLE II. (*Continued*)

Factor/activity	Description	Uniqueness to IL-3	Reference
NK cell growth factor (*Cont.*)	having cytotoxicity against adherent tumor cell lines		
Thy-1-inducing activity	Induces the expression of Thy 1 in bone marrow cell cultures or in cultures of *nu/nu* splenic lymphocytes	Major if not exclusive factor involved	Schrader *et al.* (1982); Prystowsky *et al.* (1983)
Colony-forming unit-spleen stimulating activity	Maintains stem cell in culture, which can form colonies in spleens of irradiated mice.	Not known	Schrader and Clark-Lewis (1982)

[a]CM, conditioned medium; CSF, colony-stimulating factor; NK, natural killer; P cell, persisting cell; 20αSDH, 20α-hydroxylated dehydrogenase.

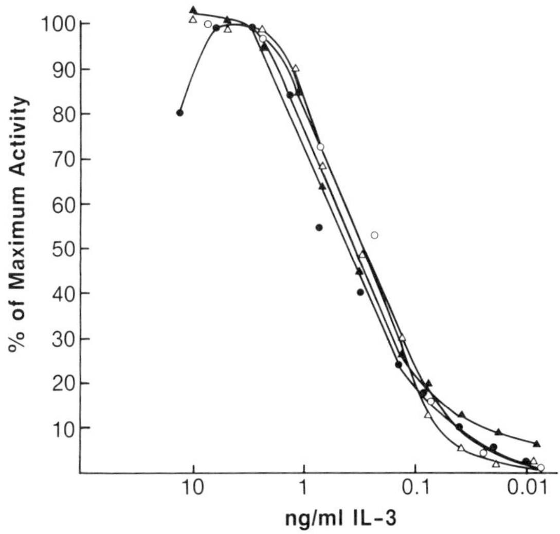

Figure 3. Dose response curves for homogeneous IL-3 in different biological assays. IL-3 was purified to homogeneity and assayed at the indicated concentrations in assays for induction of 20 αSDH in cultures of *nu/nu* splenic lymphocytes (▲—▲); induction of proliferation of an IL-3-dependent cell line derived from long-term bone marrow cultures (△—△); induction of the proliferation of cultures of mast-like cells (●—●), and induction of colony formation in soft agar of bone marrow cells.

with IL-3. In particular, during purification, the activity copurifies with IL-3 and, using complete medium, most of the activity can be inhibited by an antiserum against IL-3. Therefore, the available evidence suggests that the cell lines are uniquely dependent on IL-3 for growth in tissue culture and that in addition to the rapidity, the assays using these lines have a remarkable specificity for IL-3.

A variety of IL-3-dependent cell lines have been examined for expression of cell-surface markers that might be used to determine the lineage(s) they might represent (Ihle *et al.*, 1982c; Dexter *et al.*, 1980; Garland and Dexter, 1983). This work was particularly relevant, since some of the initial characterizations of the lines suggested that they represented a population of committed granulocyte progenitor cells (Dexter *et al.*, 1980). This conclusion was based primarily on the macroscopic morphology of colonies in soft agar. By contrast, examination of a number of the lines showed them to be negative for alkaline phosphodiesterase and nonspecific esterase markers typically associated with granulocytes. Second, none of the cell lines could be maintained in culture with proliferate or differentiate to colony-stimulating factor for granulocytes and macrophages (GM-CSF) the factor normally associated with the regulation of the myeloid lineage. In addition, a number of the lines were Thy 1^+, indicating a T-cell origin, although Lyt 1 or Lyt 2 were generally not detectable. These results, coupled with the expression of 20 αSDH, which as noted above is more characteristically associated with differentiating T-cells than with myeloid cells, suggested a more consistent T-lineage phenotype than one of normal myeloid.

A second related question regarding the IL-3 dependent cell lines is whether they represent normal intermediates in differentiation. Since such lines are relatively difficult to establish and specifically are not routinely isolated by culturing bone marrow cells in IL-3, a type of transformation can be suspected. Where examined, the cell lines do not induce tumors in mice, although the requirement for IL-3 for growth may require special immunological conditions *in vivo* in order to manifest tumorigenic potential. With regard to normal IL-3-promoted differentiation, all the lines are unique in failing to differentiate to functional cell types. We have therefore proposed that the cell lines are transformed in a manner in which transformation is manifested as an inability to differentiate terminally. In this regard, the available cell lines derived from bone marrow cultures are very similar to a number of retrovirus-induced lymphomas (see Section V).

The activities of mast-cell growth factor, persisting-cell (P-cell) stimulating factor, and histamine-producing cell-stimulating factor are related to the ability of IL-3 to promote the differentiation *in vitro*, in the absence of exogenously added factors, of a mastlike cell that has immunoglobulin E (IgE) receptors and synthesizes histamine. Among the various phenotypes of cells that are induced and that appear in cultures of cells differentiating in the presence of IL-3, it is the mastlike cell phenotype that persists the longest, such that after 2–3 weeks in culture, essentially homogeneous populations of granulated, Thy-1^-, Ly-5^+, H-11^+, Ia^+, Mac-1^-, Ig^-, 20 αSDH^+ cells are obtained. These cells progressively lose their ability to proliferate, even in the presence of IL-3 and, in our experience, do not generally give rise to continuous factor-dependent cell lines.

The relationship of the IL-3 dependent differentiation of mastlike cells to either normal mast cell differentiation or myeloid differentiation is uncertain. In particular, mastlike cells derived from IL-3-promoted differentiation of spleen cells differ from normal mast cells in the synthesis of a chrondroitin sulfate E proteoglycan in contrast to the normal proteoglycan, heparin (Razin *et al.*, 1982; Stevens *et al.*, 1983, Razin *et al.*, 1984). In addition, IL-3-derived mastlike cells produced after stimulation with aggregated IgE synthesize high levels of the leukotriene C_4 (LTC_4), whereas conventional mast cells generate relatively low amounts of LTC_4 (Razin *et al.*, 1983). In addition, a series of monoclonal antibodies have been derived that distinguish peritoneal resident mast cells from the tissue-culture-derived mastlike cells from either bone marrow or spleen (Le Blanc *et al.*, 1982; Katz *et al.*, 1983). These results suggest the existence of distinct mastlike cell subpopulations having major differences in phenotypes and potential function and the possibility that IL-3 is primarily responsible for the differentiation of one of these phenotypes.

In relationship to the above points, a relevant question is whether IL-3 is the only T-cell-derived factor involved in the differentiation of mastlike cells. According to reports of partial purifications of mast cell and P-cell growth factors (Yung *et al.*, 1981; Yung and Moore, 1982; Schrader *et al.*, 1982), the activity apparently purifies through multiple steps as though a single factor is involved. Moreover, the published partial purifications are consistent with major activity associated with IL-3. Also, as noted above, homogeneous IL-3 has been active in the mast-cell or P-cell assays of several laboratories. Therefore, unless proved to the contrary by purification to homogeneity and by sequence analysis, the available data are consistent with the major mastlike cell growth factor activity being IL-3. It should be noted, however, that it has been demonstrated that a clone of natural killer (NK) cells has the biochemical and morphological properties of basophil or mastlike cells (Galli *et al.*, 1982). This clone is dependent on IL-2 rather than on IL-3 for proliferation. Therefore, other lymphokines may regulate mastlike cells, although not constituting the major factor. Therefore, as indicated in Table II, IL-3 probably represents the major, but not necessarily the exclusive, factor for the differentiation and/or proliferation of mastlike cells.

In addition to the above activities, homogeneous IL-3 has a colony-stimulating activity. As illustrated in Fig. 3, the dose-response curve for this activity is identical to that for the other IL-3 activities. In terms of gross morphology, the colonies induced by IL-3 are similar to those described for the GM-CSF-type factors. On the basis of morphology and histochemical staining, IL-3 induces neutrophils, monocytes, mastlike cells, and megakaryocytes, as well as lymphocytes. With regard to T-cell-derived factors, however, the colony-stimulating activity of IL-3 represents approximately 1% of the total CSF activity of conditioned medium from activated cloned T-cells (Ihle *et al.*, 1983). The major

CSF activity is associated with a second protein that can be readily resolved from IL-3 by DEAE-cellulose chromatography. This factor, termed CSF-2, although generally indistinguishable from IL-3 in a standard CSF assay, is different from IL-3 in displaying none of the other IL-3 activities such as WEHI-3 growth factor activity, 20 αSDH-inducing activity, or mast-cell growth factor activity. Similarly, whereas the antiserum against IL-3 inhibits the CSF activity associated with IL-3, it exhibits no inhibitory activity against the CSF-2 activity. Finally, in cultures of Thy-1-depleted bone marrow cells, IL-3 induces Thy-1$^+$ cells, whereas CSF-2 shows no such activity. Similarly, IL-3 can induce 20 αSDH in bone marrow cultures, whereas CSF-2 does not. Therefore, although IL-3 displays colony-stimulating activity, it can be clearly distinguished biochemically, serologically, and biologically from the major T-cell-derived CSF.

Among the activities found to be mediated by homogeneous IL-3, a burst-promoting activity (BPA) is the most unusual relative to the other biological properties (Goldwasser *et al*., 1983). Burst-promoting activity (BPA) is the ability to increase the number of bone marrow colonies that, in the presence of erythropoietin, can differentiate to mature erythroid bursts. The current interpretation of BPA is that it is mediated by a protein(s) that regulates early erythroid differentiation and specifically induces the differentiation of a committed population that responds to erythropoietin (Iscove, 1978). The observation of BPA for IL-3, and thus a presumptive role in erythroid differentiation, is unusual for several reasons: (1) 20 αSDH expression is generally associated with IL-3. An examination of a variety of erythroleukemia cell lines representing early erythroid cell types has found none that express 20 αSDH or that have detectable receptors for IL-3; (2) erythroid differentiation occurs normally in *nu/nu* or neonatally thymectomized mice, which are generally unable to produce IL-3 and lack evidence of IL-3 induced differentiation (i.e., 20 αSDH expression); (3) the apparently exclusive T-cell origin of IL-3 would lead to the implication that normal erythroid differentiation is regulated by an immune response; and (4) perhaps the most relevant observation, that the assay for BPA may detect other factors, such as CSF-2, that are biologically distinct from IL-3. In particular, it is conceivable that cells responding to IL-3 or other factors could produce a BPA-type activity. Such a complication of interpretation of results can be partially overcome by using more rigorous cell cloning conditions to study biological activities. Nevertheless, because of the limitations discussed above, it is currently difficult to directly demonstrate that IL-3 regulates the differentiation of an early erythroid precursor.

In attempts to study the regulation of precursor cells for the monocyte-macrophage differentiation inducing factor CSF-1, the factor hemopoietin-2 was introduced (Bartelmez *et al*., 1984). By definition, this is a factor which can cause the differentiation or expansion *in vitro* of stem cells that have receptors for CSF-1. This population represents the precursor population, which in response to CSF-1, can be induced to differentiate to a mature macrophage-like adherent population. Homogeneous IL-3 has been found to have this activity; however, whether only IL-3 has this activity is not known. The available data appear to point to the possible existence of multiple factors that induce the differentiation of CSF-1 responsive cells. As with the BPA activity, it was initially unclear that the hematopoietin-2 activity could be accommodated within the effects known to be directly mediated by IL-3. However, more recently, several observations have provided suggestive evidence that this activity may be within the scope of IL-3-mediated effects. First, IL-3-dependent lymphoma cell lines that generate CSF-1 receptor-positive progeny have been obtained (R. Stanley and J. N. Ihle, unpublished data). More important, adherent cells that are generated in the presence of IL-3 and are a source of CSF-1 are 20 αSDH positive, in contrast to normal peritoneal adherent macrophages which are 20 αSDH negative. Therefore, the hematopoietin-2 activity, as suggested below, may constitute an important differentiation potential of the IL-3-regulated pathway, although CSF-1, as a terminal differentiation inducing factor, may be active on other lineages as well.

Among assays that might detect a functional activity, IL-3 has been shown to promote the differentiation or *in vitro* expansion of cells displaying cytolytic activity associated with cells having natural cytotoxicity (NC) (Lattime *et al.*, 1983; Djeu *et al.*, 1982). This activity, called NC activity, is distinguishable from NK cytolytic activity in a number of ways: (1) the cell-surface phenotype is distinct and is peculiar in that it lacks a variety of markers normally expressed by T cells or NK cells; (2) the spectrum of potential targets does not include lymphoid cells such as YAC, but rather appears to be more specific for adherent type targets such as the WEHI-164 cell line; and (3) the activity is not altered by interferon, whereas NK activity is increased by interferon. The relationship of the NC activity to any of the phenotypes of cells generated by IL-3 is unknown.

Perhaps the most important activity of IL-3 relative to a potential role in T-cell differentiation is the ability of IL-3 to induce Thy 1 in cultures of *nu/nu* splenic lymphocytes or in cultures of Thy-1-depleted normal bone marrow cells. The initial description of a Thy-1-inducing factor (Schrader *et al.*, 1982) involved culturing Thy-1-depleted bone marrow cells for 3–4 days in conditioned media from mitogen-stimulated lymphocytes. At 3–4 days, analysis by fluorescence-activated cell sorter showed that 20–40% of the cells had an intensity of Thy-1 expression comparable to that of the bulk of thymocytes. In addition to lymphocyte conditioned media, WEHI-3 conditioned medium was observed to have the activity, as did conditioned media from T-cell hybridomas. The activity was not correlated with either IL-2 or the major T-cell-derived CSF. It has been subsequently demonstrated that IL-3 is the major, if not exclusive, T-cell-derived factor capable of inducing Thy 1 in such cultures (Prystowsky *et al.*, 1983). Of particular significance is the inability of IL-2 to induce Thy 1 or to cause significant proliferation of bone marrow cells in the absence of mitogens, suggesting the lack of a role for IL-2 in early T-cell differentiation.

The expression of Thy 1 in cultures of Thy-1-depleted bone marrow cells has been interpreted to indicate that expression of Thy 1 may not be limited to T cells in such cultures (Schrader *et al.*, 1982). The evidences to support this conclusion are: 1) the lack of response to IL-2 and 2) the ability of Thy-1 positive populations to yield cells capable of forming macrophage and/or granulocyte colonies *in vitro* and *in vivo* based on gross morphological appearance. The implication of these results is that the differentiation of granulocytes and macrophages may be characterized by the expression of Thy 1. Since the majority of mature granulocytes and macrophages do not express Thy 1, the expression must be either transient or only occur in one of the potential pathways for the differentiation of granulocytes and macrophages. Irrespective, this observation may be useful in further defining the differentiation induced by IL-3 and relating this to normal hematopoietic stem-cell differentiation.

IV. NORMAL SEQUENCE OF DIFFERENTIATION PROMOTED BY IL-3

The sequence of events induced by IL-3 in cultures of lymphocytes illustrates the interrelationship of some of the activities described above as well as providing a possible sequence of differentiation. Our studies have concentrated on the events that occur in either bulk cultures or under cloning conditions for *nu/nu* splenic lymphocytes. The rationale for using *nu/nu* splenic lymphocytes is two fold. First, the absence of an *in vivo* source of IL-3 in *nu/nu* spleen and the lack of apparent IL-3-mediated differentiation i.e., 20 αSDH expression would suggest that precursors accumulate at a point at which IL-3 is required for further differentiation. Therefore, in tissue culture, the addition of IL-3 might be expected to give rise to a more synchronous sequence of events than if the starting population had cells at various stages of IL-3-induced differentiation. Second, the absence of a helper T-cell population in *nu/nu* spleen that would be capable of providing factors such as CSF-2 and IL-2 might be expected to minimize the number of indirect effects and thus reflect more directly the effects due to IL-3. This caveat obviously only applies to T-cell-derived factors and does not include factors such as CSF-1, which can be produced by a variety of cell types.

The first recognizable events occurring in cultures of *nu/nu* splenic lymphocytes in the presence of IL-3 are the induction of cell proliferation and of 20 αSDH. During the first week, as a consequence of cell death, induction of 20 αSDH, and proliferation of a 20 αSDH^+ population, the specific activity of 20 αSDH increases approximately 1000-fold; then, at about the end of that first week, it begins to decrease. On the basis of this observation, it has been suggested that the first progeny of IL-3-induced differentiation might be characterized by extremely high levels of 20 αSDH. Subsequent to the peak of 20 αSDH and during the first week, there is an increase in cells expressing the cell-surface markers of Ly 5 and H-11. By approximately 1 week in culture, 100% of the cells express these markers. The acquisition of these markers as part of the differentiation process is indicated by the observation that antisera against Ly 5 and complement do not remove the IL-3-inducible cell in *nu/nu* splenic lymphocytes. In contrast to Ly 5 and H-11, control markers such as surface Ig or Mac-1, although initially detectable, are not detectable after 5–7 days in culture. After 1 week, the cultures contain detectable Thy-1^+ cells that increase up to two weeks, at which time approximately 20% of the cells are positive. This value subsequently decreases with continuing culture. During the first two weeks of culture there is morphological evidence for granulocyte differentiation and the differentiation of an adherent macrophage-like cell type. After approximately one week in culture, granulated cells become detectable. With further time in culture a more homogeneous population of heavily granulated cells appears. Consistent with this, the histamine content of the cells increases from nondetectable levels at 1 week to peak values at approximately 3 weeks, after which the values decrease. The rate of proliferation of the cells during culture also varies dramatically. In the first two weeks there is a substantial proliferation occurring, based on the numbers of mitotic cells. With time, however, the rate decreases such that by 4–5 weeks little proliferation is detectable. After approximately 4–5 weeks the cultures essentially contain a homogeneous population of mastlike cells which persist in culture for another 4–5 weeks before the cultures die out. The phenotype of this persisting cell is Thy 1^-, Ly 5^+, H-11^+, Ia^+, Mac-1^-, 20 αSDH^+, and the cells contain low levels of histamine granules. Among the variety of cell types that are observed in cultures supplemented with IL-3, only the latter population can be demonstrated to be directly responsive to IL-3. Additional approaches will be necessary to demonstrate that the other phenotypes are generated as a direct consequence of the presence of IL-3.

V. IL-3-DEPENDENT LYMPHOMAS

The potential spectrum of phenotypes regulated by IL-3 has been further established by the observation that a variety of experimentally induced lymphomas in mice are IL-3 dependent for growth *in vitro*. In characterizing these lymphomas, a variety of phenotypes have been observed that have proved useful in proposing a sequence of IL-3-induced differentiation. The possible immunological basis of the etiology of lymphomas was initially recognized in studies of the immune response to Moloney leukemia virus (MoLV) (Ihle *et al.*, 1982a; Lee and Ihle, 1979; 1981a, b). This virus, when inoculated into newborn mice, induces a persistent, high-level viremia and within 3–5 months, lymphomas. The lymphomas are generally T cell or null cell and can be localized in either the thymus or the spleen. The thymic lymphomas are predominantly of the cortical TdT$^+$, 20 αSDH$^-$ thymocyte population, whereas the splenic lymphosarcomas often involve 20 αSDH$^+$ lymphocytes (Pepersack *et al.*, 1980). Associated with the ability to induce leukemia is an immune response against MoLV that is most readily demonstrable by the persistent presence of a helper T-cell population capable of producing IL-3 as well as other lymphokines in response to the virus. On the basis of these observations, it has been proposed that retroviruses, such as MoLV, induce leukemia as a consequence of a chronic immune response specifically involving the continual production of lymphokines by a virus-specific helper T cell. Consistent with this hypothesis, the preleukemic phase shows a 50- to 200-fold expansion of the cells responding to IL-3 and to other lymphokines.

One of the predictions from the above data and the general hypothesis is that some of the lymphomas induced by MoLV, and in particular the 20 αSDH$^+$ lymphomas, may be IL-3 lineage cells. In particular, excess systemic IL-3 production by viral antigen-stimulated helper T cells leads to a dramatic increase in the cells proliferating and differentiating within the IL-3 lineage. As a consequence of this increase, somatic- or viral-mediated transformation-related events might occur, thereby giving rise to IL-3 lineage-related lymphomas. To explore this possibility, the *in vitro* growth responses of primary MoLV-induced lymphomas to IL-3 were examined (J. N. Ihle, unpublished data). A typical set of responses are illustrated in Fig. 4. Among this group of 10 lymphomas, none could be established in culture in media alone in the absence of IL-3, whereas in the presence of IL-3, two of the lymphomas (65 and 68) gave continuous long-term lines; two of the lymphomas (59 and 64) could be expanded dramatically in culture, although they did not give rise to continuous cell lines; and the remainder showed only a marginal growth response to IL-3. Using the lines generated from this set of lymphomas, as well as a number of others, the phenotypes of the lymphomas have been examined.

The phenotypic properties of a number of IL-3-dependent lymphoma cell lines established in IL-3 are summarized in Table III. Among the cell lines established, three general phenotypes have been observed. One of the phenotypes is exemplified by the DA-1 line. This type of lymphoma requires IL-3 for establishment *in vitro* and continues to depend on IL-3 for growth *in vitro*. Consistent with these observations IL-3 receptors are readily detectable, as is 20 αSDH activity. The morphology of the cell line is lymphoblastic, with no detectable granulation and no detectable histamine. This particular phenotype is often observed in the IL-3-dependent cell lines established from long-term bone marrow cultures. The cell-surface phenotype is also similar, in lacking Thy-1 as well as Lyt-1, 2 or B-cell markers such as 2C2 or ThB (data not shown). However, similar to a variety of the IL-3-dependent long-term bone marrow culture lines, the DA-1 cell line is Ly 5$^+$, H-11$^+$. The second phenotype observed is IL-3 dependent for establishment and for growth *in vitro*, and is Thy 1$^-$, Ly 5$^+$, H-11$^+$, Mac-1$^-$, but differs expressing Ia. This particular phenotype is characterized by a morphologically heterogeneous

Leukemia No.	Thy1	20αSDH	cpm -	cpm +
59	+	–	135	435
60	–	–	252	1042
61	±	–	77	650
62	–	–	37	60
63	+	–	1183	5053
64	+	–	273	2473
65	–	–	257	2383
66	+	–	620	2330
67	+	–	66	166
68	+	–	250	840

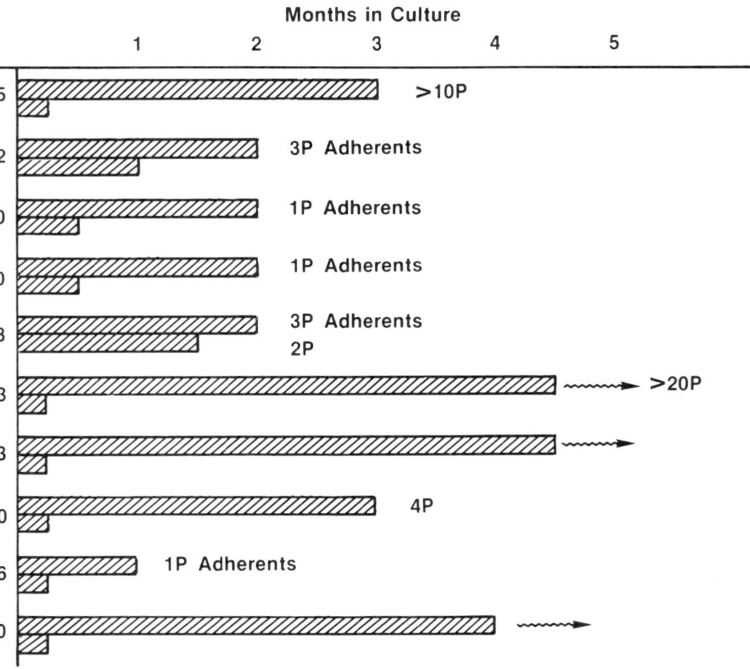

Figure 4. Establishment of lymphoma cell lines from MoLV-induced lymphomas in the presence of IL-3. BALB/c mice were inoculated with MoLV at birth. When grossly leukemic, as determined by palpation and general responses, the animals were sacrificed. The lymphoma cells from individual mice were cultured in the presence (top bar) or in the absence of IL-3 (lower bar). In addition, the lymphomas were typed for Thy and 20 αSDH expression. In the latter case, only lymphomas having high levels of activity would be detected. Responses of the lymphomas to IL-3 in a standard proliferation assay are also indicated. The number of passages of the cultures is indicated (i.e., 3P indicates three passages). See text for details.

Table III. Properties of MoLV-Induced Lymphoma Cell Lines[a]

Cell line designation	Dependence for establishment	Dependence for Growth	IL-3 receptors	Cell phenotype	20 αSDH pmole/hr/ 10^8 cells
DA-1	+	+	+	Thy 1^-, Ly 5^+, H-11^+, Mac-1^-, Ia^-	100
DA-2	+	–	–	Thy 1^+, Ly 5^+, H-11^+, Mac-1^-, Ia^-	<10
DA-3	+	+	+	Thy 1^-, Ly 5^+, H-11^+ Mac-1^-, Ia^+	3500
DA-4	+	+	+	Thy 1^-, Ly 5^+, H-11^+, Mac-1^-, Ia^+	50
DA-5	+	+	+	Thy 1^-, Ly 5^+, H-11^+, Mac-1^-, Ia^-	300
DA-6	+	+	N.D.	Thy 1^-, Ly 5^+, H-11^+, Mac-1^-, Ia^-	N.D.
DA-7	+	+	+	Thy 1^-, Ly 5^+, H-11^+, Mac-1^-, Ia^+	200
DA-8	+	–	–	Thy 1^-, Ly 5^+, H-11^+, Mac-1^-, Ia^+	100
DA-10	+	–	–	Thy 1^+, Ly 5^+, H-11^+, Mac-1^-, Ia^-	100
DA-11	+	+	+	Thy 1^-, Ly 5^+, H-11^+, Mac-1^-, Ia^+	N.D.

[a]MoLV, Moloney leukemia virus; 20 αSDH, 20 α-hydroxylated dehydrogenase.

cell population consisting of both adherent and nonadherent cells as well as some granulated mastlike cells. Consistent with the latter, some of the cells are histamine positive. A variant of this phenotype is illustrated by DA-8, which is similar in phenotype, although more lymphoblastic in morphology. The major differences are that despite its initial dependence on IL-3 for establishment *in vitro*, it is no longer dependent on IL-3 for growth and no longer has detectable IL-3 receptors. The third phenotype (DA-2, DA-11) required IL-3 for establishment of the lines, although ultimately the lines do not require IL-3 for growth and have no detectable IL-3 receptors. The phenotype of these cells is Thy 1^+, Ly 5^+, H-11^+, Mac-1^-, Ia^-, and the cells are lymphoblastic in morphology.

The above observations suggest that in some cases lymphomas involved minimally IL-3-dependent transformed cell types. Whether the other lymphomas that did not respond to IL-3 represent other lineages or require other lymphokines has not been examined in detail. Nevertheless, the cell lines differ from normal cultures of lymphocytes in IL-3 by proliferating at much higher rates and not undergoing the terminal differentiation normally observed. In these properties the lines resemble the IL-3-dependent lines established from long-term bone marrow cultures, suggesting that the latter lines may also be transformed in a similar manner. This finding is consistent with the fact that special conditions are required for their establishment and that long-term lines are relatively rare. Nevertheless, the lines from both lymphomas and from long-term bone marrow cultures display recurring properties, suggesting that they may be used to help better define the pathways involved in IL-3-induced differentiation.

VI. A PROPOSED SEQUENCE OF DIFFERENTIATION INDUCED BY IL-3

A model for the sequence of differentiation induced by IL-3 is illustrated in Fig. 5. The sequence shown is primarily based on properties predicted by IL-3-dependent cell lines and the pattern of phenotypes observed in cultures of *nu/nu* splenic lymphocytes cultured in IL-3. The initial stem cell induced to express 20 αSDH lacks any of the cell-surface markers examined. The correlation of 20 αSDH expression with the first step in the sequence is strongly suggested by the rapid induction observed in *nu/nu* splenic lymphocyte cultures. This precursor population is generally found only at low levels in the spleen in normal animals but appears to occur primarily in the bone marrow. Based on the increases observed in 20 αSDH following culture in IL-3, it can be proposed that the first progeny of IL-3-induced differentiation expresses high levels of 20 αSDH. Among the IL-3-dependent cell lines examined, one (C3H sffv) has the properties predicted by the above results—i.e., the line is Thy 1^-, Ly 5^-, H-11^-, and strongly 20 αSDH^+. Just what factors may be required for the generation of cells capable of responding to IL-3, and therefore characterized by the expression of IL-3 receptors, is unknown. Since such cells exist in *nu/nu* mice, their ontogeny is not dependent on mature T cells. The observation that the Dexter culture system can maintain such cells that subsequently give rise to long-term IL-3-dependent lines when cultured in WEHI-3 CM, suggests that some component of the bone marrow stromal element may be involved in maintenance of such a stem cell.

The proposed second phenotype in the lineage is a Thy 1^-, Ly 5^+, H-11^+, Ia^- 20 αSDH^+ cell that is absolutely dependent on IL-3 for continued proliferation and differentiation. In cultures of *nu/nu* splenic lymphocytes this is the predominant phenotype observed within 3–5 days. This particular phenotype is also the most common observed among the IL-3-dependent long-term bone marrow culture derived cell lines as well as being a common phenotype among MoLV-induced IL-3-dependent lymphomas. This type of IL-3-dependent cell line is generally not granulated nor does it contain histamine.

The third step in the sequence of differentiation appears to be a commitment to one of at least two further sequences of differentiation. In particular, a variety of IL-3-dependent cell lines exist that are Thy 1^+, Ly 5^+, H-11^+, Ia^-, 20 αSDH^+.

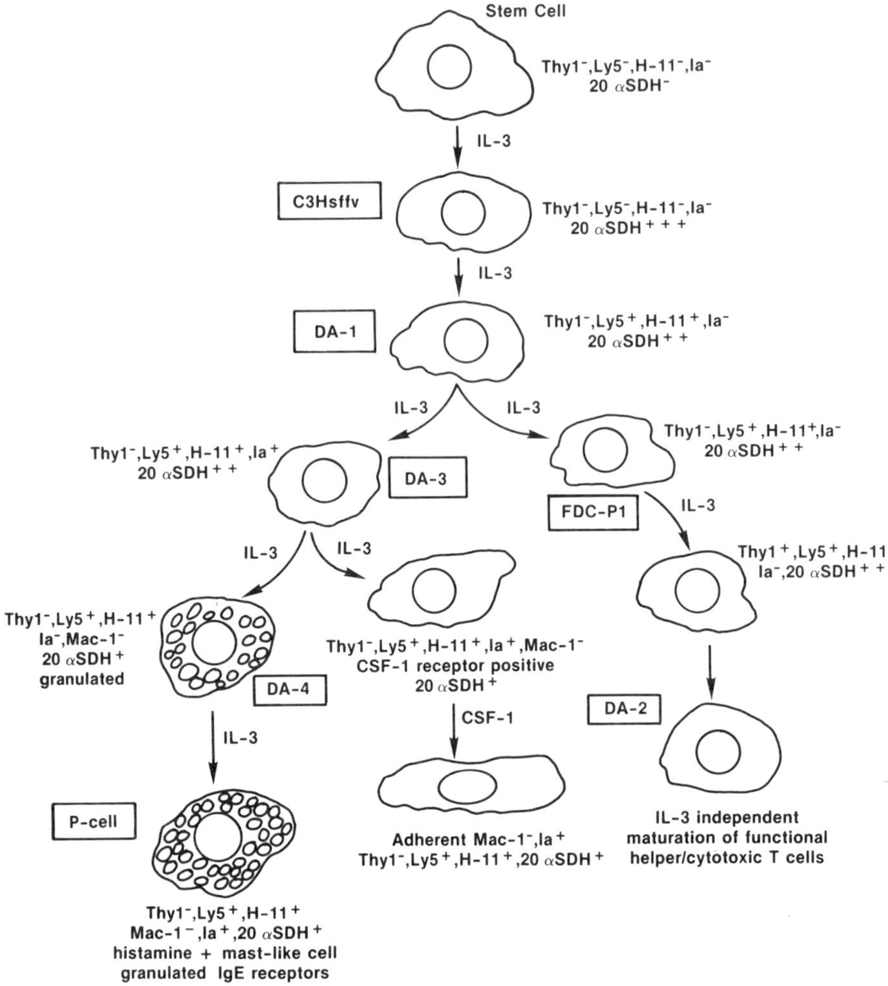

Figure 5. Proposed sequence of differentiation regulated by IL-3. Specific aspects of the proposed sequence are discussed in the text. Boxes indicate particular lymphoma cell lines or the phenotypes of bone marrow culture derived IL-3-dependent lines.

The expression of Thy 1 in these lines is interesting in that the cultures are rarely 100% Thy 1^+ cells. Cloning of the cells never gives rise to 100% Thy 1^+ lines, rather, cloning always results in lines that contain Thy 1^+ cells. Therefore, we would propose that these lines are stem-cell lines that give rise to more differentiated Thy 1^+ cells, which cannot be expanded in the presence of IL-3, but that require other unknown factors to continue their differentiation. Alternatively, the expression of Thy 1 may be transient in normal differentiation and in some cases the loss of Thy 1 may indicate a commitment to differentiation. Among the MoLV-induced lymphomas the regular occurrence of Thy 1^+ IL-3-independent cell lines from IL-3-maintained cultures could be due to the secondary transformation of such cells in that the Thy 1^+ cell now becomes factor independent. This type of occurrence could also explain the emergence of helper-like phenotype cells from IL-3-maintained cultures (Hapel *et al.*, 1981), although the frequency of generating such cell lines is much lower than indicated in the initial studies, for reasons which are not clear.

Indirect evidence for this type of precursor has been demonstrated by *in vivo* experiments. In particular, the medullary thymocyte population is Thy 1^+, Ly 5^+, H-11^+, 20 αSDH^+. This population does not contain cells that can directly proliferate in response to IL-3 or IL-2 but can respond to IL-2 after mitogen stimulation. Because of the expression of 20 αSDH, the lack of a response to IL-3 was unexpected but nevertheless suggested experiments to determine whether other factors could induce this phenotype of cell. Since the precursors for medullary thymocytes have been proposed to be the cortical population of TdT^+ 20 αSDH^- cells, the response of these cells to either IL-2 or IL-3 was examined. In neither case, with or without mitogen, was any proliferative response or induction of 20 αSDH detectable (Keller and Ihle, submitted). We have proposed an alternative (Ihle *et al.*, 1982c) that the medullary and cortical populations are distinct pathways of T-cell differentiation. The TdT^+ cells are terminally differentiated and undergoing clonal deletion, whereas the medullary cells are being processed to mature T cells. In this case, the medullary thymocyte might be anticipated to have been derived from a distinct bone marrow prothymocyte. Consistent with this, both Thy 1^+ TdT^+ and Thy 1^+ 20 αSDH^+ cells are found in the bone marrow in the large blast fractions containing the thymus-reconstituting cells. Nevertheless, for this reason it is important to note that in comparing IL-2 and IL-3, only IL-3 is capable of inducing bone marrow proliferation, 20 αSDH, as well as Thy-1 expression. Therefore, in bone marrow cultures IL-3 can generate the medullary prothymocyte phenotype. Although a similar phenotype is observed in cultures of *nu/nu* splenic lymphocytes in IL-3, it never persists. Finally, the possible role of IL-3 in the bone marrow in generating a thymocyte precursor is suggested by the observation that 20 αSDH as a marker *in vivo* is associated with T cells. Similarly, if one excludes IL-3-dependent cell lines among a wide variety of cell lines examined, 20 αSDH is uniquely associated with the TdT^- T-cell phenotype. Therefore, the acquisition of 20 αSDH as well as Thy 1 is a reasonable marker of T-cell maturation, although whether other phenotypes express these markers is an open question.

As indicated in Fig. 5, the second commitment pathway is characterized by a cell with a Thy-1^-, Ly-5^+, H-11^+, Ia^+ 20 αSDH^+ phenotype. How the expression of Ia in *nu/nu* splenic lymphocyte cultures correlates with this scheme is not known. Nevertheless, the MoLV-induced IL-3-dependent lines, such as DA-3, provide a striking illustration of this step in differentiation. In particular, an adherent population is continually generated, i.e., Ia^+, $Mac\text{-}1^-$, 20 αSDH$^+$. In addition, granulated histamine-positive cells are constantly generated in the cultures. The maintenance of this line is dependent on IL-3 and the line is characterized by the presence of receptors for IL-3.

As indicated in Fig. 5, an intermediate lymphoma phenotype also exists which is uniquely committed to the mastlike progeny. This is based on the presence of long-term IL-3-dependent lymphoma cell lines, which are granulated, although generally only having low levels of histamine, which do not generate adherent cell populations. These cells continue to require IL-3 for proliferation throughout. This phenotype is also the persisting cell (P-cell) or mastlike cell phenotype observed in long-term cultures of cells differentiating in the presence of IL-3. The above proposed scheme of IL-3-promoted differentiation is consistent with data derived from a series of initial approaches, but it is speculative in many aspects. In addition, the scheme does not consider the possible role that IL-3 may play in promoting the differentiation of granulocytes or erythropoietin responsive cells. The scheme is therefore proposed as an initial conceptual framework from which to begin a more precise documentation and study of the various progeny of IL-3-induced differentiation.

VII. CONCLUSIONS

The initial goal of identifying a factor that could induce 20 αSDH expression was to study the events associated with early T-cell differentiation. The available evidence supports the hypothesis that induction of 20 αSDH represents an early step in the differentiation of a lineage of cells that includes T cells. *In vitro*, the data provide evidence, however, only to a point in T-cell differentiation that would appear to represent a medullary prothymocyte. *In vivo*, it is well established that differentiation of the T-cell lineage beyond this stage is absolutely dependent on the thymic microenvironment. Therefore, ultimately following the differentiation of the IL-3-induced Thy-1^+, 20 αSDH$^+$ bone marrow prothymocyte will require the development of an *in vitro* system that permits this component of lymphocyte differentiation to occur. It should also be noted that T-lymphocyte differentiation may be speculated to occur in discreet stages regulated by different factors: an early bone marrow IL-3 dependent phase, a thymus-dependent phase, and a peripheral antigen and IL-2 regulated phase. These stages could be proposed to represent three phases of functional T-cell maturation: (1) commitment, (2) maturation, and (3) amplification phases. Nevertheless, the expression of 20 αSDH and its regulation by IL-3 may provide a means to approach some of the intermediate phases of T-lymphocyte differentiation *in vitro*.

In addition to T-lymphocyte differentiation, the results obtained with homogeneous IL-3 demonstrate an initially unexpected component of the lineage. In particular, the most dramatic, persistent component of IL-3-regulated differentiation *in vitro* involves a class of mastlike cells. The possible relationship of mastlike cells to the T-cell lineage had been previously noted by a number of investigators (Ishizaka *et al.*, 1976; Thiede *et al.*, 1971). It was subsequently proposed that the T-cell-lineage relationship was not due to a true lineage relationship but rather was due to the requirement for a T-cell-derived factor for proliferation of mast cells (Yung *et al.*, 1981, Schrader *et al.*, 1981). Although the factor, IL-3, is only derived from T cells, the evidence described above provides a number of provacative observations that are most readily explained by proposing that mastlike cells are derived from a lineage that includes early T-cell differentiation. Similarly, the data suggest that other functional products of this lineage may include macrophages as well as granulocytes and erythroid precursors. These cells may require additional factors such as CSF-1 or erythropoietin for continued differentiation. The availability of homogeneous IL-3 will allow continued studies which may ultimately help to better understand hematopoietic stem cell differentiation including early T-cell differentiation.

ACKNOWLEDGMENTS

This research was sponsored by the National Cancer Institute, Department of Health and Human Services, under Contract No. NO1-CO-23909 with Litton Bionetics, Inc. I would like to thank Dr. Rudolf Medicus, Dr. Richard Mural, Dr. Terry Bowlin, Dr. Edmund Palaszynski, Dr. Stephen Oroszlan, Dr. Louis Henderson, and Jonathan Keller for the many helpful discussions during the course of this work. The invaluable assistance of Dr. Herbert C. Morse III at the National Institutes of Health at Bethesda is gratefully acknowledged. I would also like to thank Allen Scott, Debbie Gilbert, and Miriam Hursey for their expert technical assistance, and Linda Brubaker for help in preparation of the manuscript.

VIII. REFERENCES

Bartelmez, S. H., Sacca, R. S., and Stanley, E. R., 1984, (submitted).

Bazill, G. W., Haynes, M., Garland, J., and Dexter, T. M., 1983, *Biochem. J.* **210**:629.

Dayhoff, M. O., 1976, *Atlas of Protein Sequence and Structure*, National Biomedical Research Foundation, Washington, DC, Vol. 5, Suppl. 2, p. 1.

Dexter, T. M., Garland, J., Scott, D., Scolnick, E., and Metcalf, D., 1980, *J. Exp. Med.* **152**:1036.

Djeu, J. Y., Lanza, E., Hapel, A. J., and Ihle, J. N., 1982, in: *NK Cells and Other Natural Effector Cells* (R. B. Herberman, ed.), p. 917, Academic Press, New York.

Dy, M., Lebel, B., Kamoun, P., and Hamburger, J., 1981, *J. Exp. Med.* **153**:293.
Fung, M. C., Hapel, A. J., Ymer, S., Cohen, D. R., Johnson, R. M., Campbell, H. D., and Young, I. G., 1984, *Nature* **307**:233.
Galli, S. J., Dvorak, A. M., Ishizaka, T., Nabel, G., Simonian, H. D., Cantor, H., and Dvorak, H. F., 1982, *Nature* **298**:288.
Garland, J. M., and Dexter, T. M., 1982, *Eur. J. Immunol.* **12**:998.
Garland, J. M., Dexter, T. M., Lanotte, M., Howarth, C., and Aldridge, A., 1983 in: *Interleukins, Lymphokines and Cytokines* (J. J. Oppenheim and S. Cohen, eds.), p. 123, Academic Press, New York.
Gillis, S., Union, N. A., Baker, P. E., and Smith, K., 1979, *J. Exp. Med.* **149**:1460.
Goldwasser, E., Ihle, J. N., Prystowsky, M. B., Rich, I., and Van Zant, G. 1983, in: *Normal and Neoplastic Hematopoiesis*, p. 301, Alan R. Liss, New York.
Greenberger, J. S., Gans, P. J., Davisson, P. B., and Moloney, W. C., 1979, *Blood* **53**:987.
Hapel, A. J., Lee, J. C., Farrar, W. L., and Ihle, J. N., 1981, *Cell* **25**:179.
Ihle, J. N., Pepersack, L., and Rebar, L., 1981, *J. Immunol.* **126**:2184.
Ihle, J. N., Enjuanes, L., Lee, J. C., and Keller J., 1982a, in: *Current Topics in Microbiology and Immunology*, **101**:31.
Ihle, J. N., Keller, J., Henderson, L., Klein, F., and Palaszynski, E. W. 1982b, *J. Immunol.* **129**:2431.
Ihle, J. N., Rebar, L., Keller, J., Lee, J. C., and Hapel, A., 1982c, *Immunol. Rev.* **63**:101.
Ihle, J. N., Keller, J., Oroszlan, S., Henderson, L., Copeland, T., Fitch, F., Prystowsky, M. B., Goldwasser, E., Schrader, J. W., Palaszynski, E., Dy, M., and Lebel, B., 1983, *J. Immunol.* **131**:282.
Iscove, N. N. 1978, in: *Hemoatopoietic Cell Differentiation* (D. W. Goldie, M. S. Cline, D. Metcalf, and C. F. Fox, eds.) p. 37, Academic Press, New York.
Ishizaka, K., and Adachi, T. 1976, *J. Immunol.* **117**:40.
Katz, H. R., LeBlanc, P. A., and Russell, S. W., 1983, *Proc. Natl. Acad. Sci. USA* **80**:5916.
Lattime, E. C., Pecoraro, G. A., and Stutman, O., 1983, *J. Exp. Med.* **157**:1070.
Le Blanc, P. A., Russell, S. W., and Chang, S.-M. T, 1982, *J. Reticuloendothel. Soc.* **32**:219.
Lee, J. C., and Ihle, J. N., 1979, *J. Immunol.* **123**:2351.
Lee, J. C., and Ihle, J. N., 1981a, *Nature* **209**:407.
Lee, J. C., and Ihle, J. N., 1981b, *Proc. Natl. Acad. Sci. USA* 78:7712.
Lee, J. C., Hapel, A. J., and Ihle, J. N., 1982, *J. Immunol.* **128**:2393.
Miller, R. A., and Stutman, O., 1983, *J. Immunol.* **130**:1749.
Nable, G., Galli, S. J., Dvorak, A. M., Dvorak, H. F., and Cantor, H., 1981, *Nature* **291**:332.
Nagao, K., Yokoro, K., and Aaronson, S. A., 1981, *Science* **212**:333.
Palaszynski, E. W., and Ihle, J. N., 1984, *J. Immunol.* **132**:1872.
Pepersack, L., Lee, J. C., McEwan, R., and Ihle, J. N., 1980, *J. Immunol.* **124**:279.
Prystowsky, M. B., Ely, J. M., Beller, D. I., Eisenberg, L., Goldman, J., Goldman, M., Goldwasser, E., Ihle, J., Quintans, H., Remold, H., Vogel, S., and Fitch, F. W., 1982, *J. Immunol.* **129**:2337.
Prystowsky, M. B., Ihle, J. N., Otten, G., Keller, J., Rich, I., Naujokas, M., Loken, M., Goldwasser, E., and Fitch, F. W., 1983, in: *Normal and Neoplastic Hematopoiesis*, Vol. 9 (D. W. Goldie and P. A. Marks, eds.), p. 369, Alan R. Liss, New York.
Razin, E., Cordon-Cardo, C., and Good, R. A., 1981, *Proc. Natl. Acad. Sci. USA* **78**:2559.
Razin, E., Stevens, R. L., Akiyama, F., Schmid, K., and Austen, K. F., 1982, *J. Biol. Chem.* **257**:7229.
Razin, E., Mencia-Huertas, J.-M., Stevens, R. L., Lewis, R. A., Liu, F.-T., Corey, E. J., and Austen, K. F., 1983, *J. Exp. Med.* **157**:189.
Razin, E., Ihle, J. N., Seldin, D., Mencia-Huerta, J. M., Katz, H. R., Leblanc, P. A., Hein, A., Caulfield, J. P., Austen, K. F., and Stevens, R. L., 1984, *J. Immunol.* **132**:1479.
Schrader, J. W., and Clark-Lewis, I., 1982, *J. Immunol.* **129**:30.
Schrader, J. W., Lewis, S. J., Clark-Lewis, I., and Culvenor, J. G., 1981, *Proc. Natl. Acad. Sci. USA* **78**:323.
Schrader, J. W., Battye, F., and Scollay, R., 1982, *Proc. Natl. Acad. Sci. USA* **79**:4161.
Stanley, E. R., and Guilbert, L. J., 1981, *J. Immunol. Methods* **42**:253.

Stevens, R. L., Razin, E., Austen, F., Hein, A., and Caulfield, J. P., 1983, *J. Immunol.* (in press).
Thiede, A., Muller-Hermelink, H.-K., Sonntag, H. G., Muller-Ruchholtz, W., and Leder I.-D., 1971, *Klin. Wochenschr.* **49**:435.
Weinstein, Y., 1977, *J. Immunol.* **119**:1223.
Weinstein, Y., Linder, H. R., and Eckstein, B., 1977, *Nature* **266**:632.
Yokota, T., Lee, F., Rennick, D., Hall, C., Arai, N., Mosmann, T., Nabel, G., Cantor, H., and Arai, K., 1984, *Proc. Natl. Acad. Sci. USA* **81**:1070.
Yung, Y.-P., and Moore, M. A. S., 1982, *J. Immunol.* **129**:1256.
Yung, Y.-P., Eger, R., Tertian, G., and Moore, M. A. S., 1981, *J. Immunol.* **127**:794.

P-Cell Stimulating Factor: Biochemistry, Biology, and Role in Oncogenesis

John W. Schrader, Ian Clark-Lewis, Richard M. Crapper, Grace H. W. Wong, and Sabariah Schrader

Immunoregulation Laboratory
The Walter and Eliza Hall Institute of Medical Research
Royal Melbourne Hospital
Victoria 3050, Australia

I. INTRODUCTION

The use of monoclonal lines of T cells in the form of T-cell hybridomas (Schrader *et al.*, 1980a,b, 1982a; Harwell *et al.*, 1980; Schrader and Clark-Lewis, 1981), T-cell lymphomas (Ralph *et al.*, 1978; Hilfiker *et al.*, 1981; Golde *et al.*, 1980; Gillis *et al.*, 1980; Clark-Lewis *et al.*, 1982a,b), and more recently T-cell lines (Staber *et al.*, 1982; Kelso *et al.*, 1982; Prystowsky *et al.*, 1982) has established conclusively that the T lymphocyte is the direct source of factors with a wide range of bioactivities. Our original observation on the induction of lymphokine synthesis by a T-cell hybridoma, 123, indicated that stimulation of a single cloned line resulted in the release of multiple bioactivities (Schrader *et al.*, 1980a). These included factors affecting B and T lymphocytes (T-cell replacing factor, TRF) and T-cell growth factor (TCGF; now referred to as Interleukin-2, IL-2) (Schrader *et al.*, 1980a,b), activities stimulating the growth and differentiation of progenitors of neutrophils, macrophages, and megakaryocytes (Schrader *et al.*, 1980a), and an activity stimulating the *in vitro* production of pluripotential hemopoietic stem cells (Schrader *et al.*, 1980a,b; Schrader and Clark-Lewis, 1982a).

The two general points that emerged from our work with T-cell hybridomas, i.e., that production of lymphokines required stimulation and that single clones usually produced multiple bioactivities, have been confirmed using T-cell lymphomas (Hilfiker *et al.*, 1981; Schrader *et al.*, 1982a), T-cell lines (Nabel *et al.*, 1981; Prystowsky *et al.*, 1982; Staber *et al.*, 1982) and short-term cultures of T-cell clones (Staber *et al.*, 1982; Kelso *et al.*, 1982). In many cases, these multiple bioactivities clearly reflect the secretion of multiple, chemically distinct lymphokines. While the available evidence does not exclude that in some instances T cells may release a single lymphokine, it is a useful rule of thumb to regard the production of one lymphokine by a T-cell source as presumptive evidence that other lymphokines are being produced in parallel. It is hazardous to regard a crude supernatant of even a culture of cloned T-cell line as a source of a single lymphokine, e.g., IL-2, as other molecules with potentially confusing activities such as Thy-1-inducing factor (TIF) (Schrader *et al.*, 1982b) will almost certainly be present (see Section II). Multiple types of assay must be used to fully characterize the products released by T-cell clones.

II. RELATIONSHIP OF P-CELL STIMULATING FACTOR TO OTHER BIOACTIVITIES PRODUCED BY T CELLS

Initially we set out to characterize in molecular terms some of the non-antigen-specific bioactivities produced by T-cell hybridomas. The first aim was to determine which bioactivities could be separated by biochemical techniques and thus shown to be the properties of distinct molecular species. While it is relatively straightforward to establish that two bioactivities are due to different molecules, as will become evident in the following discussion, it is much more difficult to establish that two bioactivities are due to the same molecule (or indeed to any given molecule). Bioassays form the basis of the definition, description, and discussion of lymphokines, therefore, before summarizing our results, it is worth reviewing briefly the limitations of some of the systems we use.

A. Assays for T-Cell Lymphokines

Assays for lymphokines present three general problems. First, in many cases the assays are not absolutely specific in the sense that multiple lymphokines can give positive results. The assays for colony-stimulating factors (CSF) are one example. In these assays (Pluznik and Sachs, 1965; Bradley and Metcalf, 1966), bone marrow cells are cultured in medium made viscous by the addition of agar or methylcellulose, and the development of discrete colonies of cells of various hemopoietic lineages, e.g., neutrophils, macrophages, megakaryocytes, erythroid cells, or sometimes mixtures of cell types, is monitored.

Consider as an example the problem of assessing the significance of an observation that a particular culture supernatant stimulated the growth of a colony of macrophages. As discussed elsewhere (Schrader, 1983), there are now known to be at least four biochemically distinct factors that can stimulate to a greater or lesser degree the growth of colonies of macrophages. These are CSF-1, also known as macrophage-CSF (M-CSF) (Stanley and Heard, 1977); granulocyte-macrophage-CSF (GM-CSF) (Burgess *et al.*, 1977); granulocyte CSF (G-CSF) (Nicola *et al.*, 1983); and P-cell stimulating factor (PSF) (I. Clark-Lewis *et al.*, 1984; Schrader *et al.*, 1983b; Schrader, 1983) (see Section IV.C). The enhancement of *in vitro* antibody-forming cell responses to sheep erythrocytes by populations of *nu/nu* spleen cells is another example of an assay in which multiple factors, e.g., T-cell replacing factor (Schimpl and Wecker, 1975), IL-2 (Watson *et al.*, 1979; Clark-Lewis and Schrader, 1982a,b), and IL-1 or B-cell activating factor (Wood, 1979) give positive responses.

Second, many assays involve heterogeneous populations of cells; thus, it is not clear whether the lymphokine under investigation is exerting its effects indirectly through a second cell rather than by a direct action on the presumptive target cell. This is a problem with any assay that does not deal with either a single, isolated cell or a homogeneous population of target cells. Methods have been developed for a single-cell approach with hemopoietic colony-forming cells (Metcalf *et al.*, 1980; also discussed in Schrader, 1983) and with B cells (Pike *et al.*, 1982). For routine purposes, however, the use of cloned cell lines as homogeneous populations of target cells have obvious practical advantages. Such cell lines form the basis of assays for gamma-interferon (γ-IFN), IL-2 (Gillis *et al.*, 1978), or PSF (Schrader, 1981).

The third general point is that single lymphokines can act in multiple assays. With complex assays that employ heterogeneous populations of cells, this can reflect the action of a lymphokine on its expected target, e.g., if IL-2 acts as a T-cell replacing factor by expanding residual T cells rather than by acting directly on B cells (Watson *et al.*, 1979; Harwell *et al.*, 1980). In other cases, however, by using factors produced from single cloned genes and cloned target populations, it has been possible to demonstrate unequivocally that a single lymphokine has multiple targets, one example being the demonstration that the T-cell factor that induces Ia antigens on macrophages, B cells, and T-dependent mast cells is identical to γ-IFN (Wong *et al.*, 1982, 1984).

B. P-Cell Stimulating Factor

P cells were first observed in the course of attempts to grow suppressor T cells from a subpopulation of spleen cells using cultures supplemented with medium conditioned by Concanavalin A (Con A)-stimulated spleen cells (Schrader *et al.*, 1980; Schrader and Nossal, 1980; Schrader, 1981). After several weeks, the cultures were dominated by a homogeneous population of round, nonadherent cells having characteristic refractile borders and occasional cytoplasmic processes. These cells shared many cytochemical properties with mast cells; the coarse, water-soluble, cytoplasmic granules stained with Alcian blue or Astra blue and metachromatically with toluidine blue and contained histamine, serotonin, acid phosphatase, and chloroacetate esterase. Present on the cell surface were Fc receptors for four classes of immunoglobulin: IgE, IgG_1, IgG2a, and IgG2b. Although many of these features are shared with mast cells, until there was definitive evidence on whether the cells were related to mast cells (see below), we elected to use an operational title, persisting cell (P cell), based on the characteristic pattern of persistent *in vitro* growth. Similar cell lines have been generated in a number of other laboratories from normal tissue (Razin *et al.*, 1981; Tertian *et al.*, 1981; Nabel *et al.*, 1981), long-term bone marrow cultures (Nagao *et al.*, 1981; Tertian *et al.*, 1981), or virus-infected cultures (Hasthorpe, 1980).

1. *P-Cell Stimulating Factor*

The growth of P cells was absolutely dependent on a specific factor produced by Con A-stimulated spleen cells. We gave this factor the operational title P-cell stimulating factor (PSF). The production of PSF by T cells was initially established by the demonstration that PSF was produced by Con A-stimulated T-cell hybridomas (Schrader *et al.*, 1980a,b, 1981a; Schrader, 1981). The same molecule, however is produced by stimulation of T-cell lines (Nabel *et al.*, 1981; Staber *et al.*, 1982; Prystowsky *et al.*, 1982; Krammer *et al.*, 1983; Schrader, 1983) and of short-term T-cell clones (Staber *et al.*, 1982). The requirement of P cells for PSF could not be replaced by the addition of either of two distinct T-cell-derived factors–IL-2 or T-cell-derived granulocyte-macrophage colony-stimulating factor (T-cell GM-CSF). Nor could PSF be replaced by other polypeptides, such as macrophage-CSF (CSF-1), mouse-lung-derived GM-CSF, epidermal growth factor, nerve growth factor, or fibroblast growth factor (Schrader, 1981; Schrader *et al.*, 1981a; R. M. Crapper *et al.*, unpublished observations).

Because P cells could be cloned, and because these populations were homogeneous in the sense that every cell in the population exhibited cytoplasmic granules, P cells formed the basis of an assay system in which the only possible target was a granulated P cell. Moreover, because the growth and survival of P cells were absolutely dependent on the presence of PSF, it was possible to design very simple and sensitive systems with which to detect and quantitate PSF.

2. *Assay of PSF*

Initially, to assay PSF, we cultured 50 P cells in 10 μl cultures in Terasaki plates and scored the growth and survival of P cells visually (Schrader, 1981;

Clark-Lewis and Schrader, 1981). In order to handle large numbers of samples, however, it was necessary to automate the assay; in our present procedure, 500 P cells are incubated together with titrated amounts of the substance under test in 10-μl cultures in inverted Terasaki plates. DNA synthesis is monitored using the uptake of [^{3}H]thymidine or [^{125}I]IUDR. This simple, miniaturized system permits accurate titration of multiple samples, one technician being able to handle several thousand individual cultures in a day.

C. Distinctions between PSF and Two Other Regulatory Glycoproteins Made by T Cells

1. Properties of Three Lymphokines Made by a T-Cell Hybridoma

Using biochemical techniques, we established that the Con A-stimulated T-cell hybridoma 123, also a second T-cell hybridoma and T6, made a minimum of three regulatory molecules. Table I summarizes the property of these three distinct proteins, all of which we showed to be glycosylated (Clark-Lewis and Schrader 1981, 1982b). It should be noted that all three of these molecules were

Table I. Properties of Three Lymphokines Produced by T Hybridoma 123[a]

	TCGF	T-cell GM-CSF	PSF
Molecular weight			
Gel filtration in saline	35,000	30,000	30,000
Gel filtration in 6 M guanidine	30,000	23,000	23,000
Hydrophobicity (phenyl-Sepharose)	++++	++	++
Lectin binding	Wheat germ agglutinin	Wheat germ agglutinin Con A	Wheat germ agglutinin Con A
pI (after neuraminidase treatment)	4.9	4.9	6.5 (mean)
C18 μBondapak HPLC column (% acetonitrile)	Not done	41%	38%
Targets	T cells	Neutrophil-macrophage progenitor	Homogeneous and heterogeneous P-cell lines Hemopoietic progenitor cells of all lineages Pluripotential hemopoietic stem cells

[a]Con A, Concanavalin A; P-cell, persisting cell; PSF, P-cell stimulating factor; TCGF, T-cell growth factor; CT-cell GM-CSF, T-cell granulocyte–macrophage colony-stimulating factor.

distinct from the fourth regulator recently shown to be a T-cell lymphokine, γ-IFN (Marcucci *et al.*, 1981; Nathan *et al.*, 1981). γ-IFN was not produced by T-cell hybridoma 123 in our hands, showing it to be distinct from the three lymphokines produced by 123. When medium conditioned by Con A-stimulated spleen cells was used as a starting material, all three factors shown in Table I could be separated from γ-IFN (Clark-Lewis *et al.*, 1982a).

2. *Distinction of PSF from TCGF*

PSF could be readily distinguished from TCGF in terms of its molecular weight, isoelectric point after neuraminidase treatment, and its affinity for phenyl Sepharose (Clark-Lewis and Schrader, 1981, 1982a,b). In Section IV.E we will discuss data indicating that TCGF and PSF have nonoverlapping target specificities. Nevertheless, their respective targets possess superficial similarities that could generate confusion. Thus both PSF and TCGF can act on cells that bear Thy-1 antigen, i.e., Thy-1^+ myeloid progenitor or stem cells, and T cells, respectively, or on cells that are cytotoxic for tumor cells, although the target specificity of the respective cytotoxic cells differ.

3. *Distinction of PSF from T-Cell GM-CSF*

PSF could be distinguished biochemically from another T-cell derived lymphokine, which like PSF, acts on a type of hematopoietic progenitor cell. We have termed this molecule T-cell-derived granulocyte-macrophage colony stimulating factor (T-cell GM-CSF) because of its T-cell origin and the type of colony it stimulates in cultures of bone marrow cells. T-cell GM-CSF entirely lacks the capacity to stimulate T cells. T-cell GM-CSF can be separated from PSF in T-cell conditioned medium by isoelectric focusing of neuraminidase treated material, as in these circumstances the pI of T-cell GM-CSF is about 4.9 (Clark-Lewis and Schrader, 1982a), while PSF focuses as a broader peak with a mean pI of 6.5 (Clark-Lewis and Schrader, 1981). T-cell GM-CSF and PSF can be more simply separated by using reverse phase high-pressure liquid chromatography. In this technique, the T-cell GM-CSF (in medium conditioned by the T-cell hybridoma 123, the T-lymphoma EL-4, the TCGF-dependent T-cell clone A3-37.4, or by Concanavalin A-stimulated spleen cells) elutes from a water C18-μ Bondapak column at 41% acetonitrile, 0.2% trifluoroacetic acid, whereas PSF elutes at an acetonitrile concentration of 38% (Clark-Lewis, Thomas and Schrader, submitted). However, the GM-CSF derived from the T-cell hybridoma T 19.1 differs from the T-cell GM-CSF from most T-cell sources and elutes an an acetonitrile concentration of 49%, resembling in this respect the GM-CSF present in medium conditioned by endotoxin-stimulated mouse lungs (Burgess *et al.*, 1981). Thus, these results suggest that there may be multiple forms of GM-CSF produced by

T cells and other cells, all of which are distinct from PSF in their biological and biochemical properties. Recent genetic experiments indicate that there is only a single GM-CSF gene in the mouse genome, and that this gene is expressed in both T cells and in the mouse lung (N. Gough *et al.*, submitted). Differences in posttranslational processing probably underlie the differences we have observed in the behavior of the various GM-CSFs on reverse-phase HPLC columns.

D. CFUs-Stimulating Activity and Thy-1-Inducing Factor: Two Factors with Molecular Properties Identical to Those of PSF

1. CFUs-Stimulating Activity

In 1974, Cerny reported that *in vitro* treatment of spleen cells with phytohemagglutinin (PHA) increased the numbers of pluripotential hemopoietic stem cells as measured by the colony-forming unit-spleen (CFU-s) assay (Till and McCulloch, 1961). We showed that both medium-conditioned Con A-stimulated spleen cells and that conditioned by Con A-stimulated T-cell hybridoma 123 cells contained a factor that stimulated the production of CFUs in cultures of bone-marrow cells (Schrader *et al.*, 1980a,b, 1981b; Schrader and Clark-Lewis, 1982a). We termed this factor CFUs-stimulating activity (CFUs-SA). Our assay for CFUs-SA involved the incubation *in vitro* of bone marrow cells 10^6 in 1-ml cultures containing either medium alone or medium supplemented with dilutions of the material under assay. After a period of 6 days, the cultures were harvested and the numbers of splenic colony-forming cells (CFUs) present were assayed by injection of aliquots of the cell suspensions into groups of lethally irradiated host mice. These mice were killed at day 7 or 8 and macroscopic colonies of erythroid and myeloid colonies in the spleen were counted (Till and McCulloch, 1961).

Using this assay, we showed that CFUs-SA was distinguishable from TCGF by its molecular weight and behavior on hydrophobic chromatography on phenyl-Sepharose, and from T-cell GM-CSF by IEF of neuraminidase-treated material (Schrader and Clark-Lewis, 1982a). Thus, while the T-cell GM-CSF had a pI of 4.9, CFUs-SA had a mean pI of 6.5. T-cell GM-CSF and CFUs-SA could also be separated by RP-HPLC, CFUs-SA eluting with PSF from a Waters C18 μBondapak column at a concentration of acetonitrile of 38%, while the T-cell GM-CSF eluted at a concentration of 41%, or in one case, 49% (Schrader *et al.*, 1983b). By contrast, CFUs-SA had the same molecular weight, behavior on phenyl-Sepharose, mean pI after neuraminidase treatment, and behavior on RP-HPLC as did PSF (Schrader and Clark-Lewis, 1982a; Clark-Lewis *et al.*, 1984 and J. Schrader and I. Clark-Lewis, unpublished data). Experiments with highly purified PSF indicate that PSF and CFUs-SA are identical (see Section IV).

2. *Thy-1-Inducing Factor*

At a time when there was great interest in the possibility that IL-2 could induce the differentiation of T cells from their precursors, we observed that cultures of bone marrow cells depleted of T cells and incubated for 3–4 days with medium conditioned by Con A-treated spleen cells contained 20–60% of cells that expressed high levels of the Thy-1 antigen (Schrader and Clark-Lewis, 1982b; Schrader *et al.*, 1982b). The factor involved, which we operationally termed Thy-1-inducing factor (TIF), was produced by the T-cell hybridoma 123, indicating a T-cell origin (Schrader *et al.*, 1982b). However, TIF was distinguishable from TCGF in terms of its lower molecular weight and in being produced by the tumor WEHI-3B, which produces neither TCGF nor T-cell GM-CSF (Schrader *et al.*, 1982b). It was further distinguishable from T-cell GM-CSF in that the latter, but not TIF or PSF, was produced by clones of the T-cell hybridoma T19.1 (Schrader *et al.*, 1982a). Pure PSF is active in the TIF assay, and the two are probably identical (see Section III).

There was no evidence that the Thy-1^+ cells generated in these cultures were T cells or T-cell precursors. TCGF would not maintain the proliferation of the Thy-1^+ cells, although a minimum of one in three proliferated in medium containing PSF (Schrader *et al.*, 1982b). Furthermore, the Thy-1^+ cells were shown to include progenitors of P cells, neutrophils, and macrophages, as well as pluripotential hemopoietic stem cells (CFUs) (Schrader *et al.*, 1982b). The demonstration that a factor distinct from IL-2 (TCGF), could induce Thy-1 antigens on non-T cells, in a situation in which Thy-1 had hitherto been accepted as a marker for the T-lymphocyte lineage, placed an important caveat on some previous work that had been interpreted in terms of the development of T cells from precursors.

III. PURIFICATION OF PSF

A. Preparation of Pure PSF from WEHI-3B

Having established that there were at least four distinct categories of T-cell-derived lymphokines, i.e., TCGF, T-cell GM-CSF, PSF, and γ-IFN, we elected to study in detail the structure of PSF, one goal being to see whether PSF could be separated from activities such as CFUs-SA and TIF, which affected pluripotential hemopoietic stem cells and hemopoietic progenitors of multiple lineages. While the demonstration that PSF was separable from other T-cell lymphokines such as TCGF, T-cell GM-CSF, or γ-IFN (Clark-Lewis and Schrader, 1981, 1982a,b; Clark-Lewis *et al.*, 1982a) required relatively small amounts of material sufficient for analysis in the very sensitive bioassays, it became evident very early in our studies that these lymphokines had very high specific activities and the molecules were present in conditioned medium in very small amounts.

To obtain sufficient material for structural analysis, it was evident that very large quantities of conditioned medium would be required; selection of a convenient source for large scale production was therefore of critical importance. Because the T-cell hybridomas, T-lymphomas, and T-cell lines we had investigated all required induction with mitogen or antigen in order to release PSF, we turned to a myelomonocytic leukemia tumor, WEHI-3B (Warner *et al.*, 1969), which had been shown to be a constitutive producer of PSF (Nagao *et al.*, 1981; Yung *et al.*, 1981; Clark-Lewis *et al.*, 1982b).

We have prepared large quantities of conditioned medium using selected clones of WEHI-3B that grow readily in ascitic form. The cells are harvested from the ascitic fluid, are washed, and are then cultured in serum-free medium, to produce starting material with a relatively high specific activity. The purification strategy involved the use of 100-liter batches of conditioned medium subjected to several high-capacity separation procedures followed by a sequence of fractionations using high-resolution, HPLC columns (Clark-Lewis *et al.*, 1984). In sequence, we used hollow-fiber pressure dialysis, ammonium sulfate precipitation, and chromatography on phenyl boronate and Sephadex G-100. The material was then treated with neuraminidase to reduce charge heterogeneity due to sialic acid (Clark-Lewis and Schrader, 1981). The first HPLC steps involved a Mono-Q ion-exchange column, the second a Waters C18 μBondapak RP column eluted with a shallow gradient of acetonitrile, and the third and fourth a TSK-3000 SW gel-permeation column operated at pH 7.0 and then at pH 2.0.

To establish the homogeneity of the purified PSF, the material was analyzed by SDS-PAGE. Although we failed to detect any bands on the gel using the sensitive silver stain, autoradiography of a gel containing ^{125}I-labeled PSF revealed a broad band which corresponded exactly to the PSF activity eluted from a parallel track of the gel (Clark-Lewis *et al.*, 1984). Analysis of the ^{125}I-labeled PSF by SDS-PAGE under reducing conditions, followed by autoradiography, indicated a broad band corresponding to a slightly higher molecular weight (32,000), suggesting that PSF was composed of a single polypeptide chain with internal disulfide bridges. The characteristically broad band of PSF seen on SDS-PAGE is probably due to glycosylation of the molecule.

B. Partial Amino Acid Sequence of PSF

In collaboration with S. Kent and L. Hood of the California Institute of Technology, we have subjected the purified PSF to microterminal amino acid sequence analysis. The material gave the following unique terminal sequence:

NH_2-Ala-Ser-Ile-Ser-X-X-Asp-Thr-His-Arg-Leu-Thr-Arg-X-Leu

This sequence was contained within the amino acid sequence predicted from the nucleotide sequence of cDNA clones that express an activity stimulating the growth of factor-dependent hematopoietic cells and that have been isolated by two groups (Fung *et al.*, 1984, Yokota *et al.*, 1984). These results, together with the biological data (Section IV), indicate that the material we have purified and sequenced is the active molecule.

Our NH_2-terminal amino acid sequence overlaps with that of Interleukin-3 as determined by Ihle and colleagues (Ihle *et al.*, 1983). However, our sequence differs in that it has 6 additional NH_2-terminal amino acids, suggesting that the Interleukin-3 purified by Ihle *et al.* had undergone further cleavage. Comparison of our sequence with that predicted from the nucleotide sequence of the cDNA clones, indicates that the signal peptide would be cleaved at the Gln–Ala bond. Cleavage at this point is largely consistent with the pattern of cleavage sites of other secreted proteins (Von Heijne, 1983). The fact that the amino acid sequence predicted from the cDNA clones isolated from WEHI3-B and from a cloned T-cell line are identical, except at one position (Fung *et al.*, 1984, Yokota *et al.*, 1984), suggests that the WEHI-3B-derived PSF is very similar to the physiological product, i.e., that of activated T cells.

C. Translation of PSF mRNA in *Xenopus* Oocytes

As a step toward cloning the PSF gene, we have examined the translation of PSF mRNA in the reticulocyte lysate and *Xenopus* oocyte systems. For reasons that are unclear, we were unsuccessful in our attempts to obtain the efficient or reproducible translation of PSF using reticulocyte lysates. In contrast, microinjection of polyadenylated mRNA from WEHI-3B into *Xenopus* oocytes resulted in the secretion of readily detectable amounts of PSF. The amounts of PSF secreted in the medium rose linearly with the amount of mRNA injected per oocyte over a range of 2–20 ng. The amounts of PSF in the medium increased over a 5-day period, reaching 5000 units per oocyte.

The medium in which mRNA-injected oocytes had been incubated also contained activity that stimulated the growth of colonies of neutrophils, macrophages, and megakaryocytes. Sucrose-gradient fractionation of the WEHI-3B mRNA demonstrated that PSF and the neutrophil-granulocyte and megakaryocyte CSFs were all translated from mRNA of the same size, a result consistent with the notion that a single polypeptide mediates all these bioactivities (Schrader, 1983; Schrader *et al.*, 1983b).

IV. BIOLOGICAL STUDIES OF PSF

A. Multiple Targets for PSF in Bone Marrow

We have found that purified PSF that is active in the PSF assay at $\leqslant 1.3 \times 10^{-13}$ M is also active in three assays that measure effects on hemopoietic bone marrow cells, i.e., the agar colony assay, the Thy-1-inducing factor assay (Schrader *et al.*,

1982b), and the CFUs-SA assay (Schrader and Clark-Lewis, 1982a). In the agar colony assay, the purified PSF eluted from the SDS gel stimulated the growth of colonies of neutrophils and macrophages and also of megakaryocytes (Fig. 1), indicating that this material added can be considered as both a GM-CSF and a megakarocyte (MK)-CSF. It should be noted that our assay system, to which erythropoietin was not added, would not detect erythroid differentiation *in vitro*.

The fact that this purified PSF acted as TIF, CFUs-SA, and an MK-CSF and GM-CSF, suggests that PSF stimulates a range of hemopoietic cells that include the pluripotential hemopoietic stem cell and progenitors of macrophages, neutrophils, and megakaryocytes. Results from other laboratories (Iscove *et al.*, 1982; R. Cutler, N. A. Nicola, and D. Metcalf, personal communication) indicate that erythroid colonies are also stimulated under appropriate conditions (see Section IV.C.3). All three assays, however, suffer from the disadvantage that they employ heterogeneous populations of cells, raising the possibility that the observed effects of the purified PSF are indirect.

B. Two Direct Targets of Purified PSF

We have evidence for the direct interaction of purified PSF with two cell types: first, the homogeneous population of P cells we originally described and

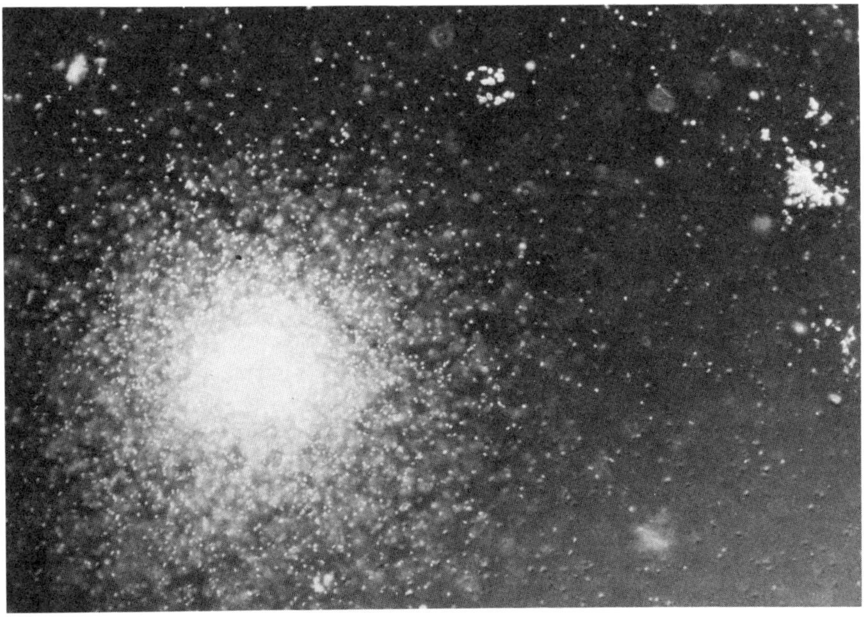

Figure 1. Colonies of neutrophils, macrophages, and megakarocytes grown in an agar culture of CBA bone marrow cells, stimulated by purified PSF.

second, progenitor cells that are bipotential, giving rise to both mast cells and megakaryocytes and occurring in PSF-dependent lines of cells that we call heterogeneous P cells, for reasons explained below.

1. PSF and Homogeneous P Cells or T-Dependent Mast Cells

Because the populations of P cells that we originally described were homogeneous in the sense that every cell, including those with mitotic figures, had mast-cell-like cytoplasmic granules, our demonstration that highly purified PSF supported the *in vitro* growth of these cell populations establishes that PSF acts directly on these cells. The significance of this fact for an understanding of physiological events, however, depends on knowing the relationship between the P cells found *in vitro* and cells that occur under natural circumstances *in vivo*.

Morphological criteria such as cytoplasmic granulation are inadequate and potentially misleading. For example, we have shown that the granulated lymphocytes of the gut mucosa characterized by cytoplasmic granules having the same staining properties as those of P cells (Guy Grand *et al.*, 1978), are not related to P cells or the mast cells of the gut mucosa and, in fact, are probably a type of T cell (Schrader *et al.*, 1983). Likewise, when cultured in the presence of supernatants conditioned by activated T cells, cytotoxic T cells and cells with natural killer (NK) cell activity can become heavily granulated (Brooks *et al.*, 1982; Kedar *et al.*, 1982; Shortman *et al.*, 1983; see also Schrader, 1983).

However, recently we conclusively identified the *in vivo* counterparts of the *in vitro* lines of homogeneous P cells that we originally described. Table II summarizes evidence supporting our original proposal (Schrader *et al.*, 1981a) that P cells correspond to the T-dependent subset of mast cells associated with lymphoid tissues and the mucosal surfaces of the gut and bronchi (Askenase, 1981). We have established correlations between the frequency in various tissues of cells able to generate P cells *in vitro* and of histologically detectable T-dependent mast cells *in vivo* (Crapper and Schrader, 1983). Both the frequency of P-cell precursors and of T-dependent mast cells can be increased by T-cell-dependent antigenic stimulation (Crapper and Schrader, 1983; Ruitenberg and Elgersma, 1976). Finally, and convincingly, when injected directly into the dermis, genetically marked P cells assume the appearance of mast cells, although they retain their dependence on PSF (Crapper *et al.*, 1984a, b). Thus as we proposed initially, PSF appears to be the T-cell lymphokine that accounts for the T-cell-dependent increases in mast cell numbers that occur in the gut and in parasitic infection (Ruitenberg and Elgersma, 1976) and probably in other sites such as the lung (Ahlstedt *et al.*, 1983) or skin as well.

2. Heterogeneous P-Cell Lines and PSF

a. Bipotential PSF-Dependent Lines of Mast Cell–Megakaryocyte Progenitors. The populations of P cells that we described originally are characteristically

Table II. Evidence That Homogeneous P Cells Correspond to the T-Dependent Subset of Mast Cells *in Vivo*[a]

In antigen-stimulated lymph nodes:
- PSF is produced
- mast cells numbers increase
- P-cell precursor numbers increase

In the mucosa of the gut of normal (but not W^f/W^f mutant) mice:
- T-dependent mastocytoses occur in response to parasitic infection
- there is a high frequency of P cell precursors

Genetically marked P cells injected intradermally into W^f/W^f mice give rise to PSF-dependent mast cells.

[a]References: Schrader *et al.* (1983b), Crapper and Schrader (1983), Crapper *et al.* (1984a,b), and Schrader (1983).

homogeneous in the sense that all cells are granulated. The homogeneous P cells grew relatively slowly with a doubling time of 36 hr or so, a fact reflected in their low cloning efficiency in agar (about 5–10%) and the small size of the resultant colonies (Schrader, 1981). Furthermore, cultures of homogeneous P cells have a finite life span of 3–6 months.

However, we have also observed that cultures of bone marrow cells supplemented with WEHI-3B-conditioned medium can give rise to lines of cells that, despite repeated cloning, form populations that are heterogeneous, both in terms of gross morphology and cytology (Schrader, 1983). In most cases, cells varied in size and shape and in the number and shape of nuclei and the presence of cytoplasmic granulation. Unlike the homogeneous lines of P cells, these heterogeneous P-cell lines grew rapidly (doubling time of about 18 hr), formed large colonies in agar with a plating efficiency of up to 50% and, unlike the homogeneous P cells, appear to be immortal. Furthermore, unlike homogeneous P-cell lines, which are diploid, the heterogeneous P-cell lines are aneuploid. We have shown that some of these lines are bipotential and that they contain single cells that give rise to both mast cells and megakaryocytes, the latter being identified by their polyploidy and by the presence of cytoplasmic acetylcholinesterase (Jackson, 1973).

b. Direct Action of Purified PSF on Isolated, Single Bipotential Progenitor Cells. Growth of these bipotential heterogeneous P-cell lines is supported by purified PSF but not by T-cell GM-CSF or M-CSF. Because of the heterogeneity of these lines, however, demonstration of the requirement for PSF for growth and survival need not necessarily imply that PSF is acting directly on the progenitor that is able to generate both mast cells and megakaryocytes. For example, this bipotential progenitor could be responding indirectly to a product of some more differentiated cell, such as histamine from a mast cell or a factor like platelet-derived growth factor from the megakaryocytes present.

To counter this objection, we plated out low numbers of cells of this line (an average of 0.15 cells/well); then, by directly identifying wells containing

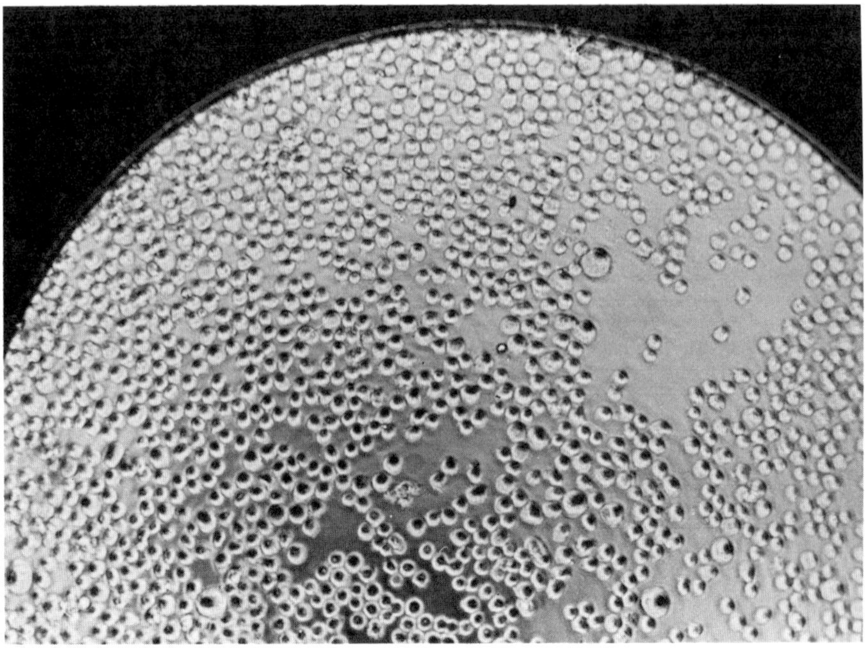

Figure 2. T-dependent mast cells and megakaryocytes grown from a single cell of a heterogeneous P-cell line (R6-X), stimulated by purified PSF.

only a single cell with an inverted microscope, we could very easily assess the effect of our purified PSF on single, isolated cells. About 50% of the single cells responded to PSF, generating clones containing both mast cells and megakaryocytes. Figure 2 shows a typical culture of heterogeneous cells grown from a single starting cell in the presence of purified PSF.

These experiments demonstrate that purified PSF stimulates the cell capable of generating both mast cells and megakaryocytes. On rare occasions, polyploid megakaryocytes were observed to divide in response to purified PSF, suggesting that at least in this cell line, polyploid megakaryocytes have receptors for PSF.

c. Lines of Factor-Dependent Hemopoietic Progenitor Cells in Other Laboratories. Dexter *et al.* (1980) and Greenberger *et al.* (1980) described continuous lines of cells having characteristics of neutrophil progenitors; these appear to depend for their growth on a factor produced by WEHI-3B that is probably identical with PSF. Greenberger *et al.* (1983) recently described a continuous line that possesses the capacity to generate both myeloid and erythroid cells; again, this appears to respond to a similar factor from WEHI-3B cells. Using single-cell techniques and lines such as described here, it should be possible to demonstrate unequivocally that purified PSF acts directly on pluripotential hemopoietic stem cells and neutrophil progenitors.

C. Relationship of PSF to Similar Factors Studied by Other Groups

While we have been studying PSF, a number of groups have used a variety of assays to study factors produced by activated T cells or by the myelomonocytic leukemia, WEHI-3B. It is becoming increasingly likely that all three groups are studying a single molecule.

1. Histamine-Producing Cell-Stimulating Factor and Mast-Cell Growth Factor

PSF is probably identical with the histamine-producing cell-stimulating factor (HCSF) studied by Dy *et al.* (1981) and the mast-cell growth factor studied by others (Yung *et al.*, 1981; Nabel, *et al.*, 1981). In some cases, there are apparent differences in biochemical properties. For example, our estimates of 30,000 M_r by gel filtration in saline and of 23,000 M_r in the presence of a denaturing agent, guanidine hydrochloride, 6 M (Clark-Lewis and Schrader, 1981), are smaller than the figures of 40,000–50,000 by gel filtration in saline reported by others (Dy *et al.*, 1981; Nabel *et al.*, 1981; Yung *et al.*, 1981). The fact that we prepared our conditioned medium in the absence of serum may account for this difference as serum components may associate with PSF and increase its apparent molecular weight. Certainly our experiments with SDS-PAGE suggest that the lower figures are closer to the correct value. The NH_2-terminal amino acid sequence of PSF is identical with the sequence predicted from the nucleotide sequence of the MCGF-cDNA cloned by Yokota *et al.* (1984), pointing to the identity of those factors.

2. Interleukin-3

IL-3 was defined as an activity that induced the enzyme 20α-hydroxysteroid dehydrogenase (20 αSDH) in a population of T-cell progenitors (Ihle *et al.*, 1981a). Initially, the molecular weight of IL-3 was reported as 41,000 by SDS-PAGE (Ihle *et al.*, 1981b, 1982a) or 40,000–50,000 by gel filtration (Ihle *et al.*, 1981a,b). However, more recently, a lower-molecular-weight version of IL-3 was reported, with a molecular weight of 28,000 as determined by SDS-PAGE (Ihle *et al.*, 1982b).

Ihle and colleagues now assay IL-3 by the support of the proliferation of continuous-factor dependent lines of cells analogous to P cells, rather than by the induction of 20 αSDH (Ihle *et al.*, 1982b), and thus the same activity is now being monitored as in the PSF assay or in the assays of Dexter and colleagues, who use similar factor-dependent myeloid lines as targets (Dexter *et al.*, 1980; Bazill *et al.*, 1983).

IL-3 is of particular significance as Ihle's group was the first to report amino acid sequence information on putatively pure material (Ihle *et al.*, 1983). Ihle has sent his highly purified material to various groups, including ours, and it has been established that this material is active in assays for PSF, CFUs-SA, and TIF, together with HCSF and CSF (Ihle *et al.*, 1983). It is interesting to note that the specific activity if the material that Ihle has used for amino acid sequence analysis is 100-fold lower than that of the material that we have purified from the same source, the tumor WEHI-3B. Thus, the material that Ihle has sequenced gives a 50% response as a concentration of about 10^{-11} M using his cell line as a target, while the most highly purified material that we have obtained gives a 50% maximal response in our PSF assay at 10^{-13} M. However, the larger quantities of material available to Ihle mean that his determinations of protein concentrations may be more accurate than ours. Other possible explanations are that his preparation has lost some bioactivity through denaturation or that our target cell line requires a lower concentration of the factor for a maximal response. It is also possible that the absence of the first six NH_2-terminal amino acids of Ihle's IL-3 preparation (see Section III.B) could affect bioactivity.

3. *Burst-Promoting Activity*

Iscove and colleagues (1982) analyzed an activity from WEHI-3B-conditioned medium that stimulates the formation of bursts of erythroid cells from bone marrow progenitors, called burst-promoting activity (BPA). These workers showed that BPA copurified through an extensive purification scheme with mixed erythroid-myeloid CSF, a GM-CSF, and a megakaryocyte CSF (Iscove *et al.*, 1982). The copurification of GM-CSF and MK-CSF from WEHI-3B agrees with our own data and suggests that a single molecule is affecting pluripotential hemopoietic stem cells, as well as granulocyte–macrophage, megakaryocyte, and mast-cell and erythroid progenitors. Similar results have been obtained with material from medium conditioned by pokeweed mitogen-stimulated spleen cells, in this case the activity being termed multi-CSF (R. Cutler, N. A. Nicola, and D. Metcalf, personal communication).

4. *WEHI-3 Factor*

Recently, Dexter's group reported the partial purification of a factor from WEHI-3 that supports the growth of continuous factor-dependent lines of myeloid progenitors (Bazill *et al.*, 1983). These investigators reported that the molecular weight of this factor, when eluted from SDS gels, was about 25,000 which is slightly lower than the mean molecular weight that we observed (Clark-Lewis *et al.*, 1984); the difference probably reflects differences in glycosylation.

Although Bazill *et al.* (1983) published a photograph of a gel in which a stained protein corresponded to the position of the biological activity, they noted that they were unable to find this band consistently in association with the biological activity. We do not find this surprising, as the amount of bioactivity they applied to the gel was more than 100-fold less than that which we have applied to gels with negligible staining at the molecular-weight position corresponding to the bioactivity. It seems likely that the band on the gel they reported on was attributable to a copurifying contaminant present in variable amounts in different preparations.

Fung *et al.* (1984) have recently isolated a cDNA clone from WEHI-3B, using growth stimulation of Dexter's factor-dependent line, FDPC-1, as an assay. The amino acid sequence predicted from this cDNA clone agrees with that determined for PSF. Furthermore, in collaborative experiments with A. J. Hapel, I. G. Young, and colleagues, we have shown that expression of this cDNA clone results in activity in the PSF, TIF, and CFUs-SA assays. Thus, PSF and the WEHI-3B factor of Dexter appear to be identical.

5. Nomenclature

As it is likely that PSF/MK-CSF/TIF/CFUs-SA/GM-CSF/IL-3/BPA/mixed-CSF/HCSF/MCGF/WEHI3 factor are one and the same molecule, is it time to rationalize the nomenclature? Given that a cDNA that probably expresses all of these activities has now been cloned, definitive answers about the spectrum of targets of the factor and the range of its physiological sources should soon be at hand. Moreover, the concomitant rapid progress in molecular analysis of other lymphokines and hematopoietic growth factors should lead to an understanding of any structural and evolutionary relationships between these molecules. It would seem prudent to wait the relatively short time required to accumulate these data. We hope that the opportunity will then be taken to design a rational system of nomenclature for these factors, based on definitive structural and functional data, that will be useful to both immunologists and hematologists.

D. Does PSF (IL-3) Act on T Cells?

From the above considerations, it appears likely from our data as well as from the data of Ihle, Iscove, Dexter, and Metcalf that a single molecule acts on progenitors of mast cells, megakaryocytes, neutrophils, macrophages, erythroid cells, eosinophils, and also pluripotential hemopoietic stem cells. However, Ihle's group has maintained that an important action of IL-3 is upon T-cell progenitors (Ihle *et al.*, 1981a, b, 1982a). This view is based on several arguments.

One argument involved the role of IL-3 in the generation of clones of helper T cells (Hapel *et al.*, 1981). However, this phenomenon appears to be less reproducible than originally thought (Ihle *et al.*, 1982a); furthermore, as these clones were not dependent on IL-3 for continued growth, there was no evidence that IL-3 interacted with them directly.

Another argument related to the induction of the enzyme 20 αSDH. This enzyme was originally thought to be restricted to the T-cell lineage (Weinstein, 1977), although Ihle's group now reports that it has also been found in mast cells, although not in myeloid cells (Ihle *et al.*, 1982a). The latter point, however, is disputed (Garland and Dexter, 1982).

Other evidence consistent with the direct affect of IL-3 or PSF on T cells is that some IL-3-dependent lines have been reported to express low levels of Lyt 1 (Ihle *et al.*, 1982a). It should be borne in mind, however, that Lyt 1 is not restricted to T cells (Hardy *et al.*, 1982).

Elsewhere we have discussed the pitfalls in the classification of cells *in vitro* (Schrader, 1983). One complication was revealed by our demonstration that TIF, which we now consider to be identical with PSF, induced the Thy-1 antigen on myeloid progenitors from normal bone marrow (Schrader *et al.*, 1982b). This observation is in accord with the expression of Thy 1 on some of the myeloid or mast-cell factor-dependent lines (Ihle *et al.*, 1982a; Dexter *et al.*, 1980); obviously, the expression of Thy 1 on an *in vitro* line is no longer acceptable as evidence that the line is of T-cell origin. Nevertheless, although there is no evidence that PSF acts on T cells, PSF does stimulate the *in vitro* growth of cells capable of repopulating the thymus (J. W. Schrader and I. Clark-Lewis, in preparation). However, further work is required to determine whether these thymus-repopulating cells are pluripotential hematopoietic stem cells or a population that includes cells committed to repopulate the thymus (i.e., prothymocytes).

E. PSF and Cell-Mediated Cytotoxicity

Another potentially confusing area involves that of cytotoxic cells, and in particular their response to lymphokines and the presence in their cytoplasm of granules. Lattime *et al.* (1983) showed that IL-3 promotes natural cytotoxic (NC) activity in population of normal cells. P cells, like peritoneal mast cells (Farram and Nelson, 1980), are cytotoxic for fibrosarcoma targets (Schrader, 1983), although not for lymphoma targets such as YAC or P815, even when coupled with antibodies (Schrader, 1983), indicating an NC pattern of specificity.

Also relevant to the question of the relationship between mast cells, T cells and NK cells are the granulated intraepithelial lymphocytes that occur in the mucosa of the gut (Guy-Grand *et al.*, 1978). These cells are characterized by a small number of cytoplasmic granules that closely resemble those of mast cells or P cells in their staining properties and in containing histamine. We have shown, however, that these granulated lymphocytes express T-cell markers such as Lyt 2 and in some cases Thy 1 (Schrader *et al.*, 1983a). Although it was proposed that the granulated lymphocytes were precursors of mast cells (Guy-Grand *et al.*, 1978) this does not appear to be the case (Schrader *et al.*, 1983a), as these cells do not respond to PSF (Schrader *et al.*, 1983a) and are probably members of the T-cell lineage. The precursors of the gut mast cells are found in high frequency in the mucosal lymphocyte population but, unlike the granulated cells, are Lyt 2^- (Schrader *et al.*, 1983). Interestingly, these granulated cells appear to have NK function (Flexman *et al.*, 1983). It would be interesting to know whether the granules in the large granular lymphocytes (LGL) associated with NK function in several species also resemble the granules of mast cells.

Finally, it should be noted that there develop in tissue culture, in the presence of IL-2 rather than PSF, T cells that are cytotoxic against multiple lymphohemopoietic targets and have a very heavily granulated cytoplasm (Brooks *et al.*, 1982; Kedar *et al.*, 1982; Schrader, 1983; Shortman *et al.*, 1983). It is our current view that the question of whether a cytotoxic cell responds to PSF or to TCGF (IL-2) is of greater value in assigning it to either the mast-cell or the T-cell–NK lineage than is the presence of cytoplasmic granulation.

F. Physiology of PSF

PSF and its presumptive synonyms have all been discovered and analyzed strictly *in vitro*. We have attempted to explore the physiological role of PSF *in vivo* using two approaches: (1) an analysis of the *in vivo* events associated with antigen induced T-cell activation, and (2) the *in vivo* effects of a PSF-producing tumor.

1. Effects of T-Cell Activation In Vivo on Targets of PSF

The results of the experiments we have performed are summarized in Table III. The correlation between the activation of T cells and increased frequencies of precursors of P cells and of histologically detectable mast cells *in vivo*, fits with the notion that PSF is acting *in vivo* (Crapper and Schrader, 1983; Crapper *et al.*, 1984a). This is strengthened by evidence that when cells from lymph nodes draining a site of immunization are cultured, PSF is spontaneously released into the medium. It should be noted that these correlations have been seen in the case of both an artificial immunization and a naturally occurring

Table III. Evidence That PSF Can Act *In Vivo* Both Locally and Systemically[a]

Immunization results in a T-dependent increase in the frequency of P-cell precursors in local lymph nodes.
Inoculation of mice with a localized PSF-producing tumor (but not a non-PSF-producing variant) results in:
–a systemic increase in mast cells, megakaryocytes, metamyelocytes and P-cell precursors
–the persistence in the dermis of mast cells derived from locally injected P cells

[a]From Crapper and Schrader (1983) and Crapper *et al.* (1984a).

pathological process that occurs in aging SJL mice and involves T-cell activation (J. W. Schrader and G. R. Johnson, unpublished data).

2. *Evidence for an In Vivo Effect of Circulating PSF*

Mast cells that develop from P cells injected into the skin did not survive for longer than 2 weeks unless the host mouse was bearing a subcutaneous PSF-producing tumor (but not a non-PSF-producing variant) (R. M. Crapper *et al.*, 1984). Likewise, in mice bearing a subcutaneous PSF-producing tumor but not a non-PSF-producing variant, there was an increase in the frequency of P-cell precursors in the bone marrow and spleen. In the spleen, histological examination also showed an increased frequency of mast cells and megakaryocytes (Crapper *et al.*, 1984a). As the PSF-producing tumor was localized in the groin and there were no signs of metastasis to the skin, bone marrow, or spleen, these results suggested that PSF could act, not only locally, but also by passing through the blood. Positive evidence that PSF was produced and released from this tumor *in vivo* was obtained in experiments in which PSF was detected in the ascites fluid, urine, and blood of mice bearing intraperitoneal PSF-producing tumors (Crapper *et al.*, 1984).

3. *Clearance of PSF In Vivo*

Experiments in which T-cell-derived or WEHI-3B-derived PSF was injected intravenously and serum was assayed for PSF at intervals, indicated that functional PSF is rapidly removed from the blood with an initial rapid clearance ($t_{1/2}$ = 3–4 min.), presumably reflecting equilibration with the extravascular fluid, followed by a second phase ($t_{1/2}$ = 40 minutes) (Crapper *et al.*, 1984a). This rapid removal of PSF from the blood may form an important control mechanism that ensures that systemic effects occur only when very large numbers of T cells are activated, e.g., during a massive infection or infestation.

4. *How Does a Multitargeted PSF Produce a Mastocytosis?*

Previously we suggested that PSF accounted for T-dependent mastocytoses (Schrader *et al.*, 1981). Given our evidence that PSF acts on multiple types of hemopoietic progenitor cells, however, why should the secretion of PSF result in the accumulation of one type of myeloid cell, namely, mast cells and not of other types of blood cells such as red cells and macrophages?

Our experiments on the gut mucosa (Schrader *et al.*, 1983a; Crapper and Schrader, 1983), the site at which T-dependent mastocytosis has been best studied (e.g., Ruitenberg and Elgersma, 1976), suggests that the answer lies in the availability of potential targets. Thus, whereas in the gut mucosa there is a relatively high frequency of cells that react to PSF by becoming P cells (or T-dependent mast cells) (Schrader *et al.*, 1983a), there are undetectable levels of progenitors of macrophages or neutrophils, or of pluripotential hemopoietic stem cells (Crapper and Schrader, 1983). It therefore seems likely that the precise effect of PSF is governed by the type of potential target cells available in a given tissue.

V. PSF AND ONCOGENESIS

A. Paradoxical Production of PSF by WEHI-3B

Our group has shown that T-cell hybridomas, T-cell lymphomas, continuous T-cell lines, and normal T cells activated *in vivo* and *in vitro* can all produce PSF (Schrader *et al.*, 1980a,b, 1981a, 1982a; Schrader and Nossal, 1980; Schrader, 1981, 1983). For these reasons, we regard PSF as essentially a T-cell lymphokine and have found the fact that a myelomonocytic leukemia WEHI-3B is a good source of this factor (Nagao *et al.*, 1981; Yung *et al.*, 1981; Clark-Lewis *et al.*, 1982b) a challenging paradox. One suggestion, that the PSF-producing sublines of WEHI-3B have been misclassified and in fact represent abnormal T cells, has been based on the fact that many of these lines express the Thy-1 antigen (Walker *et al.*, 1982). This argument is not particularly convincing, though, as we have shown that myeloid cells can express Thy 1 in the mouse (Schrader *et al.*, 1982b).

The production of PSF by WEHI-3B in fact differs from that by T cells in two important respects: (1) it is constitutive, whereas with T cells, in our experience, production must always be induced; and (2) the production of PSF by WEHI-3B occurs in apparent isolation, as WEHI-3B, unlike T-cell sources of PSF, does not simultaneously produce other lymphokines, such as TCGF, γ-IFN, or T-cell GM-CSF (J. W. Schrader and I. Clark-Lewis, unpublished observations).

We have proposed that the answer to this paradox lies in the notion that WEHI-3B arose initially from a type of heterogeneous P cell, i.e., a PSF-dependent line of neutrophil–macrophage progenitor cells that initially became autonomous when the gene for PSF was activated by some means. The expression of the Thy-1 antigen fits with this model, as we have shown that PSF induces the expression of Thy 1 on neutrophil–macrophage progenitor cells (Schrader *et al.*, 1982b), and Dexter and colleagues (1980) have reported that Thy 1 is expressed on factor-dependent lines of myeloid progenitors.

B. Concomitant Initiation of PSF Production, Autonomous Growth, and Tumorigenesis in a P-Cell Line

Recently, we obtained evidence that this sequence of events can occur, in the form of observations on a variant of a clone of heterogeneous P cells that became independent of exogenous PSF (Schrader *et al.*, 1983b; Schrader and Crapper, 1983). The key observation was that this variant line could be shown to be producing PSF. This indicated that P cells had the metabolic capacity to synthesize and secrete PSF. Furthermore, because autonomy and the production of PSF arose simultaneously in this and in an independently derived variant, it seems likely that the activation of the PSF gene accounted for the autonomy.

Concomitant with the acquisition of the ability to produce PSF and to grow autonomously *in vitro*, the variant line also became tumorigenic. Thus, while cells of the parental line had disappeared 2 weeks after injection into a syngeneic mouse, inoculation of the autonomous PSF-producing variant was followed by the development of a large tumor mass, metastases, and leukemia. A panel of autonomous variant P cells, all of which produce PSF and are leukemogenic, but which have arisen from independent events, has been generated (S. Schrader and J. W. Schrader, unpublished data) and will be used in the investigation of the mechanism of activation of the PSF gene.

We have argued that the myelomonocytic leukemia WEHI-3B arose through a similar series of events (Schrader *et al.*, 1983b, Schrader and Crapper, 1983; Schrader, 1984). In support of this view of leukemogeneis, we have recently shown that a myeloid leukemia that arose in a mouse *in vivo*, responded to PSF *in vitro* and had receptors for PSF (S. Schrader and J. W. Schrader, unpublished data).

We have suggested (Schrader, 1984) that PSF may play an autostimulatory role in oncogenesis involving the pluripotential hematopoietic stem cell and its progeny. Different disorders involving cell types responsive to PSF could correspond to the various elements of the following sequence of events: first, the PSF-driven proliferation of normal progenitor cells, second, the emergence of an immortalized PSF-dependent line analogous to the nontumorigenic, PSF-dependent heterogeneous P-cell lines (Schrader, 1983), and third, the activation of the PSF gene with consequent autonomy and tumorigenesis. A final evolutionary step may be the emergence of a clone that is no longer dependent on autologous PSF. Given that PSF stimulates a range of hemopoietic progenitor cells from the pluripotential stem cell to more committed progenitors of various lineages (Schrader, 1983), some or all of these processes could be involved in proliferative disorders, not only of the bone marrow, but also of cells derived from the bone marrow such as those involved in Hodgkin's disease. The role of PSF and the activation of the PSF gene in the initiation and progress of such diseases is the subject of ongoing investigation.

VI. CONCLUSION

We have established that PSF is directly synthesized by T lymphocytes and is released, together with a group of other lymphokines, whenever T cells are activated. Purification of this factor has indicated that PSF acts at concentrations as low as 10^{-13} M and affects cells of all nonlymphoid lineages of bone marrow-derived cells. PSF can enter and circulate in the blood *in vivo*, although there is an efficient mechanism for removal of functional PSF from the circulation. In some circumstances, PSF released locally can stimulate hemopoietic progenitors in the bone marrow and spleen and, while PSF may normally act in the immediate vicinity of the activating T cell, e.g., stimulating mast-cell progenitors in the gut wall or bronchi or multiple types of progenitor cells in granulomata, in severe infections it may act systemically and stimulate hemopoiesis in the bone marrow. PSF may have important therapeutic roles in stimulating the rapid growth of hemopoietic cells, e.g., following bone marrow grafts or therapy with cytotoxic drugs. Administration of PSF may be a useful adjunct to immunosuppressive therapy, and might ensure that the lack of T cells and their products will not impair the hemopoietic function of the bone marrow.

Finally, we now have new and striking evidence that the cells that normally respond to PSF can, under abnormal circumstances, produce PSF. As expected, the production of PSF is accompanied by emancipation from the requirement for exogeneous PSF and, in the cases we have studied, by the acquisition of the capacity for unrestrained malignant growth *in vivo*. Cloning of the PSF gene should be followed by a rapid increment in knowledge about the relationship of this factor to other regulatory molecules produced by T cells, the mechanism and regulation of its expression, and more detailed information on how abnormal activation of this gene can occur in PSF-dependent cells.

ACKNOWLEDGMENTS

This work was supported by the National Health and Medical Council, Canberra, Australia, The Bushell Trust, and The Windemere Hospital Foundation. We thank Ms. Joanne Ringham, Mrs. Debra Billingsley, and Ms. Denise Galatos for excellent assistance.

VII. REFERENCES

Ahlstedt, St., Björksten, B., Nygren, H., and Smedegard., G., 1983, *Immunology* **48**:247.
Askenase, P. W., 1981, *Springer Semin. Immunopathol.* **2**:417.
Bazill, G. W., Haynes, M., Garland, J., and Dexter, T. M., 1983, *Biochem. J.* **210**:747.
Bradley, T. R., and Metcalf, D., 1966, *Aust. J. Exp. Biol. Med. Sci.* **44**:297.
Brooks, C. G., Kuribayashi, K., Sale, G. E., and Henney, C., 1982, *J. Immunol.* **128**:2326.
Burgess, A. W., Camakaris, J., and Metcalf, D., 1977, *J. Biol. Chem.* **252**:1988.
Burgess, A. W., Bartlett, P. F., Metcalf, D., Nicola, N. A., Clark-Lewis, I., and Schrader, J. W.., 1981, *Exp. Hematol.* **9**:893.
Cerny, J., 1974, *Nature* **249**:63.

Clark-Lewis, I., and Schrader, J. W., 1981, *J. Immunol.* **127**:1941.
Clark-Lewis, I., and Schrader, J. W., 1982a, *J. Immunol.* **128**:168.
Clark-Lewis, I., and Schrader, J. W., 1982b, *J. Immunol.* **128**:175.
Clark-Lewis, I., Schrader, J. W., and McKimm-Breschkin, J. L., 1982a, *J. Immunol. Methods* **51**:311.
Clark-Lewis, I., Schrader, J. W., Wu, Y-Y, and Harris, A. W., 1982b, *Cell Immunol.* **69**:196.
Clark-Lewis, I., Kent, S. B. H., and Schrader, J. W., 1984, *J. Biol. Chem.* **259**:7488.
Crapper, R. M., and Schrader, J. W., 1983, *J. Immunol.* **131**:923.
Crapper, R. M., Clark-Lewis, I., and Schrader, J. W., 1984a, *Immunology* (in press).
Crapper, R. M., Thomas, W. R., and Schrader, J. W., 1984b, *J. Immunol.* (in press).
Dexter, T. M., Garland, J., Scott, D., Scolnick, E., and Metcalf, D., 1980, *J. Exp. Med.* **152**:1036.
Dy, M., Lebel, B., Kamour, P., and Hamburger, J., 1981, *J. Exp. Med.* **153**:293.
Farram, E., and Nelson, D. S., 1980, *Cell. Immunol.* **55**:294.
Flexman, J. P., Shellam, G. R., and Mayrhofer, G., 1983, *Immunology* **48**:773.
Fung, M. C., Halpel, A. J., Ymer, S., Cohen, D. R., Johnson, R. N., Campbell, H. D., and Young, I. G., 1984, *Nature* **307**:223.
Garland, J. M., and Dexter, T. M., 1982, *Eur. J. Immunol.* **12**:998.
Gillis, S., Ferm, M. M., Ou, W., and Smith, K. A., 1978, *J. Immunol.* **120**:2027.
Gillis, S., Scheid, M., and Watson, J. D., 1980, *J. Immunol.* **125**:2570.
Ginsberg, H., and Sachs, L., 1963, *J. Natl. Cancer Inst.* **31**:1.
Golde, D. W., Bersch, N., Quam, S. G., and Lusis, A. J., 1980, *Proc. Natl. Acad. Sci. USA* **77**:593.
Greenberger, J. S., Newberger, P. E., and Sakakeeny, M. S., 1980, *Blood* **56**:368.
Greenberger, J. S., Sakakeeny, M. A., Humphries, R. K., Eaves, C. J., and Eckner, R. J., 1983, *Proc. Natl. Acad. Sci. USA* **80**:2931.
Guy-Grand, D., Griscelli, C., and Vassalli, P., 1979, *J. Exp. Med.* **148**:1661.
Hapel, A. J., Lee, J. C., Farrar, W. C., and Ihle, J. N., 1981, *Cell* **25**:179.
Hardy, R. R., Hayakawa, K., Haaijman, J., and Herzenberg, L. A., 1982, *Nature* **297**:589.
Harwell, L., Skidmore, B., Marrack, P., and Kappler, J., 1980, *J. Exp. Med.* **152**:893.
Hasthorpe, S., 1980, *J. Cell. Physiol.* **105**:379.
Hilfiker, M. L., Moore, R. N., and Farrar, J. J., 1981, *J. Immunol.* **127**:1981.
Ihle, J. N., Pepersack, L., and Rebar, L., 1981a, *J. Immunol.* **127**:2565.
Ihle, J. N., Keller, J., Lee, J. C., Farrar, W. L., and Hapel, A. J., 1981b, in: *Lymphokine and Thymic Factors and Their Potential in Cancer Therapeutics* (A. L. A. Goldstein, M. Chirigos, eds.), Raven Press, New York.
Ihle, J. N., Rebar, L., Keller, J., Lee, J. C., and Hapel, A. J., 1982a, *Immunol. Rev.* **63**:5.
Ihle, J. N., Keller, J., Henderson, L., Klein, F., and Palaszynski, E. W., 1982b, *J. Immunol.* **129**:2431.
Ihle, J. N., Keller, J., Oroszlan, S., Henderson, L. E., Copeland, T. P., Fitch, F., Prystowsky, M. B., Goldwasser, E., Schrader, J. W., Palaszynski, E., Dy, M., and Lebel, B., 1983, *J. Immunol.* **131**:282.
Iscove, N. N., Roitsch, C. A., Williams, N., and Guilbert, L. J., 1982, *J. Cell. Physiol.* **1**:65.
Jackson, C. W., 1973, *Blood* **42**:413.
Kedar, E., Ikejiri, B., Gredni, B., Bonavida, B., and Herberman, R. B., 1982, *Cell. Immunol.* **69**:305.
Kelso, A., Glasebrook, A. L., Kanagawa, O., and Brunner, K. T., 1982, *J. Immunol.* **129**:550.
Lattime, E. C., Pecoraro, G. A., and Stutman, O., 1983, *J. Exp. Med.* **157**:1070.
Marcucci, F., Waller, M., Kirchner, H., and Krammer, P., 1981, *Nature* **291**:79.
Metcalf, D., Johnson, G. R., and Burgess, A. W., 1980, *Blood* **55**:138.

Nabel, G., Greenberger, J. S., Sakakeeny, M. A., and Cantor, H., 1981, *Proc. Natl. Acad. Sci. USA* **78**:1157.

Nagao, K., Yokowa, K., and Aaronson, S. A., 1981, *Science* **212**:333.

Nathan, I., Groopman, J. E., Quan, S. G., Bersch, N., and Golde, D. W., 1981, *Nature* **292**:842.

Nicola, N. A., Metcalf, D., Matsumoto, M., and Johnson, G. R., 1983, *J. Biol. Chem.* **258**: 9017.

Pike, B. L., Vaux, D. L., Clark-Lewis, I., Schrader, J. W., and Nossal, G. J. V., 1982, *Proc. Soc. Natl. Acad. Sci. USA* **79**:6350.

Pluznik, D. H., and Sachs, L., 1965, *J. Cell. Physiol.* **66**:319.

Prystowsky, M. B., Ely, J. M., Beller, D. I., Eisenberg, L. Goldman, J., Goldman, M., Goldwasser, E., Ihle, J., Quintans, J., Remold, H., Vogel, S. N., and Fitch, F. W., 1982, *J. Immunol.* **129**:2337.

Ralph, P., Broxmeyer, H. E., Moore, M. A. S., and Nakoinz, I., 1978, *Cancer Res.* **38**:1414.

Razin, E., Cordon-Cardo, C., and Good, R. A., 1981, *Proc. Natl. Acad. Sci. USA* **78**:2559.

Ruitenberg, E. J., and Elgersma, A., 1976, *Nature* **264**:258.

Schimpl, A., and Wecker, E., 1975, *Transplant Rev.* **23**:176.

Schrader, J. W., 1981, *J. Immunol.* **126**:452.

Schrader, J. W., 1983, *CRC Crit. Rev. Immunol.* **4**:197.

Schrader, J. W., 1984, *Lancet* **III(8395)**: 133.

Schrader, J. W., and Clark-Lewis, I., 1981, *J. Immunol.* **126**:1101.

Schrader, J. W., and Clark-Lewis, I., 1982a, *J. Immunol.* **129**:30.

Schrader, J. W., and Clark-Lewis, I., 1982b, *Curr. Top. Microbiol. Immunol.* **100**:221.

Schrader, J. W., and Crapper, R. M., 1983, *Proc. Nat. Acad. Sci. USA* **80**:6892.

Schrader, J. W., and Nossal, G. J. V., 1980, *Immunol. Rev.* **53**:61.

Schrader, J. W., Arnold, B., and Clark-Lewis, I., 1980a, *Nature* **283**:197.

Schrader, J. W., Clark-Lewis, I., and Bartlett, P. F., 1980b, in: *Biology of Bone Marrow Transplantation*, Vol. XCII (*Symposium on Molecular Cell Biology*) (R. P. Gale and C. F. Fox, eds.), pp. 443–460, Academic Press, New York.

Schrader, J. W., Lewis, S. J., Clark-Lewis, I., and Culvenor, J. G., 1981a, *Proc. Natl. Acad. Sci. USA* **78**:323.

Schrader, J. W., Bartlett, P. F., Clark-Lewis, I., and Boyd, A. W., 1981b, in: *Microenvironments in Hemopoietic and Lymphoid Differentiation* (CIBA Foundation Symposium 1984) (R. Porter and J. Whelan, eds.), pp. 130–160, Pitman Medical, London.

Schrader, J. W., Bartlett, P. F., and Clark-Lewis, I., 1982a, *Lymphokines* **5**:290.

Schrader, J. W., Battye, F., and Scollay, R., 1982b, *Proc. Soc. Natl. Acad. Sci. USA* **79**: 4161.

Schrader, J. W., Scollay, R., and Battye, F., 1983a, *J. Immunol.* **130**:558.

Schrader, J. W., Clark-Lewis, I., Crapper, R. M., and Wong, G. H. W., 1983b, *Immunol. Rev.* **76**:79.

Shortman, K., Wilson, A., Scollay, R., and Chen, W.-F., 1983, *Proc. Natl. Acad. Sci. USA* **80**:2728.

Staber, F. G., Hultner, L., Marcucci, F., and Krammer, P., 1982, *Nature* **298**:79.

Stanley, E. R., and Heard, P. M., 1977, *J. Biol. Chem.* **252**:4305.

Tertian, G., Yung., Y.-P, Guy-Grand, D., and Moore, M. A. S., 1981, *J. Immunol.* **127**:788.

Till, J. E., and McCulloch, E. A., 1961, *Radiat. Res.* **14**:213.

von Heijne, G., 1983, *Eur. J. Biochem.* **133**:17.

Walker, E. B., Lanier, L. L., and Warner, N. L., 1982, *J. Immunol.* **128**:852.

Warner, N. L., Moore, M. A. S., and Metcalf, D., 1969, *J. Natl. Cancer Inst.* **43**:963.

Watson, J. S., Gillis, S., Marbrook, J., Mochizuki, D., and Smith, K. A., 1979, *J. Exp. Med.* **150**:849.
Weinstein, Y., 1977, *J. Immunol.* **119**:1223.
Wong, G. H. W., Clark-Lewis, I., McKimm-Breschkin, J. L., and Schrader, J. W., 1982, *Proc. Soc. Natl. Acad. Sci. USA* **79**:6989.
Wong, G. H. W., Clark-Lewis, I., Harris, A. W., and Schrader, J. W., 1984, *Eur. J. Immunol.* **14**:52.
Wood, D. D., 1979, *J. Immunol.* **123**:2400.
Yokota, T., Lee, F., Rennick, D., Hall, C., Arai, N., Mossman, T., Nabel, G., Cantor, H., and Arai, K., 1984, *Proc. Nat. Acad. Sci. USA* **81**:1070.
Yung, Y. P., Eger, R., Tertian, G., and Moore, M. A. S., 1981, *J. Immunol.* **127**:794.

Mast-Cell Growth Factor: Its Role in Mast-Cell Differentiation, Proliferation, and Maturation

Yee-Pang Yung and Malcolm A. S. Moore

Department of Developmental Hematopoiesis
Sloan-Kettering Institute for Cancer Research
New York, New York 10021

I. INTRODUCTION

The mast cell was first recognized as granular cells in the unstained mesentery of frog by Friedrich von Recklinghausen early in 1863. In 1879, using a staining procedure, Paul Ehrlich termed these granular cells mast cells. The mast cell is generally considered a connective tissue cell that possesses the capacity to accumulate metachromatically staining cytoplasmic granules (Selye, 1965; Fernex and Riley, 1968). Mast cells may differ substantially in size and shape, depending on their location and state of maturation. They are widely distributed throughout the body in connective tissues, particularly around small blood vessels, nerves, glandular ducts, the submucosa of the digestive tract, oral and nasal mucosa, the lining of the respiratory tract, and in the skin. Mast cells are rarely found in the brain or in parenchymatous organs, but are present in capsular connective tissue and the stroma of various lymphatic organs and endocrine glands (Selye, 1965; Valtonen, 1961; Pretlow and Cassady, 1970). Histochemically, their cytoplasm and the granules contain a variety of biologically active compounds, the most important being the anticoagulant heparin, the mediators of allergic reactions (e.g., histamine, serotonin, and slow-reacting substance), as well as various enzymes (Selye, 1965; Buisseret, 1982). Much information is available on the mechanism of immunoglobulin E (IgE) antibody-mediated mast-cell degranulation, and on their role in allergic reactions and inflammatory responses (Pepys and Edwards, 1979; Buisseret, 1982), yet the normal physiological role of mast cells is still obscure.

Concerning the origin of mast cells, it has been reported that mast cells appear at a rather late stage during embryonic development—after the 16th day of embryonic life in the rat—and that they are derived from the mesenchyme (Fernex and Riley, 1968). Beyond this, there is still little consensus. Regarding how the mast cell system develops, it is commonly held that basophils, which resemble mast cells histochemically, are blood-borne cells and that the mast cells constitute their fixed tissue counterpart. Ehrlich (1879) suggested that mast cells did not develop from leukocytes or their precursors, but rather from fixed connective tissue cells. Others, however, disagree and believe mast cells to be of hematopoietic origin (Metcalf and Moore, 1971). It was not until recently, however, through the work of Kitamura and co-workers (Kitamura *et al.*, 1978; Hatanaka *et al.*, 1979), that the hematopoietic origin of mast cells was affirmed. By transplanting bone marrow cells from mice carrying the beige gene marker for characteristic giant mast cell granules into genetically mast cell deficient W/W^v anemic mice, these investigators demonstrated the development of mast cells from pluripotent hematopoietic stem cells of donor beige type. More recently, Nakahata and Ogawa (1982), through the use of an *in vitro* cloning technique, established the origin of mast cells from multipotential hematopoietic progenitors. Nevertheless, much controversy still exists over the lineage origin of mast cells. It is not known whether a committed mast cell progenitor exists. After observing the massive replacement of large areas of a thymus of NZB mice by mast cells, Burnet (1965) suggested a correlation between mast cells and lymphocytes. Since then, on the basis of additional circumstantial evidence, he and various other investigators have proposed a T-lymphocyte derivation of mast cells (Burnet 1965, 1977; Ginsburg and Sachs, 1962; Ginsburg *et al.*, 1978; Ishizaka *et al.*, 1976; Guy-Grand *et al.*, 1978). Despite this apparent close relationship between T cells and mast cells, the morphological and histochemical similarity between the granules of mast cells and the blood-borne basophilic leukocytes is striking. Indeed, the terms basophil and mast cell have often been used interchangeably (Selye, 1965), and more recently, on the basis of ultrastructural studies, a common origin has been proposed for basophils and mast cells (Lennert and Parwaresch, 1979; Zucker-Franklin, 1980). A common precursor has likewise been hypothesized for mast cells and macrophages on morphological grounds (Zucker-Franklin *et al.*, 1981; Czarnetsky, 1981). While there may exist different subpopulations of mast cells, it is difficult to rationalize the ability of cells of different lineages to differentiate into mast cells.

Much of our present knowledge of hematopoietic differentiation was gained through advances in tissue-culture techniques and molecular biology in recent decades. Our current concept of hematopoiesis is that of a complex, self-regulating system involving the interaction of a myriad of hematopoietically active factors and hormones with the hematopoietic cells. To cite an example, specific colony-stimulating factors (CSFs) have been identified for granulocyte macrophage and megakaryocyte colony formation (Burgess *et al.*, 1980; Stanley *et al.*, 1975, 1976; Sheridan and Metcalf, 1973; Kurland and Moore, 1977). Macrophages, in turn, produce prostaglandins that act as feedback inhibitors of myelopoiesis (Kurland *et al.*, 1979; Pelus *et al.*, 1981, 1982). Granulopoiesis and macrophage production are further inhibited by various iron-binding proteins, notably polymorphonuclear neutrophil-derived lactoferrin and monocyte–macrophage-derived acid isoferritin (Broxmeyer *et al.*, 1978, 1980, 1981; Broxmeyer, 1982a, b). Moreover, myelopoiesis can, on the other hand, be further enhanced by macrophage-derived enhancing factors (Castro-Malaspina *et al.*, 1982, 1983; Wang *et al.*, 1983b), and more recently a differentiation factor has been identified (Moore and Yung, 1982; Moore and Sheridan, 1982). It is therefore apparent that each and every step in the hematopoietic differentiation cascade is triggered as well as regulated by extremely potent and highly specific cytokines. It is conceivable that the development of the mast-cell system from the pluripotent hematopoietic stem cell will not be an exception.

Progress in studying the functional role and the ontogenesis of mast cells has been hindered by the difficulty in isolating pure populations of mast cells. Pretlow and Cassady (1970) succeeded in separating rat peritoneal mast cells by rate zonal separation and isopycnic centrifugation. They further classified mast cells according to state of maturation into four classes, with the immature mast cells being of lower density, containing fewer and larger granules that stain with Alcian blue but not safranin, and the most mature mast cells being of much higher density, densely packed with smaller granules loaded with histamine and staining positively with safranin. However, this procedure is tedious and yields a limited number of mast cells. Earlier studies involving cultured mast cells used neoplastic mast cells (Paff *et al.*, 1947). Although normal animal and human mast cells have been cultivated (Zitcer *et al.*, 1953), the usefulness of these systems has not been established. Ginsburg and Lagunoff (1967) reported that mouse mast cells developed from lymph node and thoracic duct cells cultured on fibroblast monolayers. Later, Ishizaka *et al.* (1976) adapted the system for rat mast cells. Young mast cells in this system appeared as mononuclear blasts bearing receptors for IgE and metachromatically staining cytoplasmic granules. Upon prolonged culture, the number and affinity of the receptors for IgE as well as the density of the granules increased (Ishizaka *et al.*, 1976). Nevertheless, this culture system was limited to short-term (several weeks) duration and required a feeder layer.

In recent years, *in vitro* techniques have been developed for the long-term culture as well as short-term cloning of mast cells. The purpose of this review is to summarize the available information and provide an overview of our present knowledge of the mast-cell differentiation pathway. Emphasis is placed on the molecular events and on their impact at the cellular level during mast cell development.

II. *IN VITRO* CULTURE OF MURINE MAST CELLS

A. Growth-Factor-Dependent Long-Term Culture System for Murine Mast Cells

We first reported on the growth from precursors in long-term marrow cultures of a Thy-1^- cell bearing basophilic cytoplasmic granules in mitogen-activated murine splenic leukocyte-conditioned medium (Tertian *et al.*, 1980; Yung et al., 1980). These cells were later identified as mast cells (Tertian *et al.*, 1981) on the basis of their characteristic morphology, the ultrastructure of their cytoplasmic granules, positive reactions with toluidine blue and Alcian blue, the presence of IgE receptors, and the monoamines and sulfated products contained in the cytoplasm (Table I). Various other investigators have also reported their ability to generate and maintain in a continuous proliferative state cell lines of basophil or mast cell morphology, notably with concanavalin A (Con A)-stimulated spleen cell-conditioned medium-dependent persisting (P) cells of Schrader (Schrader, 1981; Schrader *et al.*, 1981), the WEHI-3 cell-conditioned medium-dependent basophil/mast-cell-like cell of Nagao *et al.* (1981), the cloned mast cells of Nabel *et al.* (1981), and the pokeweed mitogen-stimulated spleen-conditioned medium-dependent Friend virus-infected FMP1.1 cell line described by Hasthorpe (1980). Although the origin of these latter cell lines and the sources of conditioned medium used differed, the proliferating cell types were basically similar. In addition, several investigators have reported on the establishment of WEHI-CM-dependent cell lines from virus- or carcinogen-treated cultured bone marrow cells, notably the promyelocytic cell lines of Greenberger *et al.* (1979). However, it was not established that these were not merely mast-cell lines, and that viral infection or carcinogen was necessary for their generation.

As a source of growth factor for mast cells, various types of conditioned medium (CM) have proved adequate (Table II). As some of these CM also contain Interleukin-2 (IL-2) and mitogens, the presence of T cells or pre-T cells often interferes with the establishment of mast cell lines. Thus, it becomes necessary to establish mast-cell lines using cell sources lacking or depleted of T and/or pre-T cells. Medium conditioned by the myelomonocytic leukemia WEHI-3 cells, which does not contain IL-2, or spleen conditioned medium depleted of IL-2 by DEAE-cellulose column chromatography (Yung *et al.*, 1981) provides an alternative solution. In general, several weeks of culture with biweekly passaging at 2.5×10^3-10^5 cells/ml in fresh RPMI 1640 medium supplemented with 10% fetal bovine serum (FBS) in the presence of 10–50% (depending on the source) of conditioned medium is necessary to establish the mast-cell lines. In order to ascertain the purity of the lines, cloning by limiting dilution can be performed.

Table I. Properties of Cultured Mast Cells[a]

Positive for	Negative for
IgE receptor	Thy-1 antigen
IgG Fc receptor	Surface Ig
Ly-5 antigen	Complement receptor
Ia antigen	Mac-1 antigen
Acid phosphatase	Periodic acid-Schiff
Alcian blue	Lysozyme
Toluidine blue (metachromatia)	Peroxidase
Chloroacetate esterase	Alkaline phosphatase
Histamine	α-naphthylacetate esterase
L-Dopa	TdT
Serotonin	
5-Hydroxytryptophan	
Sulfate monoamines	

[a]Cultured mast cells were analyzed for the presence (positive) or absence (negative) of various surface markers, cytoplasmic enzymes, and histochemical staining reactions. TdT, Terminal deoxynucleotide transferase.

Once established, the mast cells can be maintained in exponential growth for indefinite duration by biweekly passaging. Five- to 10-fold or more increases in cell number can often be observed at the end of each passage. The continuous presence of CM-derived mast-cell growth factor (MCGF) is absolutely necessary for both the proliferation and viability of the cultured mast cells. Cell death ensues within 24 hr in the absence of the growth factor. Various types of conditioned media have been claimed to contain mast-cell growth-promoting activity, notably, supernatant from the cloned murine T-cell line of Nabel *et al.* (1981), and medium conditioned by T cells of helminth-infected rats for rat mast cells (Haig *et al.*, 1982). MCGF has also been detected in media conditioned by spleen

Table II. Establishment of Murine Mast-Cell Lines[a]

Source of mast-cell precursors	Source of growth factor
Athymic *nu/nu* BMC	Con A/PHA-mouse spleen-CM
T-cell-depleted BMC[b]	Con A/PHA-LBRM-CM
Athymic *nu/nu* BMC	
Normal or T-cell-depleted BMC	WEHI-CM
Athymic *nu/nu* spleen cells	MCGF
Long-term cultured BMC	

[a]BMC, bone marrow-derived cells; Con A, Concanavalin A; PHA, phytohemagglutinin.

[b]Rabbit anti-mouse brain serum plus complement was found to be more satisfactory than anti-Thy 1 plus complement.

cells of mice infected with *Schistosoma* as well as Friend virus (Y.-P. Yung and M. S. Moore, unpublished observations). Mitogen-activated rat spleen or human leukocyte conditioned media, which support the growth of murine T cell lines, however, lack detectable growth-promoting activity for murine mast cells. Whether this was due to lack of the necessary growth factor, presence of inhibitors, or lack of species crossreactivity of the rat and human factor has yet to be determined.

Kitamura *et al.* (1979b) reported that mast cell precursors were present in various lymphohematopoietic tissues and that their concentration was greater in the bone marrow than in the spleen and lymph nodes. The readiness with which mast cell lines can be established from bone marrow cells supports the claim of a hematopoietic origin for mast cells (Kitamura *et al.*, 1978, 1979a,b; Hatanaka *et al.*, 1979).

B. Cloning of Murine Mast Cells in Semisolid Media

Semisolid media cloning assays have provided hematologists a means for analyzing various types of hematopoietic precursors. As mature cells lack self-renewal capability, only immature or progenitor cells can give rise to colonies in semisolid medium. While the ability of granulocyte–macrophage precursors to form colonies (GM-CFU) *in vitro* has been well established, it was not until recently, through the use of specific staining techniques, that the various types of granulocytic colonies can be differentiated from one another. Thus, Johnson and Metcalf (1980), using Luxol-fast blue stain, detected eosinophil colonies in mouse bone marrow culture. McCarthy *et al.* (1980), using Astra blue as a specific mast-cell stain, detected small numbers of mast-cell colonies in normal human bone marrow cultures. These investigators further noted elevated numbers of mast cell colonies in cultures from some patients with acute myeloid leukemia. Similarly, using toluidine blue stain, Aglietta *et al.* (1981) reported having detected basophil colonies in agar cultures of human bone marrow cells from normal as well as chronic myeloid leukemic donors.

The ability of bone marrow cells to form basophil or mast-cell colonies is dependent on the presence of either a leukocyte feeder layer (Aglietta *et al.*, 1981) or conditioned medium (McCarthy *et al.*, 1980). Presumably, a specific basophil or mast-cell colony-stimulating factor is required. Thus, while McCarthy *et al.* (1980) failed to detect murine mast-cell colonies using mouse lung conditioned medium as a source of stimulating factor, Zucker-Franklin and coworkers (1981), using a mononuclear cell feeder layer and conditioned medium successfully induced mast-cell colonies from rat peripheral blood.

The first demonstration of mouse mast-cell colonies was recently reported by Nakahata and Ogawa (1982). Using pokeweed mitogen-stimulated mouse spleen-cell conditioned medium as a source of stimulating factor(s), these investigators successfully obtained mast-cell colonies. The study provided evidence for the clonal origin of the colonies. Through recloning of mixed hematopoietic colonies, the hematopoietic origin of mast cells was established. A shared common lineage of mast cells with erythroid, granulomacrophage, and megakaryocytic differentiation was proposed. It remains to be determined as to whether mast cells in these colonies are derived from mast cell progenitors or are differentiated from pluripotent stem cells, or both. Our attempts to obtain mast-cell colonies from suspension-cultured mast cells yielded mainly clusters.

III. SOURCES AND CELLULAR ORIGIN OF MCGF

We previously addressed the question of the cellular requirement for production of mast-cell growth factor (MCGF) (Yung and Moore, 1982). While WEHI-3, a myelomonocytic leukemic cell line (Ralph *et al.*, 1976) is a constitutive producer of MCGF, normal macrophages appear to be incapable of producing MCGF. Thus, peritoneal cells or macrophage-enriched (by adherence) peritoneal cells produce GM-CSF but fail to produce detectable levels of MCGF whether stimulated by the macrophage activator lipopolysaccharide (LPS) or not. Moreover, murine splenic T cells, depleted of adherent macrophages by adherence to Sephadex G10, fail to produce IL-2 and yet still produce abundant MCGF upon stimulation with a T-cell mitogen. Thus, macrophages appear unnecessary for MCGF production. By contrast, splenic T cells are active producers of MCGF. The depletion of Thy-1^--bearing T cells or their genetic absence in athymic *nu/nu* mice greatly reduces or abrogates the production of MCGF. The requirement for T cells to produce MCGF is further substantiated by the findings that inducer Ly-1^+2^- T-cell clones release a factor that supports mast-cell growth following stimulation with Con A (Nabel *et al.*, 1981), and the thymic lymphoma LBRM-33 cells produce MCGF upon mitogen activation (Yung *et al.*, 1981).

In addition, Schrader has reported on the presence of P-cell stimulating factor in medium conditioned by Con A-stimulated T-cell hybridoma T123 cells (Schrader, 1981). Thus, T cells alone appear adequate for MCGF production provided a T-cell mitogen is added, although we cannot exclude the possibility that macrophages may be producing MCGF under special conditions, perhaps in the presence of a T cell.

IV. BIOCHEMICAL NATURE OF MCGF

A. Molecular Heterogeneity of MCGF

MCGF derived from Con A-stimulated splenic leukocyte conditioned medium (Con A-spleen-CM), is a glycoprotein with low affinity for DEAE-cellulose. It is readily separable from the bulk of the serum protein that binds avidly to DEAE-cellulose. IL-2 present in Con A-spleen-CM likewise binds avidly to DEAE-cellulose; thus, MCGF can be separated from IL-2 after the first step of purification (Yung *et al.*, 1981). Using Sephadex G150 gel-filtration chromatography, we have estimated the molecular weight of MCGF to be approximately 35,000 (Yung *et al.*, 1981) (Table III).

Using the cloned Ly-$1^{+}2^{-}$ cell line as a source of growth factor, Nabel reported a molecular weight of 45,000 and a pI of 6.0 for a factor possessing mast cell stimulating activity (Nabel *et al.*, 1981). Clark-Lewis and Schrader (1981), using a Con A-spleen-CM and a T-cell hybridoma as source of mast-cell-like P-cell stimulating factor, on the other hand, reported a M_r of 29,000 in phosphate-buffered saline and of 23,000 in 6 M guanidine hydrochloride, as well as a pI of 4–8 and of 6–8 after neuraminidase treatment. Thus, there appears to be considerable molecular heterogeneity for MCGF. This heterogeneity may in part be a function of the purification procedures used. The source of heterogeneity is most likely related to the degree of glycosylation of the protein portion. Moreover, the source of the factor may also influence the molecular heterogeneity. This is illustrated by our study with medium conditioned by Con A-stimulated LBRM-33 cells (Con A-LBRM-CM). Protein was precipitated from Con A-LBRM-CM using 80% saturation of ammonium sulfate. After extensive dialysis, concentration by ultrafiltration (Amicon YM10 membrane), and equilibration with 5 mM sodium phosphate buffer (pH 8.3), the protein sample was applied to a DEAE-cellulose (DE-52) ion-exchange chromatography column equilibrated in the phosphate buffer. As shown in Fig. 1, most of the MCGF was recovered in the load and wash fraction and was separated from the bulk of serum protein and IL-2, which were eluted only at much higher concentrations of the phosphate buffer. However, a small amount of MCGF did bind to the DEAE-cellulose. Thus, there was a slight heterogeneity with respect to affinity for DEAE-cellulose for Con A-LBRM-CM-derived MCGF that was not observed with Con A-spleen-CM.

To further analyze the biochemical nature of LBRM-derived MCGF, peak MCGF fractions from the DE-52 column were pooled, lyophilized, and resuspended in 10 ml of a 30% glycerol–water solution and layered onto an isoelectric

Table III. Properties of Murine MCGF[a]

Activates mast cells (immature and committed precursors) into cycle
Lacks affinity for DEAE-cellulose
28,000–35,000 M_r
Heterogeneous with respect to pI upon isoelectric focusing
Sensitive to trypsin and neuraminidase-sialic acid-containing glycoprotein
Relatively resistant to heat (boiling temperature, 5 min)
Induces differentiation of mast cell precursors into immature granulated mastoblasts

[a]MCGF, mast-cell growth factor.

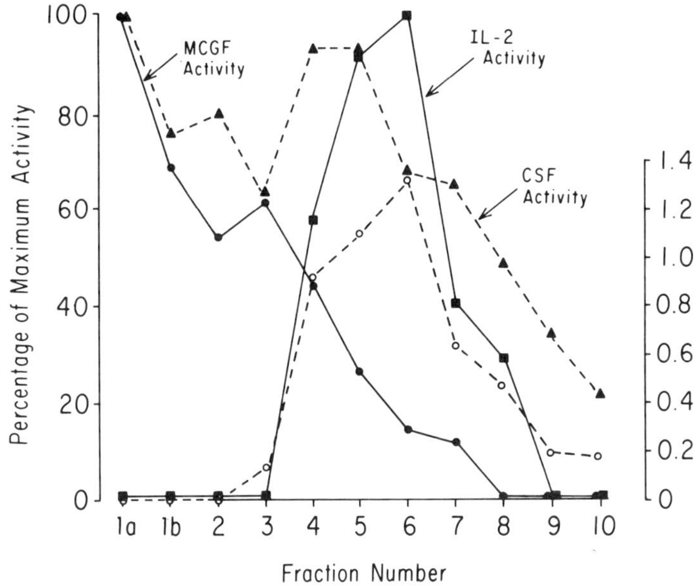

Figure 1. DEAE-cellulose (DE-52) ion-exchange chromatography of Con A-LBRM-CM. An ammonium sulfate precipitate of Con A–LBRM-CM in 5 mM sodium phosphate buffer was loaded onto a DE-52 column and eluted stepwise with increasing concentrations of sodium phosphate buffer pH 8.3. The protein concentration of individual fractions was determined by measuring the absorbance at 280 nm (o--o). Values were as indicated by the scale to the right. Con A-LBRM-CM, Con A-LBRM conditioned medium; CSF, colony-stimulating factor; IL-2, Interleukin-2; MCGF, mast-cell growth factor.

focusing column (LKB 8100) in a 5-60% glycerol density gradient, containing 3% Pharmalyte pH 3.5-10. The MCGF was applied onto an equidensity region of the gradient, and subjected to focusing at 4°C using a constant power supply (LKB 2103). At a maximum power of 10 W, a terminal voltage of 2000 V and a terminal current of 2.5 mA were attained after 26 hr of focusing. Five-ml fractions were collected and the pH of each was determined. The fractions were assayed for MCGF and CSF activity at 5% concentration. The results were shown in Fig. 2. While CSFs were detected in fractions with pI values of 3.0-5.0, MCGF showed substantial molecular heterogeneity with respect to pI, with a range of 4.5-9.5, and two major peaks at 5.5 and 7.8.

Fractions 6-10 (i.e., pI 7.8 peak) and fractions 11-15 (pI 5.5 peak) were separately pooled and loaded onto a precalibrated Ultrogel AcA 52 chromatography column in the presence of added bovine serum albumin (BSA) for stabilization. The pI 7.8 peak pool yielded two peaks of MCGF activity upon gel filtration corresponding to M_r of 29,000 and 14,000, respectively (Fig. 3), whereas the pI 5.5 peak pool yielded only a single 29,000-M_r peak (not shown).

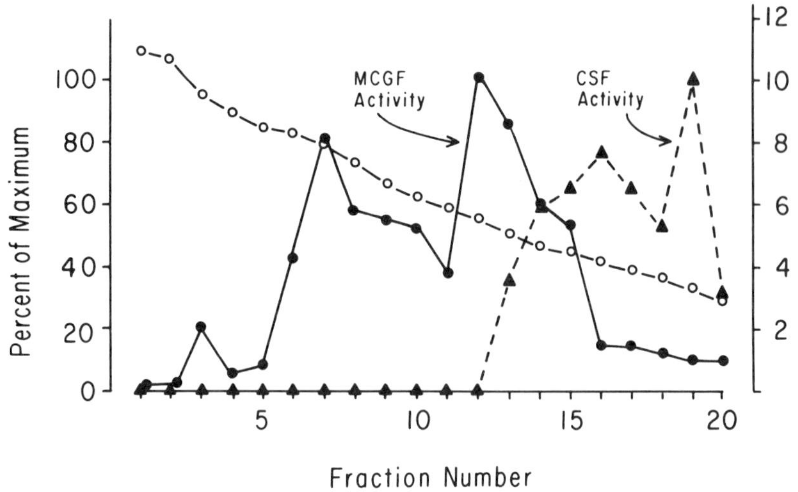

Figure 2. Isoelectric focusing of DE-52 MCGF-rich fraction. See Section IV. B for details. CSF, colony-stimulating factor.

B. Distinction of MCGF from the CSFs

A variety of lymphokines are present in mitogen-activated murine splenic leukocyte conditioned medium and in medium conditioned by the myelomonocytic leukemia WEHI-3 cell line (Moore and Yung, 1982). It is thus of great importance to establish MCGF as unique for mast cells and different from other known hematopoietic growth factors. We have shown that MCGF is different

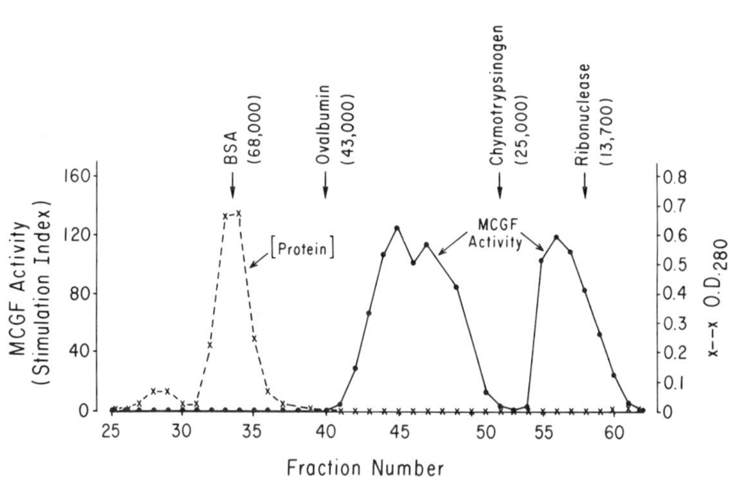

Figure 3. Ultrogel AcA 54 gel filtration of IEF-separated MCGF. See Section IV.b for details.

from IL-2 (Yung *et al.*, 1981). L-cell conditioned medium, which is rich in macrophage colony-stimulating factor (M-CSF), does not stimulate mast-cell growth. This fact and the observation that the M-CSF-rich fraction of WEHI-CM also fails to stimulate mast cell growth, provide evidence that MCGF is also different from CM-CSF (Yung *et al.*, 1981). However, MCGF shares a number of properties with granulocyte colony-stimulating factor (G-CSF) (Table IV). While no G-CSF activity could be detected in MCGF-rich fractions of Con A-spleen-CM (Yung *et al.*, 1981), both MCGF and G-CSF are present in WEHI-CM and Con A-LBRM-CM. Both factors are sensitive to trypsin and resistant to boiling temperature. NZB mice that fail to respond to WEHI-3 G-CSF also fail to respond to MCGF. Nevertheless, MCGF can be distinguished from G-CSF by several criteria (Yung *et al.*, 1982) (Table VI). While MCGF is sensitive to neuraminidase treatment, G-CSF is relatively resistant. Lactoferrin, an inhibitor of macrophage CSF production, suppresses G-CSF production by WEHI-3 cells without affecting MCGF production, and peritoneal cells produce G-CSF but not MCGF when stimulated with LPS. Thus, it is unlikely that MCGF and G-CSF constitute separate functional determinants of the same molecule, and studies using Procion red agarose affinity chromatograph (Fig. 4) seem to bear this out. While both MCGF and CSF activities fail to bind to blue agarose (Fig. 4a), MCGF appears to bind preferentially to procion red agarose (Fig. 4b). Most of the CSFs elute in the wash, and only a small fraction of them bind to the agarose and copurify with MCGF. Differential analysis of the colony morphology further reveals most of G-CSF to be in the wash (fraction 2) and less in the MCGF-rich fraction.

In a study by Clark-Lewis and Schrader (1981) on the nature of P-cell stimulating factor (PSF), it was reported that PSF could be distinguished from mixed granulocyte-macrophage colony-stimulating factor (GM-CSF). Endotoxin-stimulated mouse lung conditioned medium, which is rich in GM-CSF, had no detected

Table IV. Similarities and Differences between MCGF and G-CSF

	MCGF	G-CSF
Presence in WEHI-3 conditioned medium	Present	Present
Presence in Con A–LBRM-conditioned medium	Present	Present
Affinity to DEAE-cellulose	Lacking	Lacking
Molecular-weight range	Same	Same
Sensitivity to trypsin	Relatively same	Relatively same
Response to boiling temperature	Resistant	Resistant
Responsiveness of NZB mice	Lacking	Lacking
Response to neuraminidase	Sensitive	Resistant
Influence of lactoferrin on production by WEHI-3 cells	Not inhibited	Inhibited
Presence in peritoneal cell-CM	Present	Absent
Presence in Con A-spleen-CM	Present	Not detectable

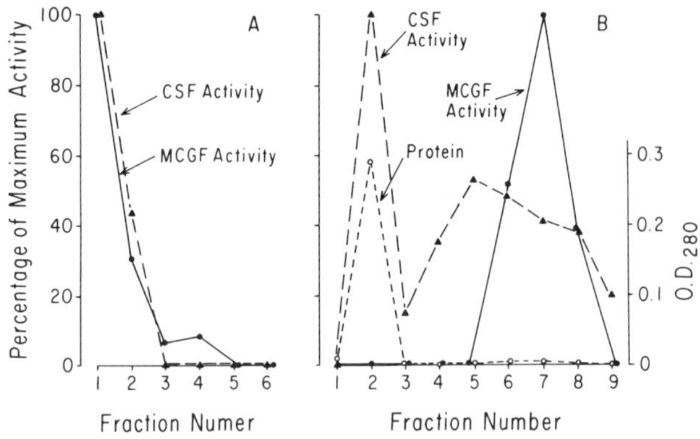

Figure 4. Affinity column chromatography of AcA 54-separated MCGF on (A) Blue agarose and (B) Procion red agarose. Columns were equilibrated with phosphate-buffered saline (PBS) and the samples were eluted with PBS containing increasing concentrations of NaCl. abbreviations as in Figs. 1 and 2.

PSF activity. Furthermore, after neuraminidase treatment, GM-CSF showed a pI of 4.7, whereas PSF was recovered within the pI range of 6–8.

While molecular purity of MCGF preparations is as yet unattainable, available data provide strong evidence that MCGF is distinct from granulocyte and macrophage CSFs.

C. Relationship with Various Other Hematopoietic Factors

Several other hematopoietically active factors have been reported over the past several years. Of special interest are a differentiation factor (DF) for myelomonocytic leukemic cells, an erythroid burst-promoting activating factor (BPA), a stem-cell stimulating factor (CFU-SF), and Interleukin-3 (IL-3). These four factors have been claimed either to copurify with G-CSF or P-cell stimulating factor (PSF) or to exhibit MCGF activity. It is thus of interest to evaluate these various factors within the context of their relationship to MCGF.

A mouse active DF that induces the terminal differentiation of the myelomonocytic leukemia WEHI-3B D^+ subline was originally detected in postendotoxin serum (Burgess and Metcalf, 1980; Moore and Yung, 1982; Moore and Sheridan, 1982). According to Burgess and Metcalf (1981), DF present in postendotoxin serum copurifies with a type of G-CSF. Because of the similarities between G-CSF and MCGF, we have examined this issue further. Analyses of a partially purified DF from endotoxin serum for MCGF activity and of a G-CSF-rich fraction of WEHI-3 conditioned medium for DF activity were both negative (Y.-P. Yung and M. A. S. Moore, unpublished data). Thus, it is unlikely that DF is the same as G-CSF or MCGF.

The purification of erythroid BPA from WEHI-3 cells by Iscove and coworkers (1982), showed that after exhaustive purification procedures, BPA remained associated with molecules that stimulate pluripotential cells, early cells committed to granulocyte, macrophage, and megakaryocyte production, and mast-cell growth (N. N. Iscove, personal communication). These investigators proposed the presence of a single lineage-indifferent factor active on pluripotential hematopoietic precursor cells as well as their early committed progeny. According to this model, growth and maturation down any particular pathway will require the participation of at least two factors, one operating early in the pathway, the other late. Thus, while the mast-cell stimulating activity of this multipotential factor could be due to actual identity with MCGF, it might also be due to the activity of the multipotential factor on a subpopulation of early committed mast-cell progenitors.

Schrader and Clark-Lewis (1982a) reported on a T-cell-derived factor (CFU-SF) that allowed for long-term (up to 4 weeks) maintenance of multipotential murine hematopoietic stem cells capable of forming spleen colonies in lethally irradiated mice. These investigators (Schrader and Clark-Lewis, 1982b) further showed that CFU-SP copurified with PSF. Typical cultures thus consisted of both P cells and CFUs. While it is unlikely for P cells and multipotential stem cells to be identical, as the latter cells can be maintained for only up to 4 weeks, several questions still remain to be answered. It is not clear if the failure to maintain the stem cells beyond 4 weeks is due to loss of or limited self-renewal capacity of the stem cells, or to P cells overgrowing the stem cells, or to differentiation of stem cells into P cells. As the P cells cannot be separated from the stem cells, there remains a possibility for stem-cell maintenance to be secondary to P-cell growth, resulting in the apparent copurification of CFU-SF with PSF. Thus, the existence of a separate T-cell-derived CFU-SF remains to be established.

Another lymphokine, Interleukin-3 (IL-3), has been reported (Lee *et al.*, 1982; Ihle *et al.*, 1982a, b). IL-3 was identified originally as a factor derived from the myelomonocytic WEHI-3 cell line that stimulated the expression of an enzyme 20α-deoxysteroid dehydrogenase on the surface of pre-T cells present in spleens of athymic *nu/nu* mice (Lee *et al.*, 1982). A significance of the enzyme as a T-cell marker was proposed, although the enzyme was later found also to be expressed on cells of non-T lineages, notably mast cells (Ihle *et al.*, 1982a). As IL-3 was found to be derived from mitogen-stimulated T cells, these investigators suggested IL-3 to be a T-cell-derived factor (Ihle *et al.*, 1982a). Moreover, proponents of IL-3 also found that IL-3 had several other functions (Ihle *et al.*, 1982b; J. N. Ihle, personal communication), e.g., support of proliferation of several WEHI-CM-dependent cell lines, PSF and CFU-SF activities, activation of natural cytotoxic cells, and Thy-1 antigen-inducing activity. Thus, IL-3 appeared to be an omnipotent lymphokine.

We recently had the opportunity to test a highly purified IL-3 preparation (Ihle *et al.*, 1982c, courtesy of J. N. Ihle) for MCGF, CSF, and DF activities. As shown in Table V, this WEHI-3-derived IL-3 lacked DF activity. However, substantial CSF activity was detectable (Table VI). In fact, the IL-3 was enriched for CSF when compared with the crude WEHI-CM. Furthermore, the lack of colony formation by NZB bone marrow cells suggested that the colonies were of the G-CSF variety. As we have demonstrated earlier, the nonidentity between G-CSF and MCGF, and as IL-3 has been claimed to have PSF and MCGF activities (Ihle *et al.*, 1983), we further tested IL-3 for MCGF activity. Comparison was made with a partially but substantially purified sample of LBRM-33 cell-derived MCGF (Table VII). It can be seen that while IL-3 has MCGF activity, this activity is much lower than that present in our MCGF preparation, and is not compatible in terms of purity with molecules active at molar concentrations of 10^{-13} or lower. Thus, there exists a possibility of multiple factors present in the "pure" IL-3 preparation having very similar biochemical properties. The conglomerate of CSFs perhaps is a good example. Although highly similar in biochemical properties and isolated from one another only with difficulty (Burgess *et al.*, 1980), these molecules remain recognizable as separate functional entities. The failure to obtain clear-cut separation may reflect a great degree of similarity of amino acid sequence or hetergeneity conferred by glycosylation. Moreover, we must not overlook the importance of the glycosidic portions. Single monosaccharide residues have proved to result in differences in blood group antigen specificity (Kobata *et al.*, 1968). A possible role of the glycosylation process in conferring specificity must be entertained.

Table V. Influence of IL-3 on Cloning and Differentiation of WEHI-3 (D+) Leukemic Cells[a]

Dilutions of 1:100 IL-3	WEHI-3 (D+) Colonies/300 cells	WEHI-3 (D+) % Control	WEHI-3 (D+) Colonies differentiated
1:2	68	86	16
1:4	79	101	14
1:8	76	97	13
1:16	78	99	12
1:32	82	105	9
1:64	80	101	7
1:128	80	102	9
PBS	79	100	16
GM-DF	37	47	68

[a] 300 cells of the differentiation-inducible WEHI-3 leukemic cell line cloned in agar in the presence of serial dilutions of 1:100 IL-3 preparation. Total colonies scored at 6 days, differentiated colonies scored as colonies converting from compact to diffuse in gross morphology. GM-DF: a partially purified preparation of leukemia differentiation-inducing protein obtained from murine post-endotoxin serum.

Table VI. G-, M-, and GM-CSF Activity of Purified Interleukin-3[a]

Dilutions of 1:100 IL-3	Colonies per 10^5 marrow cells	
	$B6D2F_1$	NZB
0.15 ml	25 ± 1	0.7 ± 0.2
0.10 ml	19 ± 4	0.7 ± 0.2
1:2	19 ± 5	0.7 ± 0.2
1:4	33 ± 9	0
1:8	11 ± 5	0
1:16	13 ± 3	0
1:32	6 ± 3	0
1:64	4 ± 2	0
1:128	2 ± 1	0
PBS	0	0
Control W-3 CM 1:2	67 ± 8	24 ± 1

[a] A 1:100 dilution of IL-3 titrated in 1 ml agar cultures of normal $B6D2F_1$ or NZB bone marrow. Colonies scored at day 7 in triplicate plates. Control CSF is a concentrated (X10) CM of WEHI-3 not subjected to purification.

Table VII. Mast-Cell Growth Factor Activity of Purified IL-3

Dilution	$[^3H]$TdR Incorporation (cpm and S.I.)[a] of BDF_1 mast cells in					
	CM DE-52 Fr. 1 MCGF (~7 μg protein/ml)		CM AcA-54 MCGF[b] (~1 ng Protein/ml)		Purified IL-3 (1:1000 dil.)	
1:2	135339.7	170.3	ND[c]		9315.3	12.0
1:4	119648.7	153.9	23245.0	29.9	2061.7	2.7
1:8	89397.0	115.9	49074.7	63.1	635.0	0.8
1:16	54674.3	70.3	28058.0	36.1	612.0	0.8
1:32	29144.0	37.5	12622.7	16.2	490.7	0.6
1:64	9314.3	12.0	6677.7	8.5	464.3	0.6
1:128	ND		1212.0	1.6	451.0	0.6
1:512	ND		697.7	0.9	ND	

[a] BDF_1 mast cells were cultured in the presence of various dilutions of the test samples for 3 days prior to pulsing with $[^3H]$TdR (1 μCi/well) in a 4-hr $[^3H]$TdR incorporation assay.
[b] Median isoelectric point of this preparation is about 5.5; M_r about 29,000. CM: Con A-LBRM-conditioned medium.
[c] ND, not done.

Pfizenmaier *et al.* (1982) recently demonstrated, through the use of a T-cell hybridoma, that IL-2 and helper T-cell replacing factor (TRF) once regarded as the same molecule, are in fact different molecular entities. There are apparently a number of highly potent hematopoietically active factors that fall within the same molecular-weight range with very similar biochemical properties. More stringent criteria than the mere homogeneity in a silver-stained gel will be needed to demonstrate their purity. Perhaps hybridoma and gene-cloning techniques will provide us the means to resolve these seemingly identical molecules.

V. NATURE OF MAST-CELL PRECURSORS

The elegant *in vivo* transplantation studies of Kitamura and co-workers (1978, 1979b; Hatanaka *et al.*, 1979) employing the W/W^v mast-cell-deficient mice have provided firm evidence for a hematopoietic origin of mast cells. By contrast, the *in vitro* cloning studies of Nakahata and Ogawa (1982), demonstrated a shared common precursor of mast cells with erythroid, granulomacrophage, and megakaryocytic differentiation. These investigators proposed that mast cell colonies grown in methylcellulose in the presence of pokeweed mitogen-stimulated spleen-cell conditioned medium could be divided into two types: those derived from committed mast-cell progenitors and those derived from multipotential hemopoietic precursors. It was recently reported by Fauser *et al.* (1982) that T lymphocytes were present in multilineage hematopoietic colonies (CFU-GEMM) of patients with Hodgkin's lymphoma, thus providing evidence for a common progenitor of myeloid and lymphoid cells. As various investigators have suggested a close relationship between mast cells and T cells (Burnet, 1965, 1977; Ginsburg and Sachs, 1962; Ginsburg *et al.*, 1978; Ishizaka *et al.*, 1976; Guy-Grand *et al.*, 1978), we have further analyzed the relationship between MCGF-responsive mast-cell precursors and IL-2-responsive T cells and/or pre-T cells present in fresh as well as Dexter-type long-term cultured bone marrow cells (Yung *et al.*, 1983). An $[^3H]$thymidine incorporation assay was established to monitor the proliferation of cells responsive to substantially purified MCGF and IL-2. Morphologically recognizable mast cells were normally not present in fresh marrow, and Dexter-type long-term cultured marrow cells were devoid of mast cells prior to 6 weeks of culture and of matured T cells after 1 week of culture (Tertian *et al.*, 1981; Moore and Sheridan, 1982). Mast cells and T cells can nevertheless be differentiated from fresh marrow and long-term marrow cultures (LMC) (Tertian *et al.*, 1981; Jones-Villeneuve and Phillips, 1980). Bone marrow cells derived from fresh bone marrow and from LMC were subjected to buoyant-density gradient separation or velocity sedimentation at unit gravity fractionation. In-

Table VIII. Summary of Buoyant Density and Velocity of Sedimentation Characterization of Bone Marrow MCGF- and IL-2-Responding Cells[a]

		Density distribution[b] (g/ml)		VS distribution[c] (mm/hr)	
Type of factor	Cell source	Range	Peak value	Range	Peak value (±SD)
MCGF	Fresh marrow	1.018–1.033	~1.033	5.5–8.5	6.21 ± 0.31 7.18 ± 0.24
	Cultured marrow	1.018–1.049	~1.033	4.5–7.0	5.91 ± 0.33 7.58 ± 0.12[b]
IL-2 + Con A	Fresh marrow	1.068–1.087	~1.075	2.0–4.0	3.27 ± 0.31 2.29 ± 0.44
	Cultured marrow	1.068–1.087	~1.075	2.0–3.0	2.53 ± 0.05

[a] LMC, long-term marrow culture; MCGF, mast-cell growth factor; VS, velocity of sedimentation.
[b] Data presented represent the average of three to five separate determinations.
[c] This second minor peak is sometimes not observed and may represent a more differentiated stage that gets diluted out upon long-term *in vitro* culture in LMC.

dividual fractions were analyzed for the presence of mast cell precursors or T cells and T-cell precursors (Table VIII). Additional studies were performed to determine the velocity sedimentation distribution of macrophage-granulocyte colony-forming cells in cultured bone marrow.

These studies showed that mast-cell precursors responsive to MCGF belong to a subpopulation of marrow cells characterized by low density ranging from 1.018 to 1.049 g/ml, and rapid rate of sedimentation ranging from 5 to 8 mm/hr. They are thus distinct from IL-2-responsive T cells or pre-T cells normally found in the density range of 1.068–1.087 and sedimenting at much slower rates of 2.0–4.0 mm/hr (Table VIII). Ginsburg *et al.* (1982) reported that mast cells derived from lymph node cells were Thy 1^-. Our studies are in support of their finding and further provide evidence for the existence of separate progenitors for mast cells and T cells.

Analysis of GM-CFU present in LMC by velocity of sedimentation showed great heterogeneity in their distribution, ranging from 3 to 8 mm/hr. Nevertheless, pure macrophage colony-forming cells (M-CFU) were found at the high end of the spectrum with a peak rate of 8 mm/hr. M-CFU are thus likely to be distinct from the majority of MCGF-responsive cells present in cultured marrow. However, mast-cell precursors could not be separated from most mixed GM-CFU. Thus, it remains to be determined whether a common progenitor exists for mast cells, granulocytes, and macrophages.

VI. MAST-CELL MATURATION IN LONG-TERM MARROW CULTURES

The long-term marrow culture system developed by Dexter and Lajtha (1976) in the mouse and subsequently adapted for sustained hematopoiesis in other species, including humans (Moore, 1982), has proved effective in initiating sustained mast-cell proliferation and differentiation in the absence of addition of any exogenous factors. Long-term cultures of marrow from many murine strains consistently exhibited production of cells with Alcian blue-positive granules, beginning 6–11 weeks after initiation of the cultures (Table IX and Fig. 5).

In addition to morphological and cytochemical features, biosynthesis of histamine and response to degranulating agents identified these cells as mast cells. The onset of mast-cell production coincided with an increase in the proportion of macrophages and a decline in the numbers of mature neutrophils and neutrophil progenitors (GM-CFU) (Table IX). Continuous production of macrophages and mast cells in murine marrow cultures has been observed for >1 year with weekly demidepopulation of culture suspension cells. Prolonged mast-cell production was also evident after 7–9 weeks of culture of murine spleen cells (Fig. 5) under conditions comparable to those used for murine long-term marrow cul-

Table IX. Influences of Strain on Duration of CFU-GM Production and Onset of Mast-Cell Production in Mouse Bone Marrow Cultures

Mouse strain	Time till (weeks): Loss of CFU-GM	Time till (weeks): Appearance of Mast Cell	Duration of observation (weeks)
DBA/2	20.1 ± 5.5	8.9 ± 2.1	25.3 ± 6.7
B6D2F$_1$	17.3 ± 6.0	8.9 ± 3.8	28.3 ± 10.0
C57BL/6	10.4 ± 2.7	5.8 ± 1.6	27.0 ± 8.5
AKR	11.3 ± 3.2	7.3 ± 2.5	13.0 ± 2.6
CBA	9.0 ± 7.0	4.5 ± 0.7	13.0 ± 1.4
BALB/c	12.7 ± 3.0	8.8 ± 1.0	22.0
(BALB/c × B6) F$_1$	10.3 ± .58	5.3 ± 0.58	15.0 ± 0
A	14.5 ± 1.5	5.8 ± 0.96	22.0
C3H	9.0	5.0	12.0
(C57BL/6 × CE) F$_1$	11.0	9.0	11.0
(CBA × NZB) F$_1$	14.0	6.0	14.0
(NZB × NZW) F$_1$	15.5 ± 2.1	11.5 ± 2.1	15.5 ± 2.1
NZW	12.0	11.0	12.0
NZB	4.5 ± 1.3	None	13.0 ± 4.1
NZC	5.0	None	10.0
C58	3.0	None	7.0
W/W^v	9.4 ± 4.2	None	16.0 ± 10.1
Sl/Sl^d	9.0 ± 7.1	None	15.0 ± 0.0

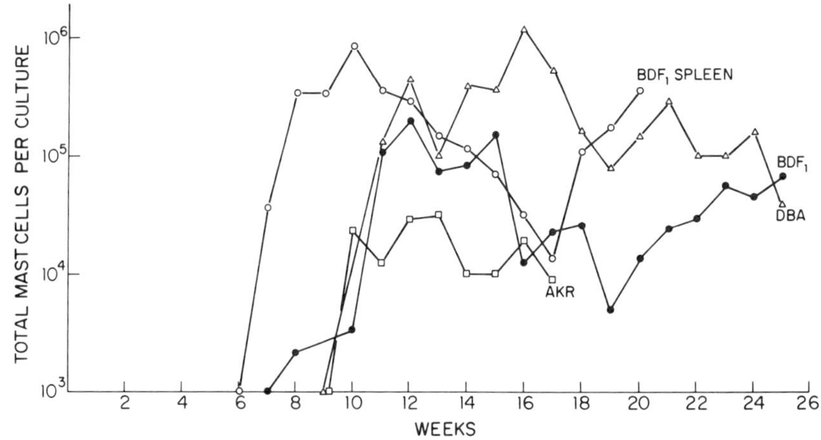

Figure 5. Mast-cell production by mouse bone marrow and spleen cultures.

ture. Spontaneous differentiation and proliferation of marrow-derived mast cells was also a feature of long-term cultures established from the prosimian tree shrew, *Tupia glis* (Moore, 1982). Marrow cultures established from this primate have exhibited sustained production of GM-CFU, differentiating neutrophils, and mast-cell production for >30 months. Periodicity of myelopoiesis and mast-cell production was evident in tree shrew marrow cultures with a close correlation between GM-CFU production and mast-cell incidence. Cultures initiated with 10^7 marrow cells produced 10^5 mast cells and approximately 10^6 mature neutophils per week, indicating that in contrast to the murine system, prolonged neutrophil production is not incompatible with generation of mast cells. While a correlation between mast-cell production and GM-CFU was evident in tree shrew cultures, morphological analysis of GM-CFU-derived colonies revealed only macrophages and neutrophils. Clonal proliferation of mast cells in semisolid agar was only evident in murine long-term marrow cultures after the decline of neutrophil/macrophage colony formation and then only as clusters of less than 40 cells after 7–10 days culture in the presence of an exogenous source of MCGF.

Comparison of long-term marrow cultures from various normal or genetically defective mice has revealed significant variations in the duration of GM-CFU production, neutrophil granulopoiesis, and onset of mast-cell production (Table X). Generally, the longer the duration of GM-CFU production, the more delayed the onset of mast-cell production. An unexpected observation was that marrow cultures established from NZB mice of all ages and independent of autoimmune status exhibited a very brief duration of GM-CFU and neutrophil production (Table X), displaying no evidence of mast-cell development over many months of observation. This finding is in marked contrast to the normal to hyperactive *in vivo* production of mast cells seen in this strain. We have observed defective

Table X. Comparison of Mast-Cell and Neutrophil Production in Long-Term Cultures of NZB, CBA, and (CBA × NZB) F_1 Marrow

Weeks of culture	CBA		NZB		(CBA × NZB) F_1	
	Mast[a] × 10^{-4}	PMN[a] × 10^{-4}	Mast[a] × 10^{-4}	PMN[a] × 10^{-4}	Mast[a] × 10^{-4}	PMN[a] × 10^{-4}
1–2	0	14.4	0	105.3	0	85.5
3–4	0	122.3	0	0	0	209.0
5–6	39.2	353.4	0	0	24.0	631.5
7–8	4.9	21.3	0	0	4.3	89.9
9–10	5.3	1.1	0	0	4.1	0.5
11–12	4.9	0	0	0	4.2	0
13–14	1.4	0	0	0	19.0	0

[a] Total mast cells and mature neutrophils (PMNs) per culture.

in vitro myelopoiesis and mast-cell production in certain other strains, such as NZC, RF, and C58, but not in cultures of marrow from related strains such as NZW or in F1 hybrids between NZB and NZW or CBA (Tables IX and X).

As reported elsewhere in this review, Sl/Sl^d and W/W^v genetically anemic mice have an *in vivo* defect in mast-cell production that can be corrected by marrow transplantation from *Sl* to *W* recipients. As shown in Table XI, mast-cell production was never observed in long-term marrow cultures of either W/W^v or Sl/Sl^d. In an attempt to duplicate the *in vivo* reconstitution experiments, we used long-term marrow coculture, a technique that we have shown to be effective in "curing" the hematopoietic stem-cell defects or hematopoietic microenvironmental abnormalities associated with these genetically anemic mice (Moore and Dexter, 1978). In Table XI the results of a series of such coculture experiments are shown. The coculture of equal numbers (5×10^6) of W/W^v, Sl/Sl^d, or NZB marrow with normal DBA marrow resulted in normal appearance of mast cells with sustained replication. This observation suggests that failure of mast cell development in NZB and other strains is not due to a suppressor mechanism. The combination of W/W^v (stem-cell defective) with Sl/Sl^d (microenvironment defective) did not reconstitute mast-cell production, but as predicted, the reverse combination resulted in a normal pattern of mast-cell development. Of considerable interest was the observation that W/W^v marrow, when used as a source of adherent microenvironment, was capable of inducing mast-cell development when NZB marrow was added, while neither mouse strain could produce mast cells *in vitro* when cultured on their own. This would suggest some type of accessory or microenvironmental abnormality in NZB mice. This contention is sup-

Table XI. Reconstitution of Mast-Cell Production by Marrow Coculture

Mouse strain	Time of loss of CFU-C (weeks)	Time of appearance of mast cells (weeks)	Duration of observation (weeks)
$W/W^v + W/W^v$	9.4 ± 4.2	None	16.0 ± 10.1
W/W^v + C57BL/6	12.0	7.0	33.0
W/W^v + DBA/2	15.0 ± 0.0	8.5 ± 2.1	24.0 ± 12.7
NZB + NZB	4.5 ± 1.3	None	13.0 ± 4.1
W/W^v + NZB	10.5 ± 6.4	4.0 ± 1.4	11.0 ± 5.7
NZB + DBA/2	13.0	11.0	15.0
$W/W^v + Sl/Sl^d$	6.0	7.0	15.0
$Sl/Sl^d + W/W^v$	4.0	None	15.0
$Sl/Sl^d + Sl/Sl^d$	9.0 ± 7.1	None	15.0 ± 0.0
Sl/Sl^d + NZB	4.0	None	15.0
Sl/Sl^d + DBA/2	15.0	9.0	15.0

Table XII. Hematopoietic Activity in 12-Week Suspension Cultures of NZB Bone Marrow in the Presence or Absence of Various Types of Macrophages[a]

	Total per culture × 10^5			Total per cultures		
				CFU-C		
Culture Type	Cells	Granulocytes	Mast cells	W-3CM	L-CCM	CFU-S[b]
NZB marrow	22.0	0.0	0.0	0	0	0
NZB marrow + AKR sup. Mφ	15.0	0.0	0.0	0	0	0
NZB marrow + peritoneal Mφ	5.5	0.0	0.0	0	0	0
NZB marrow + W/W^v sup. Mφ	20.0	0.0	1.0	0	0	0
NZB marrow + W/W^v ADH. Mφ	44.0	26.8	5.3	38,140	37,410	157

[a] Mφ, macrophage.
[b] CFU-S assayed at 11 weeks.

ported by the observation that the microenvironmentally defective Sl/Sl^d marrow was incapable of sustaining mast-cell development when seeded with NZB bone marrow (Table XI). In preliminary attempts to identify the adherent hematopoietic microenvironmental cell that is possibly defective in the *in vitro* NZB marrow culture system, we cocultured NZB marrow in the presence of 10^6 macrophages obtained from suspension cultures of AKR or W/W^v marrow or with allogeneic resident peritoneal macrophages. These cell sources failed to induce NZB mast-cell production (Table XII). Adherent W/W^v cells from prolonged marrow cultures and morphologically predominantly of macrophage type were, however, effective in restoring NZB mast-cell production even though the suspension macrophages from the same cultures were not (Table XII). Further biological, biochemical, and genetic analyses of these interesting murine models should throw light on the complex cellular and humoral regulation of mast-cell differentiation and proliferation.

VII. MAST-CELL DEFICIENCY IN W/W^v AND Sl/Sl^d ANEMIC MICE

As detailed in Section VI, the deficient mast-cell production in mice of the W/W^v and Sl/Sl^d genotypes could be reproduced *in vitro* in Dexter-type LMC. Studies in which bone marrow cells from the various strains were mixed in culture provided evidence in support of the theory that the mast-cell defect in $W/$

W^v anemic mice was due to a defect in mast-cell progenitors, whereas that in Sl/Sl^d anemic mice was due to a defective microenvironment.

With our ability to detect the MCGF and to generate and propagate mast cells *in vitro* in the presence of MCGF, we have further analyzed the cause of mast-cell deficiency in these defective mouse strains. Our studies provided some interesting information. Spleen cells from W/W^v and Sl/Sl^d mast-cell-deficient mice when stimulated *in vitro* with Con A produced as much MCGF as their normal littermates or other normal mouse strains (see Table XIII) (Yung and Moore, 1982). Thus, mast-cell deficiency in W/W^v and Sl/Sl^d mice, and more specifically the microenvironmental defect ascribed to Sl/Sl^d mice, was not the consequence of failure to produce MCGF. Cultures of bone marrow cells in the presence of MCGF further showed that mast-cell lines could be generated from W/W^v and Sl/Sl^d mice, although W/W^v mast cells appeared to grow less well than $W/+$ (Yung and Moore, 1982). Thus, mast cell precursors were present in W/W^v mice despite the presence of a stem-cell defect; Sl/Sl^d mice likewise did not lack mast-cell precursors. Similar studies involving the use of cultured marrow cells from LMC of the various strains showed identical results, i.e., while mast cells failed to mature in LMC of W/W^v and Sl/Sl^d mice, mast-cell precursors were nevertheless present and maintained for long periods in these LMCs (see Table XIII) (Yung *et al.*, 1983). Bartlett (1982) recently reported that pluripotential hemopoietic stem cells, detectable in a spleen colony (CFUs) assay, while deficient in the marrow of W/W^v anemic mice were nevertheless present in the brain in large numbers. It was also reported, by Hara *et al.* (1982), that despite lack of microscopically evident colony formation in the spleen of irradiated mice, hematopoietic cells of W/W^v mice did produce macroscopically evident mixed colonies containing erythroid, macrophage, and megakaryocytic cells (CFU-mix) *in vitro*, having number, size, and constitution comparable to those derived from $+/+$ mice. Thus, stem-cell deficiency in W/W^v mice was not due to total absence of stem cells. Our results with mast-cell precursors provide an interesting corollary.

Table XIII. Mast-Cell Deficiency in *W* and *Sl* Mice

Type of deficiency	W/W^v	$W/+$	$W/+$ W/W^v	Sl/Sl^d	$Sl/+$	$Sl/+$ Sl/Sl^d
Mature mast cells						
In vivo	Yes	No	No	Yes	No	Yes
In LMC	Yes	No	No	Yes	No	Yes
Mast-cell precursors						
In vivo	No	No	No	No	No	No
In LMC	No	No	No	No	No	No
MCGF production by spleen cells						
In vitro (+Con A)	No	No	ND[a]	No	No	ND

[a] ND, not done.

As pointed out by Hara *et al.* (1982), *in vivo* hematopoiesis in the W/W^v mice, although obviously deficient, is nevertheless sufficient for survival. Deficiency is thus more quantitative than qualitative in nature.

VIII. *IN VITRO* MATURATION OF LONG-TERM CULTURED MAST CELLS

A. Induction by LMC-Adherent Layers

The appearance of mature mast cells in LMC during the 6–12 weeks of culture prompted us to investigate whether LMC-adherent layers might be providing the environment necessary for mast-cell maturation. Cultured mast cells were introduced onto LMC-adherent layers depleted of suspension cells in the absence of MCGF (Yung and Moore, 1983). After 3 days of culture, morphologically mature mast cells could be detected in Wright's stained smear. Such mast cells resembled mature connective tissue mast cells, with dense, dark-staining cytoplasmic granules covering most of the cytoplasm. In the absence of the adherent layers and MCGF, cultured mast cells died within 24 hr. Moreover, in the presence of the adherent layers, 50% or more of the cells remained viable. Direct contact with the adherent layers appeared unnecessary, as the cultured mast cells could be separated from the adherent layers by means of a layer of 0.5% soft agar. Maturation appeared to be independent of the presence of MCGF, as at no time was MCGF detected in LMC supernate. In fact, supernate from LMC of various strains obtained at different times of culture appeared to have a partially inhibiting influence on mast-cell proliferation, although the supernates by themselves lacked maturation-inducing activity even when used undiluted. Thus, maturation could not be due to mere inhibition of the proliferative stimulus. Ultrastructurally, immature mast cells showed granules as homogeneous electron-dense membrane-bound inclusions or as membrane-bound vesicles (Fig.6). After culture on LMC adherent layers, reorganization of mast-cell granules was evident (Fig. 7A, B). Characteristic spiral lamellae or very electron-dense scrolls (Fig. 8) as described by Selye (1965) could be observed. Maturation was accompanied by a substantial increase in histamine content (from 0.2 to 2–3 pg/cell), increased density of surface IgE receptors, increased level of the enzyme chloracetate esterase, and acquisition of positive staining with safranin (Table XIV). It is of interest to point out that many of the mature mast cells contained lipid inclusions in their cytoplasm, and occasionally, clusters of mast cells could be observed to adhere to an adipocyte that presumably came loose from the adherent layer at the time the agarose was introduced onto the layer (Fig. 9). Rat mast-cell colonies had been observed to develop (Zucker-Franklin *et al.*, 1981) on top of lipid-containing macrophage colonies, and that lipid inclusions could be detected within such mast cells. Earlier studies (Potter and Wright, 1980) provided suggestive evidence for an active role of marrow lipids in murine hematopoiesis *in vivo* and in LMC. It thus appears that mast-cell maturation may be dependent on the presence of lipid or lipid-containing cells. Indeed, only well-formed LMC-adherent layers containing abundant lipid-containing cells were effective in inducing mast-cell maturation. LMC-adherent layers prior to 3 weeks of culture with no lipid accumulation, or degenerated adherent layers, failed to induce maturation. It was recently reported from our laboratory that lipid-containing cells present in LMC were of two different types: the classical fibroblast-derived adipocyte and a macrophage-derived lipid-containing cell (Castro-Malaspina *et al.*, 1982; Wang *et al.*, 1984a,b). The role of these lipid-containing cells on mast cell maturation is currently being analyzed.

Induction of maturation by LMC-adherent layers was not limited to cultured MCGF-dependent mast-cell lines. P815 murine mastocytoma cells, maintained in culture for long periods with no detectable mast-cell granule production, could nevertheless be induced to mature and acquire characteristic mature mast-cell granules (Fig. 8) (Yung and Moore, unpublished data). Mast-cell granule production in P815 mastocytoma cells has been reported by Mori *et al.* (1979, 1980). Using sodium butyrate as an inducing agent, these investigators demonstrated the formation of characteristic mast-cell granules in P815 cells. However, the granules formed were typed as the immature variety. More recently, Galli *et al.* (1982) reported on the maturation of cloned factor-dependent cultured mast cells induced by sodium butyrate, resulting in increased histamine production. It is as yet difficult to assess the importance of sodium butyrate on mast cell maturation. Further analysis of the ultrastructural and other histochemical changes would likely provide greater insight.

B. Mast-Cell Maturation on *Sl*/*Sl*^{d} LMC-Adherent Layers

In vivo mast-cell deficiency in *Sl*/*Sl*^{d} mice has been demonstrated to be due to a defect in the ability of stromal cells to support the differentiation of mast cells (Matsuda and Kitamura, 1981). Our data with LMC showing the lack of mast cell development from *Sl*/+ marrow introduced onto *Sl*/*Sl*^{d}-adherent layers appear to bear this out. Since LMC-adherent layers have been shown to induce maturation of MCGF-dependent cultured mast cells, it became of interest to determine whether failure of mast cells to appear in *Sl*/*Sl*^{d} LMC was due to failure to induce the terminal differentiation of mast cells. Cultured mast cells from various strains, as well as the mastocytoma P815 cells, when introduced onto *Sl*/*Sl*^{d} LMC-adherent layers overlaid with a layer of agar, gave rise to mature mast cells, as did adherent layers from the normal littermates (Yung and Moore, 1983). Thus, the *in vitro* *Sl*/*Sl*^{d} defect was not due to an inability of the marrow adherent cells to induce terminal mast-cell differentiation.

To recapitulate, while mast cells are deficient *in vivo* in *W*/*W*^{v} and *Sl*/*Sl*^{d} mice, these mice do not lack mast-cell precursors responsive to MCGF *in vitro*.

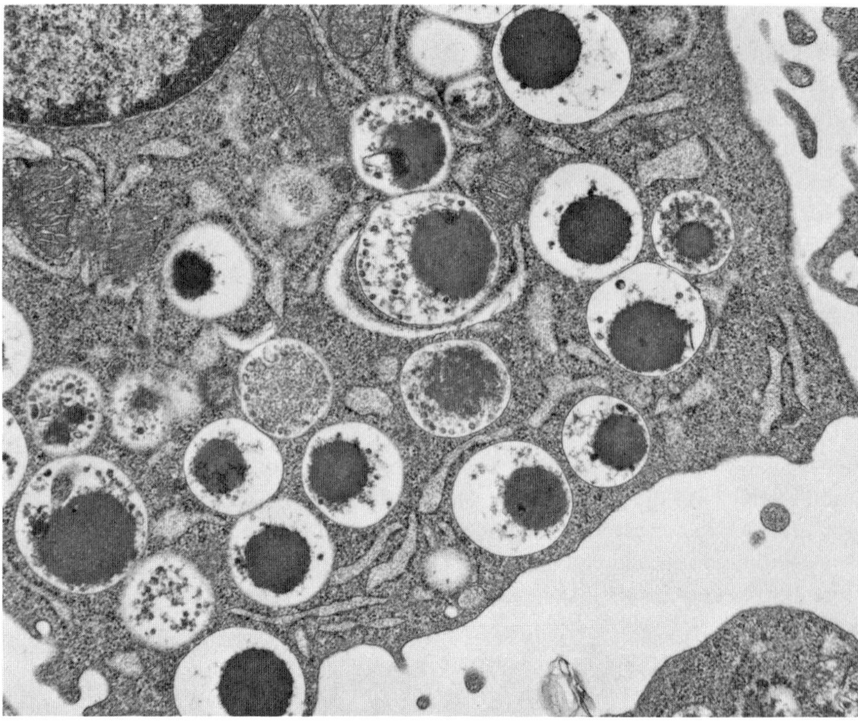

Figure 6. Ultrastructure of immature cultured mast cells showing membrane-bound granules containing electron-dense homogeneous and vesicular material.

LMC of both strains fail to generate mast cells even upon extended culture, but nevertheless maintain MCGF-responsive mast-cell precursors. LMC-adherent layers of W/W^v mice support mast-cell differentiation from $W/+$ or Sl/Sl^d marrow, but Sl/Sl^d-adherent layers failed to support mast-cell differentiation from $Sl/+$ marrow. Sl/Sl^d-adherent layers, nevertheless, can induce maturation of MCGF-dependent mast cells like any other normal strains (see Table XIII). These findings may seem contradictory, as on the one hand they indicate a mast-cell deficiency *in vivo* and *in vitro* (in LMC), and yet indicate no lack of mast-cell precursors, no lack of ability to induce terminal mast-cell differentiation, and, as pointed out earlier, no defect in the ability of the animals to produce MCGF. One should bear in mind, however, that while Sl/Sl^d and W/W^v mice are anemic, hematopoiesis was nevertheless adequate to enable them to survive. Deficiencies in these mice are thus likely to be quantitative in nature. While mast cells are deficient *in vivo* and in the environment of the LMC, under the selective advan-

Figure 7. (A, B) Electron micrographs showing ultrastructural changes of mast-cell granules after culture on agar overlaid LMC-adherent layers for 3 days.

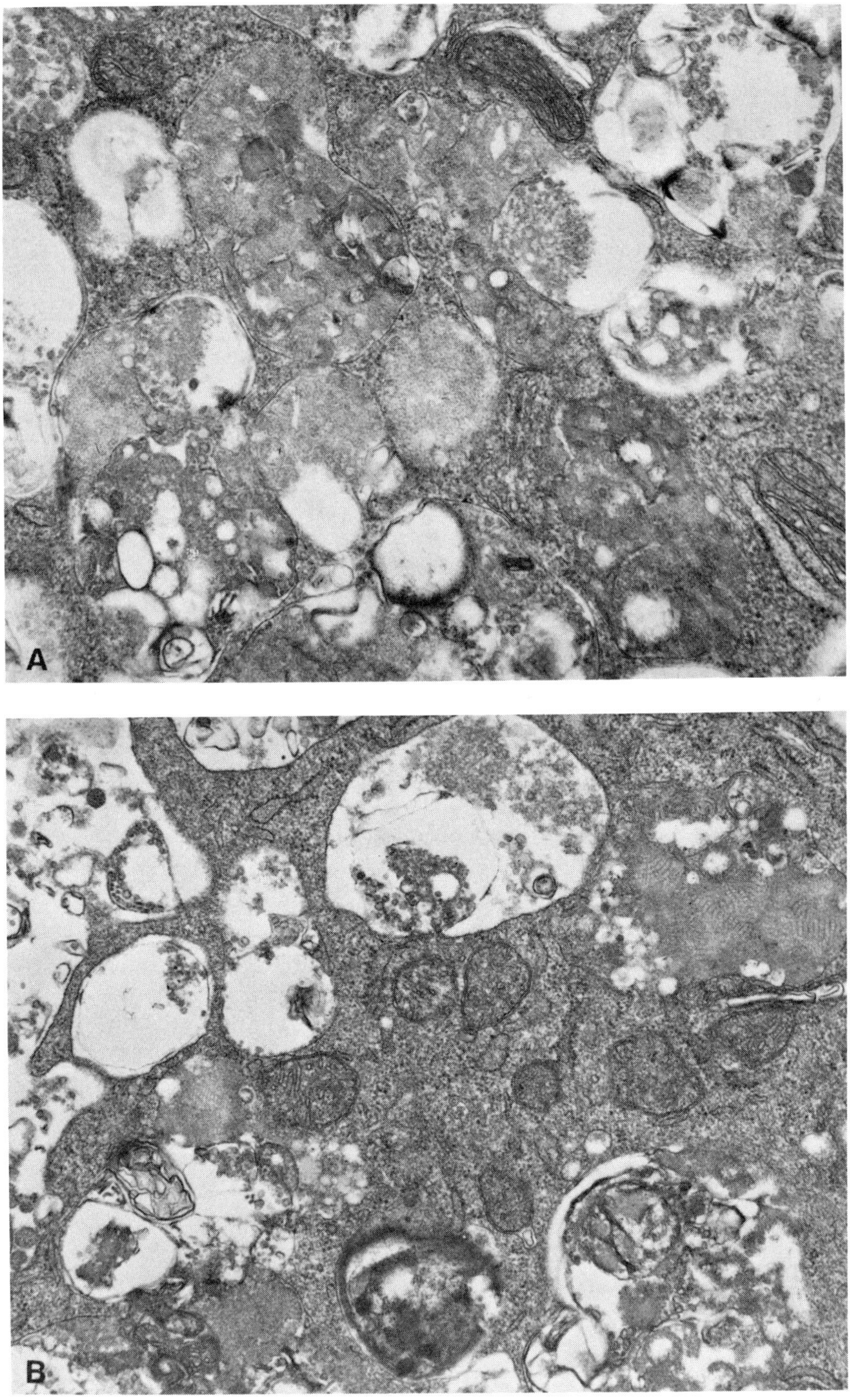

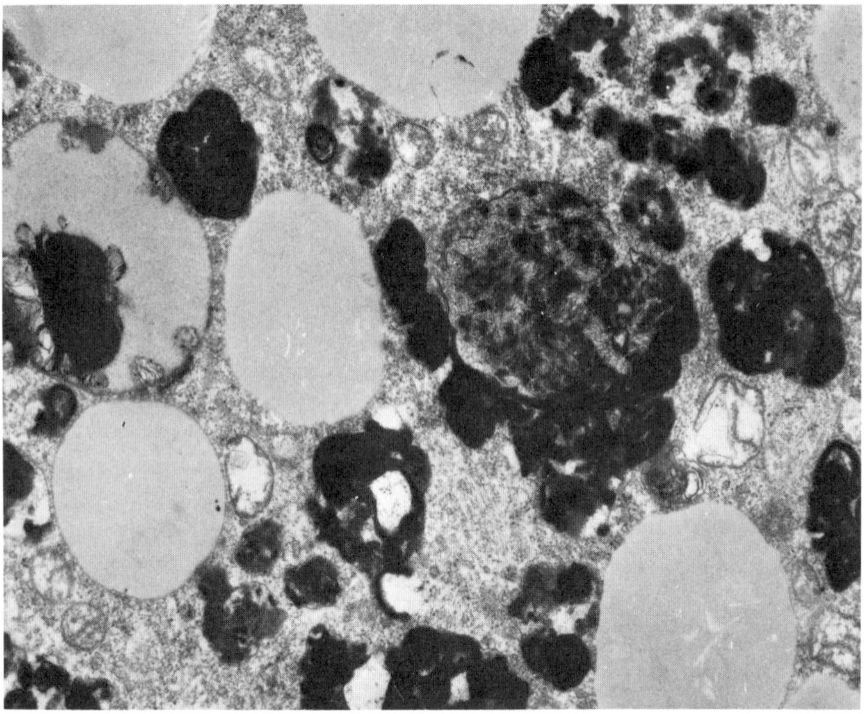

Figure 8. Electron micrograph showing ultrastructure of P815 mastocytoma cell granules formed after culture on agar overlaid LMC-adherent layers. Note electron dense ropy and scroll-like material, and presence of lipid inclusions in the cytoplasm.

Table XIV. Effects of LMC-Adherent Layers on MCGF-Cultured Mast Cells[a]

Type of marker	Assay method	No. days of culture on LMC-Adherent layer	Total histamine per 10^6 cells (ng)	Percent positive cells
Ia	Immuno-	0	–	16.5 ± 0.7
	fluorescence	3	–	43.7 ± 5.1
FcRa	Immuno-	0	–	33
	fluorescence	3	–	76.5 ± 6.4
Histamine	OPT reaction[b]	0	850	<1
		3	2800 ± 530	46.3 ± 7.5
Chloracetate	Histochemical	0	–	48.5 ± 3.5
esterase	staining	3	–	77.7 ± 14.0

[a] LMC, long-term marrow culture; MCGF, mast-cell growth factor; OPT, *o*-phthalaldehyde.
[b] Detected by fluorescence under UV light according to the method described by Guy-Grand *et al.* (1978).
[c] Total histamine content was determined by the method described by Breithaupt and Haberman (1969).

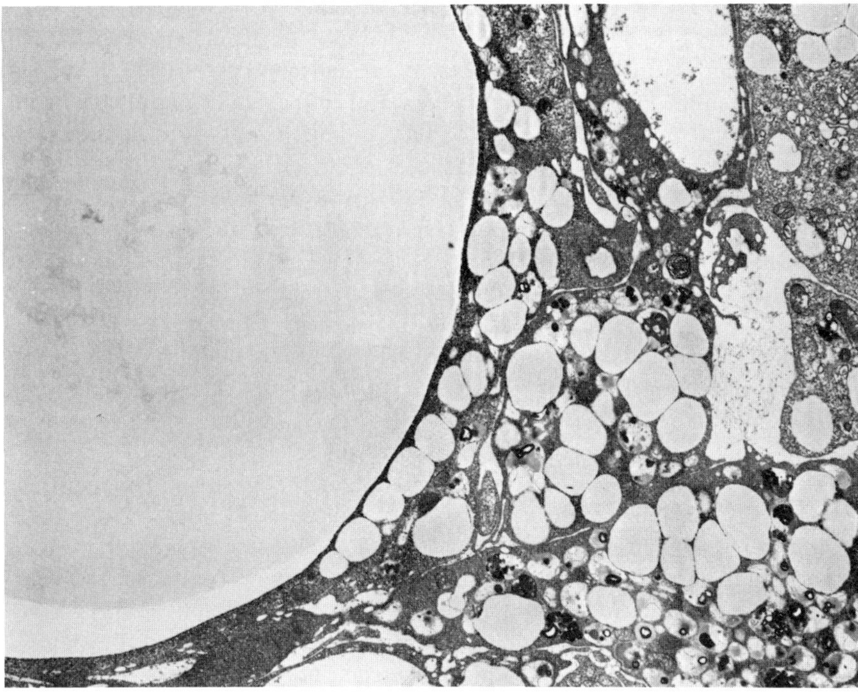

Figure 9. Electron micrograph showing adherence of maturing P815 mastocytoma cells onto a large adipocyte.

tage of the culture condition provided by the presence of MCGF, the mast-cell precursors present in these mice and in the LMC can differentiate and proliferate and, provided the right microenvironmental conditions are present, can mature fully.

IX. ARE CULTURED MCGF-DEPENDENT MAST CELLS MUCOSAL MAST CELLS?

Ginsburg *et al.* (1982) reported the existence of two types of mast cells, one derived from lymphoid tissue, referred to as mucosal mast cells, and the other found in connective tissue, was termed connective tissue mast cells. According to their studies, mucosal mast cells proliferate rapidly in the presence of T-cell-derived factor (Ginsburg *et al.*, 1981, 1982), are smaller in size, with sparse, large, metachromatic granules, low histamine content, low density of surface IgE receptors, and short life span. In contrast, connective tissue mast cells have slow growth rate, are independent of T-cell-derived factor, larger in size, possess tiny homogeneous metachromatic granules that fill most of the cytoplasm, have high histamine content, dense surface IgE receptors, and a long life span. The ability of T cells to support the growth of rat mucosal mast cells was recently reported

(Haig *et al.*, 1982). A T-cell origin for mucosal mast cells was suggested by Guy-Grand *et al.* (1978) after observing the presence of characteristic mast cell granules in mouse gut T lymphocytes. Befus and co-workers (1982) isolated mast cells from the intestinal lamina propria and epithelium of rats infected with *Nippostrongylus brasiliensis* and noted their morphological, histochemical, and functional differences from peritoneal mast cells. Razin *et al.* (1982) demonstrated the presence of a chondroitin sulfate proteoglycan distinct from heparin synthesized by cultured bone marrow-derived mast-cell lines. Similar findings were made by Galli *et al.* (1982). Ruitenberg and Elgersma (1976) reported on the absence of intestinal mast cell response in congenitally athymic mice during parasitic infection. Wlodarski *et al.* (1982), however, observed greater numbers of mast cells in popliteal lymph nodes of homozygous nude (*nu*/*nu*), and in phenotypically normal heterozygous (+/*nu*) BALB/c mice than in normal (+/+) BALB/c mice; they also noted that nude mice infected with hepatitis virus accumulated many more mast cells than did healthy mice.

While all these findings may appear to support the presence of two distinct types of mast cells, we nevertheless believe that a different interpretation must be considered. The *in vivo* studies of Kitamura and co-workers (1979a) clearly demonstrated a marrow origin for both mucosal and connective tissue mast cells. Their studies with Sl/Sl^d mutant mice (Matsuda and Kitamura, 1981) further demonstrated a requirement for an accessary cell of stromal origin for supporting the differentiation of circulating precursors into mature mast cells. Their studies suggest that mature mast cells as well as stromal cells do not normally migrate to the skin. Migration of stromal cells occurs in the presence of a wound, and differentiation of circulating precursors into mast cells occurs only at the site of the wound. Thus, tissue mast cells represent more a state of maturation than a separate lineage of mast cells. Our *in vitro* studies appear to support this model of mast cell differentiation. Thus, bone marrow-derived precursors in the presence of MCGF differentiate into immature mast cells. In the presence of a marrow stromal element, as provided by an LMC-adherent layer, such immature mast cells or mastoblasts differentiate terminally into mature mast cells. The failure to detect heparin in cultured mast-cell lines may reflect an *in vitro* artifact. Moreover, it may also reflect a maturation as well as a functional state. As mast cells are widely distributed throughout the mammalian body, there are likely to be subpopulations reflecting functional diversity and specialization, which must be distinguished from differences in lineage origin.

X. CONCLUDING REMARKS

Much of the mystery surrounding the mast-cell system has been unveiled during the past few years. It is now clear that this connective tissue cell has its origin in the hematopoietic system and that it shares a common ancestor with the rest of the hematopoietic cells, i.e., the pluripotential stem cell. Moreover, a committed mast-cell progenitor, distinct from T-lymphocyte precursors, and possibly different from myeloid progenitors, exists. While the early events leading to the commitment toward the mast-cell pathway remain obscure, the role of MCGF in the subsequent differentiation and proliferation of mast cells or mastoblasts from the precursors is apparent. Studies with long-term marrow cultures point to a role of marrow-adherent cells in the induction of mast-cell maturation, although the precise mechanism has yet to be elucidated. Results obtained from the study of W/W^v and Sl/Sl^d mast-cell-deficient mouse strains may appear contradictory; they nevertheless provide suggestive evidence for the presence of other levels of regulation of the mast cell system. The deficiency, but not total absence of mast cells in these mice, may perhaps indirectly be a hint to the hitherto obscure physiological importance of the mast cell system. The question regarding the identity or lack of identity of MCGF and other hematopoietic factors is an important one and hinges on our current concept of hematopoietic regulation by target-specific factors. With advances in molecular genetics, this issue will likely be resolved in the near future.

XI. REFERENCES

Aglietta, M., Camussi, G., and Piacibello, W., 1981, *Exp. Hematol.* 9:95.

Bartlett, P. F., 1982, *Proc. Natl. Acad. Sci. USA* 79:2722.

Befus, A. D., Pearce, F. L., Gauldie, J., Horsewood, P., and Bienenstock, J., 1982, *J. Immunol.* **128**:2475.

Broxmeyer, H. E., 1982a, *J. Clin. Invest.* 69:632.

Broxmeyer, H. E., 1982b, *J. Immunol.* **129**:1002.

Broxmeyer, H. E., Smithyman, A., Eger, R. R., Meyers, P. A., and DeSousa, M., 1978, *J. Exp. Med.* **148**:1052.

Broxmeyer, H. E., Ralph, P., Bognacki, J., Kincade, P. W., and DeSousa, M., 1980, *J. Immunol.* **125**:903.

Broxmeyer, H. E., Pelus, L. M., Gillis, S., Kincade, P., DeSousa, M., and Moore, M. A. S., 1981, in: *Heterogeneity of Mononuclear Phagocytes* (M. Landy and O. Forester, eds.), pp. 153–155, Academic Press, New York.

Buisseret, P. D., 1982, *Sci. Am.* **247**:86.

Burgess, A. W., Metcalf, D., Russell, S. H. M., and Nicola, N. A., 1980, *Biochem. J.* **185**:301.

Burgess, A. W., and Metcalf, D., 1980, *Blood* **56**:947.

Burnet, F. M., 1965, *J. Pathol.* 89:271.

Burnet, F. M., 1977, *Cell Immunol.* **30**:358.

Breithaupt, H., and Haberman, E., 1969, *Naunyn Schmiedebergs Arch. Pharmacol.* **261**:252.

Castro-Malaspina, H., Wang, S. Y., Lee, J. S., and Moore, M. A. S., 1982, *Blood* **60** (Suppl. 1) abst. 349.

Clark-Lewis, I., and Schrader, J., 1981, *J. Immunol.* **127**:1941.

Czarnetzki, B. M., 1981, *Fed. Proc.* **40**:1026 (abst.).

Dexter, T. M., and Lajtha, L. G., 1976, *Bibl. Haematol.* **43**:1.

Ehrlich, P., 1879, *Arch. Anat. Physiol.* (Lpz) *Physiol. Abt.* 166.

Fauser, A. A., Neuman, H. A., Bross, K. G., Kanz, L., and Lohr, G. W., 1982, *Blood* **60**: 1317.

Fernex, M., 1968, *The Mast-Cell System, its Relationship to Atherosclerosis, Fibrosis, and Eosinophils*, Williams and Wilkins, Baltimore.

Galli, S. J., Dvorak, A. M., Marcum, J. A., Ishizaka, T., Nabel, G., Simonian, H. D., Pyne, K., Goldin, J. M., Rosenberg, R. D., Cantor, H., and Dvorak, H. F., 1982, *J. Cell Biol.* **95:** 435.

Ginsburg, H., and Lagunoff, D., 1967, *Cell Biol.* **35:**685.

Ginsburg, H., and Sachs, L., 1962, *J. Natl. Cancer Inst.* **31:**1.

Ginsburg, H., Nir, I., Hammel, I., Eren, R., Weissman, B.-A., and Naot, Y., 1978, *Immunology* **35:**485.

Ginsburg, H., Olson, E. C., Huff, T. F., Okudaira, H., and Ishizaka, T., 1981, *Int. Arch. Allergy Appl. Immunol.* **66:**447.

Ginsburg, H., Ben-Shahan, D., and Ben-David, E., 1982, *Immunology* **45:**371.

Greenberger, J. S., Gano, P. J., Davisson, P. B., and Moloney, W. C., 1979, *Blood* **53:**987.

Guy-Grand, D., Griscelli, C., and Vassalli, P., 1978, *J. Exp. Med.* **148:**1661.

Haig, D. M., McKee, T. A., and Jarrett, E. E. E., 1982, *Nature* **300:**188.

Hara, H., Ohe, Y., Noguchi, K., Tsuyama, K., and Kitamura, Y., 1982, *Cell Tissue Kinet.* **15:**25.

Hasthorpe, S., 1980, *J. Cell. Physiol.* **105:**379.

Hatanaka, K., Kitamura, Y., and Nishimune, Y., 1979, *Blood* **53:**142.

Ihle, J. N., Rebar, L., Keller, J., Lee, J. C., and Hapel, A., 1982a, *Immunol. Rev.* **63:**5.

Ihle, J., Keller, J., Greenberger, J. S., Henderson, L., Yetter, R. A., and Morse, H. C., 1982b, *J. Immunol.* **129:**1377.

Ihle, J., Keller, J., Henderson, L., Klein, F., and Palaszynski, E., 1982c, *J. Immunol.* **129:** 2431.

Ihle, J., Keller, J., Oroszlan, S., Henderson, L. E., Copeland, T. D., Fitch, F., Prystowsky, M. B., Goldwasser, E., Schrader, J. W., Palaszynski, E., Dy, M., and Lebel, B., 1983, *J. Immunol.* **131:**282.

Iscove, N. N., Roitsch, C. A., Williams, N., and Guilbert, L. J., 1982, *J. Cell. Physiol. Suppl.* **1:**65.

Ishizaka, T., Okudaira, H., Mauser, L. E., and Ishizaka, K., 1976, *J. Immunol.* **116:**747.

Johnson, G. R., and Metcalf, D., 1980, *Exp. Hematol.* **8:**549.

Jones-Villeneuve, E. V., and Phillips, R. A., 1980, *Exp. Hematol.* **8:**65.

Kitamura, Y., Go, S., and Hatanaka, K., 1978, *Blood* **52:**447.

Kitamura, Y., Matsuda, H., and Hatanaka, K., 1979a, *Nature* **281:**154.

Kitamura, Y., Shimada, M., Go, S., Matsuda, H., Hatanaka, K., and Seki, M., 1979b, *J. Exp. Med.* **150:**482.

Kobata, A., Grollman, E. F., and Ginsburg, V., 1968, *Biochim. Biophys. Res. Commun.* **32:** 272.

Kurland, J., and Moore, M. A. S., 1977, in: *Experimental Hematology Today* (S. J. Baum and G. D. Ledney, eds.), pp. 51–62, Springer-Verlag, New York.

Kurland, J. I., Pelus, L. M., Ralph, P., Bockman, R. S., and Moore, M. A. S., 1979, *Proc. Natl. Acad. Sci. USA* **76:**2326.

Lee, J. C., Hapel, A. J., and Ihle, J. N., 1982, *J. Immunol.* **128:**2393.

Lennert, K., and Parwaresch, M. R., 1979, *Histopathol.* **3:**349.

McCarthy, J. H., Mandel, T. E., Garson, O. M., and Metcalf, D., 1980, *Exp. Hematol.* **8:**562.

Matsuda, H., and Kitamura, Y., 1981, *Exp. Hematol.* **9:**38.

Metcalf, D., and Moore, M. A. S., 1971, *Hematopoietic Cells*, Elsevier–North-Holland, Amsterdam.

Moore, M. A. S., 1982, in: *Recent Advances in Haematology* (A. V. Hoffbrand, ed.), pp. 109–142, Churchill Livingstone, New York.

Moore, M. A. S., and Dexter, T. M., 1978, *Transplant Proc.* **10:**83.

Moore, M. A. S., and Sheridan, A. P., 1982, in: *Maturation Factors and Cancer* (M. A. S. Moore, ed.), pp. 361–376, Raven Press, New York.
Moore, M. A. S., and Yung, Y. P., 1982, in: *Expression of Differentiated Functions in Cancer Cells* (R. F. Revoltella, G. M. Pontieri, C. Basilico, G. Rovera, R. C. Gallo, and J. H. Subak-Sharpe, eds.), pp. 213–221, Raven Press, New York.
Mori, Y., Akedo, H., Tanaka, K., Tanigaki, Y., and Okada, M., 1979, *Exp. Cell. Res.* **118**: 15.
Mori, Y., Akedo, H., Tanigaki, Y., Tanaka, K. M., Okada, M., and Nakamura, N., 1980, *Exp. Cell. Res.* **127**:465.
Nabel, G., Galli, S. J., Dvorak, A. M., Dvorak, H. F., and Cantor, H., 1981, *Nature* **291**:332.
Nagao, K., Yokoro, K., and Aaronson, S. A., 1981, *Science* **212**:333.
Nakahata, T., and Ogawa, 1982, *Proc. Natl. Acad. Sci. USA* **79**:3843.
Paff, G. H., Bloom, F., and Reilly, C., 1947, *J. Exp. Med.* **86**:117.
Pelus, L. M., Broxmeyer, H. E., and Moore, M. A. S., 1981, *Cell Tissue Kinet.* **14**:515.
Pelus, L. M., Saletan, S., Silver, R. T., and Moore, M. A. S., 1982, *Blood* **59**:284.
Pepys, J., and Edwards, A. M. (eds.), 1979, *The Mast Cell: Its Role in Health and Disease*, Pitman Medical, New York.
Pfizenmaier, K., Rollionghoff, M., and Wagner, H., 1982, *Curr. Top. Microbiol. Immunol.* **100**:203.
Potter, J. E. R., and Wright, E. G., 1980, *Am. J. Hematol.* **8**:361.
Pretlow, T. G., and Cassady, I. M., 1970, *Am. J. Pathol.* **61**:323.
Ralph, P., Moore, M. A. S., and Nilsson, K., 1976, *J. Exp. Med.* **143**:1828.
Razin, E., Stevens, R. L., Akiyama, F., Schmid, K., and Austen, K. F., 1982, *J. Biol. Chem.* **257**:7229.
Ruitenberg, E. J., and Elgersma, A., 1976, *Nature* **264**:258.
Schrader, J. W., 1981, *J. Immunol.* **126**:452.
Schrader, J. W., and Clark-Lewis, I., 1982a, *J. Immunol.* **129**:30.
Schrader, J. W., and Clark-Lewis, I., 1982b, *Curr. Top. Microbiol. Immunol.* **100**:221.
Schrader, J. W., Clark-Lewis, I., and Culvenor, J. G., 1981, *Proc. Natl. Acad. Sci. USA* **78**: 323.
Selye, H., 1965, *The Mast Cells*, Butterworths, Washington.
Sheridan, J. W., and Metcalf, D., 1973, *J. Cell. Physiol.* **81**:11.
Stanley, E. R., Hansen, G., Woodcock, J., and Metcalf, D., 1975, *Fed. Proc.* **34**:2272.
Stanley, E. R., Cifone, M., Hear, P. M., and Defendi, V., 1976, *J. Exp. Med.* **143**:631.
Tertian, G., Yung, Y.-P., and Moore, M.A.S., 1980, *J. Supramol. Struct.* **13**:533.
Tertian, G., Yung, Y.-P., Guy-Grand, D., and Moore, M. A. S., 1981, *J. Immunol.* **127**:788.
Valtonen, E. J., 1961, *Acta. Pathol. Microbiol. Scand. Suppl.* 151, pp. 1–96.
Wang, S. Y., Castro-Malaspina, H., and Moore, M. A. S., 1984a (submitted).
Wang, S. Y., Castro-Malaspina, H., Lu, L., and Moore, M. A. S., 1984b, *Blood* (in press).
Wlodarski, K., Morrison, K., and Rose, N. R., 1982, *Scand. J. Immunol.* **15**:105.
Yung, Y.-P., and Moore, M.A.S., 1982, *J. Immunol.* **129**:1256.
Yung, Y.-P., Tertian, G., and Moore, M. A. S., 1980, *Fourth International Congress of Immunology* (abst.) 13.3.19.
Yung, Y.-P., Eger, R., Tertian, G., and Moore, M. A. S., 1981, *J. Immunol.* **127**:794.
Yung, Y.-P., Wang, S. Y., and Moore, M. A. S., 1983, *J. Immunol.* **130**:2843.
Zitcer, E. M., Elsasser, W. H., and Kirk, P. L., 1953, *Growth* **17**:111.
Zucker-Franklin, D., 1980, *Blood* **56**:534.
Zucker-Franklin, D., Grusky, G., Hirayama, N., and Schnipper, E., 1981, *Blood* **58**:544.

Soluble-Factor Induction of B-Cell Growth

Maureen Howard

Laboratory of Microbial Immunity
National Institute of Allergy and Infectious Diseases
National Institutes of Health
Bethesda, Maryland 20205

I. INTRODUCTION

Despite a detailed knowledge of the antigen-specific receptor expressed on the membrane of B lymphocytes, the precise mechanism by which B lymphocytes are activated during an antigenic encounter has remained an area of controversy. Contending viewpoints originally attributed induction of proliferation to the delivery of signals at membrane-bound immunoglobulin (Ig) itself, at membrane-bound Ia molecules, or at uncharacterized membrane-bound mitogen receptors. However, the recent discovery of soluble factors specifically involved in B-cell proliferation has undermined such simplistic models. Now a more tenable hypothesis would seem to be that occupancy of membrane Ig (or mitogen receptors) by antigen and/or cognate T-cell interactions involving the Ia antigens of resting B cells results in functional expression of receptors for soluble proliferation cofactors and that it is these factors that in turn stimulate B cells to replicate. This chapter discusses the biological and biochemical nature of such B-cell-specific proliferation cofactors (B-cell growth factors) and considers what is currently known of their role in B-cell activation and development.

II. EVIDENCE FOR UNIQUE B-CELL PROLIFERATION COFACTORS

The concept that both antigenic and mitogenic activation of resting B cells results in functional expression of receptors for soluble proliferation and/or differentiation cofactors was initially proposed by Andersson, Melchers, and colleagues in light of experiments using either antigen-activated B cells or lipopolysaccharide (LPS) blasts together with factor-containing supernatants from antigen-stimulated long-term helper T-cell lines (Andersson and Melchers, 1981; Andersson *et al.*, 1980). While the expression of growth-factor receptors on B cells is yet to be directly demonstrated experimentally, the general notion is supported by numerous subsequent reports. A particularly valuable system for addressing such events has been the stimulation of B cells with affinity purified anti-Ig antibodies as polyclonal analogs for antigen. First developed in the rabbit system by Sell and Gell (1965) and adapted to mouse lymphocytes by Parker (1975) and Weiner *et al.* (1976), anti-Ig stimulation combines the advantages that it acts on the receptors for antigen for virtually all B cells and that the resultant activation is restricted to DNA synthesis without development of antibody-forming cells (Kishimoto and Ishizaka, 1975; Parker *et al.*, 1979). Using this system, Parker provided convincing evidence that soluble T-cell-derived factors, which had no apparent effect on resting B cells, enhanced anti-Ig-induced B-cell proliferation particularly when relatively low concentrations of anti-Ig were used (Parker, 1980, 1982). More recently, definitive proof that antigen-induced B-cell proliferation requires soluble cofactors has been provided by Nossal and colleagues (Vaux *et al.*, 1981; Pike *et al.*, 1982). Using the elegant single-cell cloning assay of Wetzel and Kettman (1981), they cultured individual affinity-purified hapten-specific B cells and showed that antigen-specific B-cell proliferation was only obtained in the presence of exogenously supplied cofactor-rich supernatants.

A major problem in precisely identifying factors involved in B-cell proliferation has been the lack of simple functional assays in which contaminating accessory cells capable of mediating secondary effects have been excluded. Even some B-cell cloning assays do not escape this dilemma, as they often depend on filler cell supplements. In an attempt to overcome this problem, we have developed a short-term B-cell costimulator assay (Howard *et al.*, 1982) in which highly purified B cells are cultured at low cell density, greatly reducing the possibility of accessory and T-cell contamination. The B-cell purification method of choice is one of negative selection (Leibson *et al.*, 1981) and yields a population of small lymphocytes, 98-99% of which express membrane Ig. In order to trigger a large proportion of these cells, affinity-purified anti-IgM antibodies are used as a polyclonal stimulus, with proliferation monitored after 3 days' culture via uptake of [^{3}H]thymidine. Others have shown that approximately 50% of resting splenic B cells can be induced to synthesize DNA in this type of assay (DeFranco *et al.*, 1982). This subset is often referred to as the Lyb-5$^+$ population of normal mouse B cells (Ahmed *et al.*, 1977).

Using this low-cell-density B-cell costimulator assay, we found that three separate stimuli were required to cause the Lyb-5$^+$ subset of small B lymphocytes to enter the S phase of the cell cycle: (1) a signal delivered by antibodies specific for the Ig receptor expressed on the B-cell membrane, (2) a signal delivered by a T-cell-derived factor that we initially designated B-cell growth factor (BCGF), and (3) a signal delivered by the macrophage-derived factor Interleukin-1 (IL-1) (Howard *et al.*, 1982, 1983b). BCGF and IL-1 act in an antigen-nonspecific, synergistic manner. Full details of our current progress in characterization of this BCGF are provided in the following sections. Identification of IL-1 as the macrophage product involved is based on correlation of B-cell and thymocyte costimulating activities following a series of biochemical purification procedures (Howard *et al.*, 1983b). Both murine IL-1 purified to apparent homogeneity (Mizel and Mizel, 1981) and human IL-1 pruified to high specific activity (Lachman *et al.*, 1977, 1980) showed excellent B-cell costimulating activity in this assay system. Indeed, in the final step in the mouse IL-1 purification scheme, B-cell and thymocyte costimulatory activity exhibited identical migration patterns. While our data provide compelling support for the notion that BCGF and IL-1 are B-cell-specific proliferation cofactors, ultimate proof of these agents acting directly on B cells will await either single-cell assays driven by these factors or reagents capable of demonstrating specific factor–receptor binding.

These results on factor involvement in B-cell proliferation are consistent with many previously reported observations, in addition to helping resolve some areas of conflict. In particular, the involvement of accessory cells in anti-IgM-induced B-cell proliferation had previously been a matter of controversy. It had been proposed by some laboratories that anti-Ig-induced proliferation proceeded independently of T cells and other accessory cells, as vigorous depletion of such cell types failed to prevent activation (Parker, 1975; Sieckmann *et al.*, 1978). However, involvement of macrophages had been reported by Mongini *et al.* (1978), and Parker's more recent work on T-cell-derived factors suggested a need for T cells (Parker, 1980, 1982). It would now appear that failure to observe the need for one or both cell types reflects the use of assay conditions in which small numbers of one or both accessory cells are present with consequent endogenous factor production. Our own experiments showed a need for both exogenous BCGF and IL-1 only at low cell densities ($\leqslant 2 \times 10^4$ cells/wells), despite the rigorous B-cell purification procedure employed. It would thus appear that very small numbers of accessory cells can provide B-cell-stimulatory cofactors.

Recently, a second murine B-cell growth factor has been introduced into the literature, with roman numeral suffixes adopted as the system of nomenclature (Swain *et al.*, 1983). To date, BCGF-II is distinguished from the BCGF-I described above simply on the basis of differential responsiveness in a variety of functional assays (Swain *et al.*, 1983). However, preliminary biochemical characterization of BCGF-II appears to distinguish these two lymphokines further (S. Swain and R. Dutton, personal communication; M. Howard, unpublished data). As yet, the relationships and/or interactions between these two growth factors are unclear. In view of the limited information currently available on BCGF-II, it will not be discussed further here.

III. BIOLOGICAL CHARACTERISTICS OF MOUSE BCGF-I

In cultures of mouse B lymphocytes, the term BCGF-I is currently used to designate the T-cell-derived B-cell costimulator that synergizes with affinity-purified anti-IgM antibodies to induce polyclonal B-cell proliferation (Howard *et al.*, 1982, 1983a). Although IL-1 is not generally added to these cultures, the conditions employed probably permit its endogenous production (refer to Section II). BCGF-I is found in culture supernatants of a subline of the thymoma, EL4, following stimulation with phorbol myristate acetate (PMA) (Howard *et al.*, 1982) and in antigen-induced supernatants from normal T-cell helper lines (Howard *et al.*, 1983a) propagated in long-term culture as described by Kimoto and Fathman (1980). An example of a standard BCGF-I assay showing the relative BCGF-I activity in these two supernatants is given in Fig. 1. Surprisingly, BCGF-I is not detected in supernatants of spleen cells cultured for 24 hr with Concanavalin A (Con A) or phytohemagglutinin (PHA). BCGF-I has little or no apparent action on resting B cells, and its effect on anti-IgM-activated B cells is polyclonal, genetically unrestricted, and seemingly limited to DNA synthesis without the production of antibody-forming cells (Howard *et al.*, 1982). It also acts as a proliferation costimulator for at least some B cells activated with LPS. When cultures are supplemented with additional differentiation cofactors, BCGF-I is found to be an essential component of both antigen-specific (Howard *et al.*, 1982) and polyclonal anti-Ig-induced (Nakanishi *et al.*, 1982) AFC responses. Preliminary experiments have indicated that BCGF-I is required for antigen-specific proliferation of affinity-purified hapten-specific B cells stimulated by hapten conjugated to the semisynthetic polysaccharide Ficoll (M. Howard, Pillai, Scott, and W. E. Paul, work in progress).

BCGF-I can be separated from Interleukin-2 (IL-2) by several different methods, including gel filtration, phenyl Sepharose chromatography, sodium dodecylsulfate-polyacrylamide gel electrophoresis (SDS-PAGE), Tris-glycinate-PAGE, and isoelectric focusing, as well as by cellular absorption (Howard *et al.*, 1982; Farrar *et al.*, 1982, 1983). It can be distinguished both functionally and by molecular weight from other previously described T-cell factors, e.g., T-cell replacing factor (TRF) (Dutton *et al.*, 1971; Schimpl and Wecker, 1975; Schimpl *et al.*, 1980; Watson *et al.*, 1979), colony-stimulating factor (Nicola *et al.*, 1979), and B-cell differentiation factor (BCDFμ) (Pure *et al.*, 1982). It does not cause proliferation of PHA-stimulated thymocytes, indicating that it is also distinct from IL-1 (Lachman *et al.*, 1977). The proportion of B cells responsive to BCGF-I has not yet been established. However, the levels of proliferation ob-

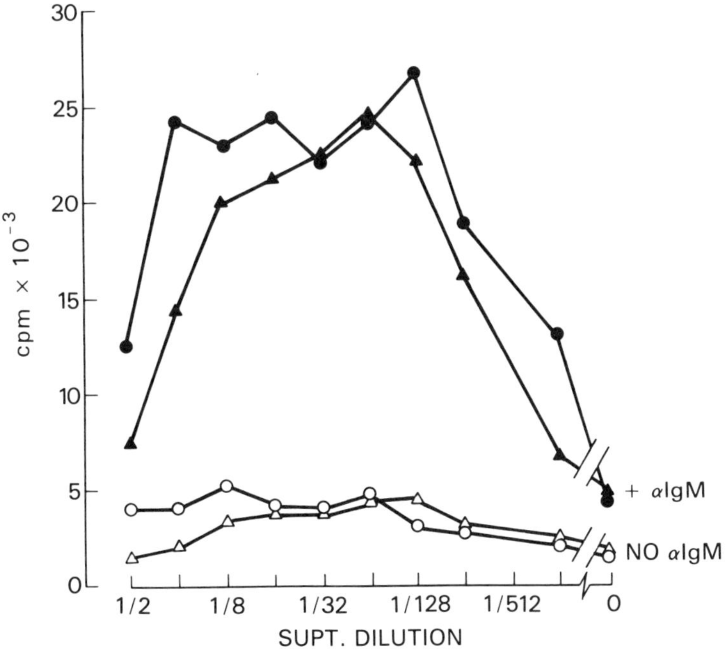

Figure 1. BCGF activity in PMA-induced EL4 supernatant (•) and antigen-activated helper T-cell line supernatant (▲). Purified B cells were cultured at 5 × 10^4 per microtiter well, with (•, ▲) or without (○, △) anti-IgM at 5 μg/ml, and various dilutions of supernatant. Cells were cultured for 3 days with a final 16-hr pulse of [^{3}H] thymidine to assess proliferation. BCGF, B-cell growth factor; PMA, phorbol myristate acetate.

tained in B-cell costimulator experiments are consistent with involvement of the entire anti-IgM responsive B-cell pool, a pool recently shown to consist of approximately 50% of normal B cells (DeFranco *et al.*, 1982). Splenic B cells from *xid* mice fail to synthesize DNA in response to the combination of anti-IgM and BCGF-I (Howard *et al.*, 1983a). Confirmation of the existence of murine BCGF-I with similar physical and biological properties to those outlined above has recently been provided by Leanderson *et al.* (1982), Lernhardt *et al.* (1982), and Pure *et al.* (1983).

IV. PHYSICOCHEMICAL PROPERTIES OF MOUSE BCGF-I

In studying the physicochemical properties of mouse BCGF-I, Farrar *et al.* (1982, 1983) and Howard *et al.* (1982) have shown that mouse BCGF-I is a glycoprotein by virtue of its trypsin and neuraminidase sensitivity. When produced by PMA-induced EL4 cells in serum-containing media, it is readily separated from the bulk of proteins in such culture supernatants by ammonium sulfate precipitation. More than 90% of the mouse BCGF-I activity is precipitated between 80% and 100% saturated ammonium sulfate; only 5-9% of the total protein is found in this fraction. By conventional gel filtration on ACA 54 in neutral solution, mouse BCGF-I elutes as a broad peak between 13,000 and 20,000 daltons. Analysis of mouse BCGF-I by SDS-PAGE shows the presence of two components that exhibit biological activity after extraction from the gels and dialysis. One has a monomeric M_r of 11,000, the other 15,000. A degree of microheterogeneity is also observed when mouse BCGF-I is examined by electrofocusing. Two major peaks of mouse BCGF-I activity are observed migrating with isoelectric points of 6.4–6.7 and 7.4–7.6, respectively. These resolve to one peak of pI 9.3 after neuraminidase treatment. Mouse BCGF-I can be completely separated from the growth factor for T cells, IL-2, by a combination of ammonium sulfate precipitation, phenyl Sepharose column chromatography, and Tris-glycine gel electrophoresis (Farrar *et al.*, 1983). Surprisingly, mouse BCGF-I displays lower electrophoretic mobility than does IL-2 on Tris-glycine gels, despite its lower molecular weight, probably due to the alkaline isoelectric points of mouse BCGF-I. Although mouse BCGF-I has not been purified to homogeneity, it has been brought to high specific activity by a sequential purification procedure involving ammonium sulfate precipitation, phenyl Sepharose chromatography, Tris-glycinate PAGE, and SDS-PAGE (Farrar *et al.*, 1983). In this sequential purification procedure, significant mouse BCGF-I activity could be recovered from the final SDS-PAGE. Surprisingly, no band of appropriate size could be observed when this final gel was stained using the highly sensitive silver nitrate procedure. As this staining procedure is capable of detecting nanogram amounts of protein, this implies that 1 unit of BCGF-I activity corresponds to less than nanogram amounts of protein.

V. HUMAN B-CELL PROLIFERATION COFACTORS

B-cell growth factors have also been described in the human system by four independent groups, namely, Sredni *et al.* (1981); Ford *et al.* (1981) and Maizel *et al.* (1982); Kishimoto *et al.* (1982) and Yoshizaki *et al.* (1982); and Fauci and co-workers (Muraguchi and Fauci, 1982; Muraguchi *et al.*, 1982; Butler *et al.*, 1983). The experimental systems used in these laboratories vary, and it is not yet clear whether the same factor is being investigated by each of the groups or whether the human BCGFs are analogous to the mouse factors. Nevertheless, some uniform conclusions regarding the nature of human BCGF(s) have emerged. The term human BCGF is currently used to designate either a material that costimulates with anti-Ig or other polyclonal B-cell activators to cause DNA synthesis by normal or leukemic human B cells (Kishimoto *et al.*, 1982; Yoshizaki *et al.*, 1982; Muraguchi *et al.*, 1982; Butler *et al.*, 1983) or alternatively a material that maintains the proliferation of activated purified human B lymphocytes in suspension culture (Sredni *et al.*, 1981; Ford *et al.*, 1981; Maizel *et al.*, 1982). Obviously, these two functions may well be mediated by different moieties. Human BCGF defined by both assays can be found in supernatants of lectin-activated normal T lymphocytes and also in T-cell hybridoma supernatants. Three of the groups have independently estimated the molecular weight of human BCGF to be 17,000, namely, Maizel *et al.* (1982), Yoshizaki *et al.* (1982), and Muraguchi *et al.* (1982). Human BCGF can be distinguished from human IL-2 by its relatively delayed appearance after lectin stimulation of human T cells and by cellular absorption studies using either normal human T-cell blasts or long-term IL-2-dependent T-cell lines (Sredni *et al.*, 1981; Kishimoto *et al.*, 1982; Yoshizaki *et al.*, 1982; Muraguchi *et al.*, 1982; Butler *et al.*, 1983). Such cells remove IL-2 but do not diminish BCGF activity in culture supernatants. The recent development of T hybridomas that secrete BCGF and not IL-2 (Kishimoto *et al.*, 1982; Butler *et al.*, 1983) and of conditioned media lacking one or other activity (Sredni *et al.*, 1981) verifies the distinction between the two mediators.

Recently, Kishimoto and colleagues reported a second distinct human B-cell growth factor produced by an IL-2-dependent allospecific T-cell clone upon stimulation with cells bearing the alloantigen for which the T cells are specific (Yoshizaki *et al.*, 1982). This factor stimulates proliferation of normal B cells cultured with anti-Ig or of leukemic B cells cultured with anti-idiotype antibody. It has a M_r of 50,000 by gel filtration. In 4 M urea, its M_r falls to 19,000. Both size estimates distinguish it from the human BCGF that the same group had described in supernatants of peripheral blood T cells stimulated with PHA. The latter showed a M_r of 17,000 by conventional gel filtration and of 12,000–14,000 in a 4 M urea. Normal T cells stimulated with the combination of PHA and PMA produced both the 17,000- and 50,000-M_r BCGFs. Most interestingly, these two BCGFs showed a synergistic effect on the proliferation of anti-Ig-stimulated B cells. This finding suggests that the larger BCGF is not simply an aggregated form of the smaller and that both factors probably act on the same B-cell subpopulation.

VI. ROLE OF MOUSE BCGF-I IN B-CELL ACTIVATION

The recent explosion of information on B-cell proliferation cofactors outlined in the preceding sections promises to clarify the controversial area of B-cell activation. It must be remembered, however, that the events of DNA synthesis and mitosis may be far removed from those signals operating at the resting (G_0)

lymphocyte level. For this reason, some groups have attempted to devise experimental systems to analyze the activation events preceding entry into the S phase of the cell cycle. One such approach was recently provided by DeFranco *et al.* (1982), who used size enlargement as an index of early cell activation events. Their studies demonstrated that the initial round of anti-IgM-induced B-cell replication takes approximately 42 hr and that few cells enter S phase before 30 hr. By manipulating the dose of anti-Ig, DeFranco and associates also identified two distinct components of the G_1 phase: an initial component lasting approximately 20 hr, and a final component of approximately 10 hr. Low doses of anti-IgM were capable of driving all splenic B cells through the first component of G_1, but only those 50% of B cells belonging to the Lyb-5^+ subset could be driven by high doses of anti-IgM through the second component of G_1 and onto S phase.

The studies of DeFranco *et al.* (1982) prompted speculation that one or both of the soluble helper factors we had shown to be critical to anti-IgM stimulation of DNA synthesis (i.e., BCGF-I and IL-1) might regulate the second control point, i.e., the transition of early G_1 B cells to late G_1 and S phase. Careful kinetic experiments were designed to test this hypothesis (Howard and Paul, 1983). Anti-IgM and one cofactor were added to B cells at the initiation of the culture, with the second cofactor being added at various times over the course of 30 hr. In light of the findings of DeFranco *et al.* (1982), [^{3}H]thymidine was added at 30 hr, and cultures were terminated at 42 hr, so that most of the thymidine uptake would represent B cells that had entered S phase for the first time. The results indicated that the cofactor IL-1 could be added 16–20 hr after initiation of culture without any significant decrease in final thymidine uptake; it therefore seems likely that this factor corresponds to the second control agent suggested by DeFranco's studies. In contrast, the effectiveness of BCGF-I as a costimulator declined rapidly and linearly as its addition was delayed. If its addition was delayed beyond 10 hr, it was essentially without effect, with little thymidine uptake resulting at 30–42 hr. This observation suggests that BCGF-I acted either on G_0 B cells or during the early (excitation) portion of the G_1 phase of the cell cycle. This time of action and biological function of BCGF-I makes it a prime candidate for the second signal of the original Bretscher–Cohn hypothesis (Bretscher, 1975; Bretscher and Cohn, 1970). Whether BCGF-I acts directly on the resting G_0 B cell or on the early G_1 B cell, its precise role in B-cell activation and its possible role in B-cell tolerance are the subjects of current investigation.

On the basis of the various experiments described above, we have proposed the following model, summarized schematically in Fig. 2, for the activation and proliferation of Lyb-5^+ B cells. Resting B cells that bind anti-IgM through their membrane IgM enter the G_1 phase of the cell cycle. This process presumably requires crosslinking of mIg; multivalent antigens would be expected to have the same effect on those resting B cells that possess receptors specific for that

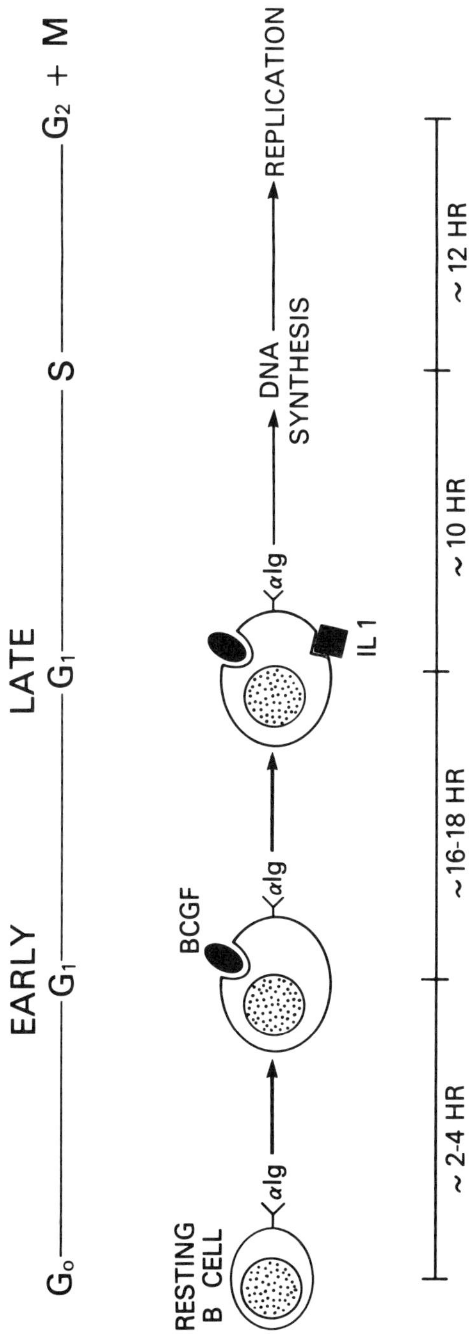

Figure 2. Model for the activation of Lyb-5^+ B cells.

antigen. BCGF-I acts either together with anti-IgM to cause the G_0–G_1 transition or acts upon the early G_1 cell. It is known that anti-IgM is required continuously during early G_1 (1982); whether BCGF-I is also needed continuously or acts at a single point in early G_1 (or G_0) is unknown. As a result of these two stimulants, the B cell progresses through early G_1 and reaches a point, at about 16–20 hr, when it requires IL-1. The presence of IL-1 permits the cell to continue to progress through G_1 and then to enter S phase. The first cells to enter S phase do so at about 30 hr after initial stimulation. From the work of DeFranco *et al.* (1982), it appears that anti-IgM is not required for cells to progress through late G_1 and to enter S phase. The need for BCGF-I in late G_1 has not been established. It seems likely that the time of action of BCGF-I and IL-1 correlates with the time that receptors for them are expressed on the B-cell surface, just as T-cell sensitivity to IL-2 appears to correlate with the expression of receptors for IL-2 on T cells that have been stimulated with lectins or antigen (Robb *et al.*, 1981). We emphasize, however, that no direct evidence for receptors for BCGF-I or IL-1 on activated mouse B cells has yet been obtained.

Thus, the overall concept for activation of Lyb-5$^+$ cells is similar to models proposed for T-cell activation (Lafferty *et al.*, 1978, 1980; Larson and Coutinho, 1979; Larsson *et al.*, 1980; Andersson *et al.*, 1979). Lafferty in particular has emphasized that antigen plus on costimulator acts on the resting T lymphocyte to induce an excited or receptive state and that this excited lymphocyte proliferates when it receives a second costimulator signal (Lafferty *et al.*, 1978, 1980).

VII. ROLE OF MOUSE BCGF-I IN AFC PRODUCTION

B cells stimulated with anti-IgM and BCGF-I proliferate but fail to develop into Ig-secreting cells as monitored by staining cells for cytoplasmic (c) IgM with a fluoresceinated monoclonal anti-IgM antibody (Nakanishi *et al.*, 1983). Others had previously shown that antigen- and anti-Ig-driven differentiation into antibody secretion requires additional factors, such as T-cell replacing factor (TRF) and/or IL-2 (Kishimoto and Ishizaka, 1975; Parker, 1980; Leibson *et al.*, 1981; Takatsu *et al.*, 1980; Swain *et al.*, 1981). Using B-cell costimulator assays similar to that described above, we recently showed that the development of specific plaque-forming cells by B cells stimulated with sheep erythrocytes (Howard *et al.*, 1982) and the appearance of cIgM$^+$ cells in cultures of anti-IgM-stimulated B cells (Nakanishi *et al.*, 1983) requires the addition of three distinct T-cell-derived factors: (1) BCGF-I, purified from induced EL4 supernatants by either isoelectric focusing (IEF) or phenyl Sepharose chromatography; (2) a supernatant obtained from the T-cell hybridoma B151K12 (Takatsu *et al.*, 1980b),

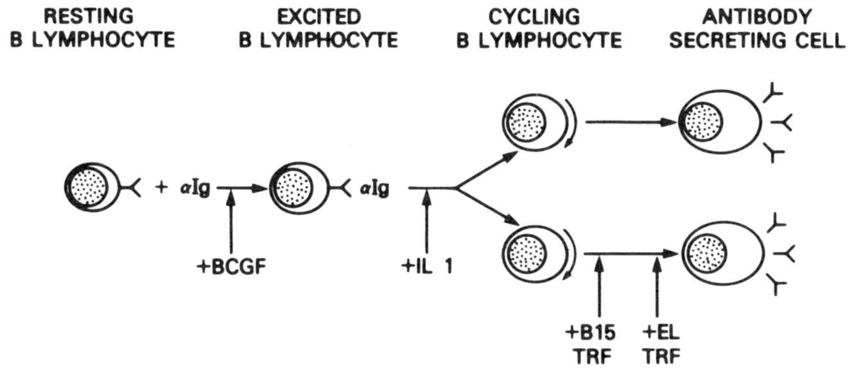

Figure 3. Model illustrating soluble factor involvement in B-cell development.

designated B151K12-TRF [B15-TRF]; and (3) the 4.5-pI fraction from the IEF gel of an induced EL4 supernatant, designated EL4 pI 4.5, or EL-TRF. The addition of any one or two of these factors to cultures of B cells stimulated with anti-IgM produced few, if any, cIgM$^+$ cells (Nakanishi *et al.*, 1983). Interestingly, while neither B15-TRF nor EL-TRF caused proliferation of anti-IgM-activated B cells, B15-TRF substantially enhanced both proliferative levels and final cell yields in cultures also containing anti-IgM and BCGF-I (Nakanishi *et al.*, 1983). The relative roles of these three cofactors in B-cell development were investigated in kinetic analyses. The results showed that BCGF-I and B15-TRF are required early in the culture, while EL-TRF appears to be a late-acting differentiation factor. Although EL-TRF preparations contain IL-2, we believe the B-cell differentiation factor is a separate entity, since other preparations rich in IL-2 fail to replace EL-TRF in these assays.

From the above data, we have proposed a model, illustrated in Fig. 3, for the action of various factors that regulate the activation, proliferation, and differentiation of Lyb-5$^+$ B cells. We suggest that agents that can crosslink membrane Ig receptors in an appropriate manner, such as anti-Ig antibodies and certain antigens, cause resting B cells to become activated and to enter the G_1 phase of the cell cycle. As a result of this activation, these G_1 B cells become sensitive to certain lymphokines, and interaction with these agents induces the cells to enter S phase. The sensitivity of G_1 B cells to such growth factors is most likely determined by the expression of growth factor receptors on the cell membrane. Lyb-5$^+$ B cells stimulated to enter G_1 by anti-IgM were sensitive to the action of BCGF-I, a T-cell-derived factor, as well as to the macrophage-derived factor IL-1. The differentiation of these cells into antibody-secreting cells requires two additional factors: B15-TRF, which apparently also acts as a growth factor; and a late-acting differentiation factor in EL4 supernatant (EL-TRF).

VIII. REFERENCES

Ahmed, A., Scher, I., Sharrow, S. O., Smith, A. H., Paul, W. E., Sachs, D. H., and Sell, K. W., 1977, *J. Exp. Med.* **145**:101.

Andersson, J., and Melchers, F., 1981, *Proc. Natl. Acad. Sci. USA* **78**:2497.

Andersson, J., Gronvik, K., Larsson, E., and Coutinho, A., 1979, *Eur. J. Immunol.* **9**:581.

Andersson, J., Schreier, M. H., and Melchers, F., 1980, *Proc. Natl. Acad. Sci. USA* **77**:1612.

Bretscher, P., 1975, *Transplant. Rev.* **23**:37.

Bretscher, P., and Cohn, M., 1970, *Science* **169**:1042.

Butler, J., Muraguchi, A., Lane, A., and Fauci, A., 1983, *J. Exp. Med.* **157**:60.

DeFranco, A., Raveche, E., Asofsky, R., and Paul, W. E., 1982, *J. Exp. Med.* **155**:1523.

Dutton, R. W., Falkoff, R., Hirst, J. A., Hoffman, M. Kappler, J. W., Kettman, J. R., Lesley, J. F., and Vann, D., 1971, *Prog. Immunol.* **1**:355.

Farrar, J., Benjamin, W., Hilfiker, M., Howard, M., Farrar, W., and Fuller-Farrar, J., 1982, *Immunol. Rev.* **63**:129.

Farrar, J., Howard, M., Fuller-Farrar, J., and Paul, W. E., 1983, *J. Immunol.* (in press).

Ford, R., Mehta, S., Franzini, D., Montagna, R., Lachman, L., and Maizel, A., 1981, *Nature* **294**:261.

Howard, M., and Paul, W. E., 1983, *Annu. Rev. Immunol.* **1**:307.

Howard, M., Farrar, J., Hilfiker, M., Johnson, B., Takatsu, K., Hamaoka, T., and Paul, W. E., 1982, *J. Exp. Med.* **155**:914.

Howard, M., Malek, T., Matis, L., Kell, W., Cohen, D., Nakanishi, K., Johnson, B., and Paul, W. E., 1983a, *J. Exp. Med.* **158**:2024.

Howard, M., Mizel, S. B., Lachman, L., Ansel, J., Johnson, B., and Paul, W. E., 1983b, *J. Exp. Med.* **157**:1529.

Isakson, P., Pure, E., Vitetta, E., and Krammer, P., 1982, *J. Exp. Med.* **155**:734.

Kimoto, M., and Fathman, C. G., 1980, *J. Exp. Med.* **152**:759.

Kishimoto, T., and Ishizaka, K., 1975, *J. Immunol.* **114**:1177.

Kishimoto, T., Yoshizaki, K., Okada, M., Miki, Y., Nakagawa, T., Yoshimura, N., Kishi, H., and Yamamura, Y., 1982, *UCLA-ICN Symp.* In press.

Lachman, L. B., Hacker, M. P., and Handschumacher, R. E., 1977, *J. Immunol.* **119**:2019.

Lachman, L. B., Page, S. O., and Metzgar, R. S., 1980, *J. Supramol. Struct.* **13**:457.

Lafferty, K., Warren, H., Woolnough, J., and Talmage, D., 1978, *Blood Cells* **4**:395.

Lafferty, K., Andrus, L., and Prowse, S., 1980, *Immunol. Rev.* **51**:279.

Larsson, E., and Coutinho, A., 1979, *Nature* **280**:239.

Larsson, E-L., Iscover, N. N., and Coutinho, A., 1980, *Nature* **283**:644.

Leanderson, T., Lundgren, E., Ruuth, E., Borg, H., Persson, H., and Coutinho, A., 1982, *Proc. Natl. Acad. Sci. USA* **79**:7455.

Leibson, H., Marrack, P., and Kappler, J., 1981, *J. Exp. Med.* **154**:1681.

Lernhardt, W., Corbel, C., Wall, R., and Melchers, F., 1982, *Nature* **300**:355.

Maizel, A., Sahasrabuddhe, C., Mehta, S., Morgen, C., Lachman, L., and Ford, R., 1982, *Proc. Natl. Acad. Sci. USA* **79**:5998.

Mizel, S. B., and Mizel, D., 1981, *J. Immunol.* **126**:834.

Mongini, P., Friedman, S., and Wortis, H., 1978, *Nature* **276**:709.

Muraguchi, A., and Fauci, A., 1982, *J. Immunol.* **129**:1104.

Muraguchi, A., Kasahara, T., Oppenheim, J., and Fauci, A., 1982, *J. Immunol.* **129**:2486.

Nakanishi, K., Howard, M., Muraguchi, A., Farrar, J., Takatsu, K., Hamaoka, T., and Paul, W. E., 1983, *J. Immunol.* **130**:2219.

Nicola, N., Burgess, A., and Metcalfe, D., 1979, *J. Biol. Chem.* **254**:5290.

Okada, M., Sakaguchi, N., Yoshimura, N., Hara, H., Shimizu, K., Yoshida, N., Yoshizaki, K., Kishimoto, S., Yamamura, Y., and Kishimoto, T., 1983, *J. Exp. Med.* **157**:583.
Parker, D. C., 1975, *Nature* **258**:361.
Parker, D., 1980, *Immunol. Rev.* **52**:115.
Parker, D. C., 1982, *J. Immunol.* **129**:469.
Parker, D. C., Fothergill, J. J., and Wadsworth, D. C., 1979, *J. Immunol.* **123**:931.
Pike, B., Vaux, D., Clark-Lewis, I., Schrader, J., and Nossal, G., 1982, *Proc. Natl. Acad. Sci. USA* **79**:6350.
Pure, R., Isakson, P., Kappler, J., Marrack, P., Krammer, P., and Vitetta, E., 1983, *J. Exp. Med.* **157**:583.
Robb, R., Munck, A., and Smith, K., 1981, *J. Exp. Med.* **154**:1455.
Schimpl, A., and Wecker, E., 1975, *Transplant. Rev.* **23**:176.
Schimpl, A., Hubner, L., Wong, C., and Wecker, E., 1980, *Behring Inst. Mitt.* **67**:221.
Sell, S., and Gell, P. G., 1965, *J. Exp. Med.* **122**:423.
Sieckmann, D. G., Scher, I., Asofsky, R., Mosier, D. E., and Paul, W. E., 1978, *J. Exp. Med.* **148**:1628.
Sredni, B., Sieckmann, D., Kumagai, S., House, S., Green, I., and Paul, W. E., 1981, *J. Exp. Med.* **154**:1500.
Swain, S., Dennert, G., Warner, J., and Dutton, R., 1981, *Proc. Natl. Acad. Sci. USA* **78**:2517.
Swain, S., Howard, M., Kappler, J., Marrack, P., Watson, J., Booth, R., Wetzel, M., and Dutton, R., 1983, *J. Exp. Med.* **158**:822.
Takatsu, K., Tominaga, A., and Hamaoka, T., 1980a, *J. Immunol.* **124**:2414.
Takatsu, K., Tanaka, K., Tominaga, A., Kumahara, Y., and Hamaoka, T., 1980b, *J. Immunol.* **125**:2646.
Vaux, D. L., Pike, B. L., and Nossal, G. J. V., 1981, *Proc. Natl. Acad. Sci. USA* **78**:7702.
Watson, J., Gillis, S., Marbrook, J., Mochizuki, D., and Smith, K. A., 1979, *J. Exp. Med.* **150**:849.
Weiner, H. L., Moorehead, J. W., and Claman, H., 1976, *J. Immunol.* **116**:1656.
Wetzel, G. D., and Kettman, J. R., 1981, *J. Immunol.* **126**:723.
Yoshizaki, K., Nakagawa, T., Fukunaga, K., Kaieda, T., Maruyama, S., Kishimoto, S., Yamamura, Y., and Kishimoto, T., 1982, *J. Immunol.* **130**:1241.

Role of Interleukin-1 in Human B-Cell Activation

Peter E. Lipsky

Rheumatic Diseases Unit
Department of Internal Medicine
University of Texas Health Science Center
Southwestern Medical School
Dallas, Texas 75235

I. INTRODUCTION

Mononuclear phagocytes (Mϕ) play an essential role in both T- and B-cell activation (Unanue, 1972). Thus, Mϕ have a critical function both as antigen-presenting cells and as cells that provide a focus for effective B- and T-cell collaboration. In addition to activities carried out by means of direct contact between Mϕ and responding lymphocytes, a number of other functions of Mϕ appear to be accomplished by secreted factors. The best studied of these factors is Interleukin-1 (IL-1), a Mϕ-derived factor of 12,000–16,000 daltons that has a variety of amplifying effects both on immunological reactivity and on inflammatory responses in general (Oppenheim and Gery, 1982). While the immunoregulatory role of IL-1 has been well described in a number of murine models of T- and B-cell activation, the function of this molecule in human immune responsiveness has been less well described. The studies presented in this chapter were therefore undertaken, to examine the role of IL-1 in the regulation of antibody production in humans. Specifically, the *in vitro* generation of immunoglobulin-secreting cells (ISC) triggered by the T-cell-dependent polyclonal B-cell activators, pokeweed mitogen (PWM) and formalinized *Staphylococcus aureus*, was used as a model system for dissecting in detail the immunomodulatory potential of IL-1. The data support the conclusion that IL-1 plays a necessary role in the generation of ISC in humans. Moreover, the results indicate that IL-1 delivers a requisite differentiation signal directly to the B-cell, without which subsequent responsiveness to T-cell-derived helper factors and maturation to Ig-secreting cells do not occur.

II. MATERIALS AND METHODS

A. Cell Preparation

Peripheral blood mononuclear cells were obtained from healthy adult volunteers by centrifugation of heparinized venous blood over sodium diatrizoate/Ficoll gradients. In some experiments, peripheral blood mononuclear cells were depleted of monocytes by sequential incubations on glass petri dishes. The characteristics of the resulting nonadherent cells were previously reported (Rosenberg and Lipsky, 1979). B- and T-cell-enriched populations were prepared from the nonadherent cells by rosetting with neuraminidase-treated sheep erythrocytes as previously detailed (Rosenberg and Lipsky, 1979).

B. Silica Treatment to Remove Phagocytic Mϕ

In some experiments, T cells were treated with silica to remove the contaminating Mϕ. This was accomplished by two sequential incubations with silica, each followed by density-gradient separation of silica and silica-containing cells from the T cells as previously described (Thiele and Lipsky, 1982).

C. Culture Conditions for Generation of ISC

Cells were cultured in microtiter plates. Routine cultures were carried out in triplicate with each microwell containing 1×10^5 peripheral blood mononuclear cells or nonadherent cells in 0.2 ml culture medium. The culture medium was RPMI 1640, supplemented with penicillin G (200 units/ml), gentamicin (10 μg/ml), L-glutamine 0.3 mg/ml, and 10% fetal bovine serum. Mitogen dissolved or suspended in Hanks' balanced salt solution (HBSS) or an equivalent volume of HBSS (0.02 ml) as control was added to the wells. They were incubated for 5–7 days at 37°C in a humidified atmosphere of 5% CO_2 and 95% air. At the end of the incubation, cells from triplicate wells were pooled, washed, and suspended in HBSS for assay. Cultures of separated B and T cells were similarly carried out, with each microwell containing 2.5×10^4 B cells alone, or supplemented with various numbers of T cells. The mitogens employed included formalinized *Staphylococcus aureus* purchased from the Calbiochem Behring Corporation and used at a final concentration of 1:10,000 (v/v) and PWM obtained from Grand Island Biological Company and used at a final concentration of 10 μg/ml.

D. Detection of ISC

ISC were detected using a reverse hemolytic plaque assay previously described in detail by Ginsburg *et al.* (1978) and Rosenberg and Lipsky (1979). For this assay, the indicator cells were *Staphylococcus aureus* protein A-coupled sheep erythrocytes, the developing antiserum was an anti-human Ig (IgA + IgM + IgG), and the complement source was an appropriate dilution of guinea pig serum that had previously been absorbed with sheep erythrocytes. For each experimental point, cells from three individual microwells were pooled and replicate determinations were carried out. All data were expressed as the mean number of ISC per 10^6 responding cells initially cultured.

E. Conditions for Generation of Mϕ Factor

Mϕ supernatants were generated as previously described by Rosenberg and Lipsky (1980). Peripheral blood mononuclear cells were suspended in medium with 10% fetal bovine serum. One ml cell suspension (2×10^6 cells/ml) was added to each well of flat bottom well tissue culture plates (Multiwell 3008, Falcon Division of Becton Dickinson and Co., Oxnard California). After a 1-hr incubation at 37°C, nonadherent cells were removed by three washes with warm medium. Next, 0.5 ml culture medium containing 10% fetal bovine serum was added to each well, and the adherent cells were cultured for 24 hr at 37°C in a humidified atmosphere of 95% air and 5% CO_2. Supernatants were then aspirated, pooled, centrifuged free of cells, filtered with a 0.45-μm filter, and stored at − 70°C. Before use, the ability of each Mϕ supernatant to augment PWM-induced ISC responses was verified as previously described by Rosenberg and Lipsky (1980).

In addition, two preparations of highly purified human IL-1 were used, prepared as previously described (Lachman *et al.*, 1980; Wood, 1979b). Each preparation exhibited similar activity when tested for the ability to augment the generation of PWM-stimulated ISC (Rosenberg and Lipsky, 1981).

F. Culture Conditions for Generation of T-Cell Supernatants

T cells, prepared by rosetting with neuraminidase-treated sheep erythrocytes followed by nylon column passage, were suspended in medium containing 10% fetal bovine serum at a concentration of 5×10^6/ml. They were then incubated with PWM (10 μg/ml) for 2 hr at 37°C. Afterward, the cells were washed three times with HBSS and resuspended in fresh culture medium at a concentration of

5×10^6/ml. Two ml of cell suspension were incubated in 17×100-mm round-bottomed polypropylene tubes for 48 hr at 37°C. Supernatants were then aspirated, centrifuged free of cells, and stored at −70°C until use. Each T-cell supernatant was shown to exhibit helper T-cell activity, indicated by the capacity to support the generation of ISC in B-cell cultures completely depleted of T cells.

G. Antiserum to Leukocytic Pyrogen (anti-LP)

Antiserum to leukocytic pyrogen (anti-LP) was produced as previously described by Dinarello *et al.* (1977). Briefly, human LP-containing Mϕ supernatants were produced *in vitro* by stimulating peripheral blood Mϕ with heat-killed staphylococci. The LP content of the Mϕ supernatants was verified by testing for the induction of fever in rabbits. Antiserum was obtained from rabbits after multiple immunizations with crude LP emulsified in Freund's complete adjuvant. The globulin fraction of the crude antiserum was prepared by precipitation with 40% saturated ammonium sulfate. Unwanted antibodies were deleted by passage over a variety of solid-phase immunoabsorbents. These were prepared by coupling various materials onto cyanogen bromide-activated Sepharose 4B (Pharmacia Fine Chemicals). The materials coupled included (1) supernatants obtained from Mϕ after incubation with staphylococci for only 30 min, a time period not adequate to produce LP; (2) supernatants from Mϕ stimulated and cultured in the presence of low concentrations of cycloheximide to prevent the synthesis of LP; and (3) fresh human AB serum. After four to six absorptions, the nonbinding globulin was assayed to confirm anti-LP activity.

Controls were either normal rabbit serum or serum obtained from rabbits immunized with an irrelevant antigen (keyhole limpet hemocyanin). Some experiments employed preimmune serum obtained from the animals subsequently used to generate the anti-LP.

III. RESULTS

A. IL-1-Augmented Generation of ISC from Human Peripheral Blood Lymphocytes

The initial experiments documented that crude Mϕ supernatants could augment the generation of ISC from cultures of human peripheral blood B cells. For these experiments, partially T-cell-depleted B cells were prepared and stimulated with PWM. This approach was taken because it had been previously shown in experiments using murine spleen cells that an effect of IL-1 on the generation of antibody forming cells was most easily detected in partially T-cell-depleted B-cell cultures (Wood and Cameron, 1975; Koopman *et al.*, 1978; Wood, 1979a). As can be seen in Table I, only a few ISC were generated in these T-cell-deficient cultures owing to the small number of contaminating T cells. The addition of Mϕ supernatants markedly increased the number of ISC generated. As can also be seen in Table I, the Mϕ supernatant itself was not a polyclonal activator in that it did not directly stimulate the generation of ISC. A marked increase in the number of ISC was only observed when a polyclonal B-cell activator such as PWM was present as well. Additional experiments demonstrated that the active factor in the Mϕ supernatants was genetically unrestricted in that Mϕ supernatants obtained from one individual were active on cells of many other individuals, regardless of histocompatibility type. In addition, the material was nonspecific in an immunological sense, demonstrating comparable activity when tested with a variety of polyclonal B-cell activators, including PWM and soluble staphylococcal protein A. Finally, Mϕ supernatants did not stimulate B-cell proliferation directly.

The active factor in the Mϕ supernatant could not replace the need for T cells in supporting T-cell-dependent polyclonal B-cell responses (Rosenberg and Lipsky, 1980). Thus when the responding population was rigorously depleted of T cells, the capacity of Mϕ factor to augment the generation of ISC was abolished. When B-cell cultures were supplemented with as few as 5–10% T cells, Mϕ factor-mediated augmentation of responsiveness was restored. Of interest, the capacity of Mϕ factor to increase the generation of ISC was most marked in cultures containing suboptimal numbers of T cells. In cultures containing larger numbers of T

Table I. Augmentation of the Generation of Ig-Secreting Cells by Mϕ Supernatants[a,b]

Addition to cultures	Generation of ISC (ISC per 10^6 B cells × 10^{-3})		
	Expt. 1	Expt. 2	Expt. 3
Medium	0.1	0.8	1.0
PWM	1.8	1.6	1.9
Mϕ sup	0.4	0.4	1.0
PWM + Mϕ sup	20.7	7.9	16.4

[a]B cells prepared by a single depletion of T cells with neuraminidase-treated sheep erythrocytes were cultured in microtiter plates (2.5 × 10^4/well). PWM (10 μg/ml) and/or Mϕ supernatant at a final dilution of 50% were added where indicated. After a 6-day incubation, the number of ISC was determined. The B-cell population was contaminated with 1–5% T cells.

[b]Ig, immunoglobulin; ISC, immunoglobulin-secreting cells; Mϕ, monocyte; PWM, pokeweed mitogen.

Table II. Interleukin-1-Augmented Generation of Ig-Secreting Cells[a,b]

Addition to NAC cultures	PWM-Induced ISC (ISC per 10^6 cells $\times 10^{-3}$) Expt. 1	Expt. 2
Medium	0	0
IL-1	0	0
Mϕ	1.4	1.3
Mϕ + IL-1	9.0	4.2

[a]Nonadherent cells were cultured in microwells (5×10^4/well) with PWM and with or without autologous Mϕ. In addition, purified IL-1 (a gift of D. D. Wood) was also added where indicated. Generation of ISC was measured after a 6-day incubation.
[b]IL-1, Interleukin-1; NAC, nonadherent cells. Other abbreviations as in Table I.

cells, thereby supporting more maximal responses, Mϕ factor augmentation of responsiveness was much less marked.

The activity of Mϕ supernatants appeared to be accounted for by their IL-1 content. Thus, highly purified IL-1 exhibited the same activity observed as crude Mϕ supernatants (Table II). In these experiments, the responding population used was nonadherent cells (NAC), a mixture of T and B cells that had been rigorously depleted of Mϕ by glass adherence. As shown in Table II, PWM stimulated the generation of no ISC in this population unless the cells were cocultured with Mϕ. Interleukin-1 itself also supported the generation of no ISC in these cultures. However, when the responding NAC cultures were supplemented with both Mϕ and IL-1, a dramatic augmentation in the number of ISC was observed. These results indicate that IL-1 is the factor in Mϕ supernatants that is able to augment the generation of ISC. However, IL-1 itself did not appear to be sufficient to support the generation of ISC. Rather, intact Mϕ also appeared to play a necessary role in supporting this response.

These results indicated that IL-1 had the capacity to augment the generation of ISC. However, a number of issues remained unclear. Although it was apparent that IL-1 exerted an amplifying effect on the differentiation of ISC, results did not enable us to determine whether it was playing a necessary role in B-cell activation. IL-1 appeared to be active in the presence of small numbers of T cells and Mϕ but could not replace either. Moreover, it was not capable of acting as a polyclonal B-cell activator. Thus, it remained possible that IL-1 was playing a nonspecific amplifying role, but was not delivering a signal required for the generation of ISC. Finally, the mechanism by which IL-1 augmented the generation of ISC remained unclear.

B. Necessary Role of IL-1 in Generation of ISC in Humans

A number of experiments were undertaken to determine whether IL-1 plays a necessary role in the generation of ISC in humans. The first series of experiments made use of the observation that human peripheral blood Mϕ secreted IL-1 for only the first 24–48 hr of *in vitro* incubation and thereafter released little additional material spontaneously into the surrounding medium (Rosenberg and Lipsky, 1981). As can be seen in Table III, Mϕ supernatants harvested after a 48-hr incubation were able to augment the generation of ISC in PWM-stimulated cultures. However, supernatants obtained from the same Mϕ after the subsequent 24 hr (48–72 hr) displayed no such augmentative activity. In additional experiments, these culture supernatants were shown not to contain suppressive factors but rather lacked detectable IL-1 activity. It should be pointed out that in these experiments the release of IL-1 was stimulated only by glass adherence and fetal bovine serum. When more rigorous stimuli were used, such as phorbol myristate acetate (PMA) or formalinized *Staphylococcus aureus*, some IL-1 activity could be detected in the supernatants of aged Mϕ, but much less than that found in the supernatants of fresh Mϕ stimulated with the same materials. Of importance, PWM did not stimulate the release of detectable IL-1 from human Mϕ preincubated for 48 hr *in vitro*. Thus, it was reasoned that an examination of the capacity of preincubated Mϕ, which produced markedly reduced amounts of IL-1, to support the generation of ISC should provide insight into whether this Mϕ-derived factor played a necessary role in the generation of ISC. Table IV shows that preincubated Mϕ were unable to support the generation of ISC. These preincubated Mϕ remained viable and phagocytically active and expressed HLA-Dr

Table III. Absence of Spontaneous Release of IL-1 by Preincubated Mϕ[a, b]

Incubation used to generate Mϕ supernatant (hr)	PWM-induced ISC (ISC per 10^6 B cells × 10^{-3})		
	Expt. 1	Expt. 2	Expt. 3
No sup	14.8	11.6	0.2
0–48	42.0	29.2	4.6
48–72	14.0	14.8	0.8

[a] Mϕ were cultured for 48 hr, after which cell free supernatants were harvested. After washing, the Mϕ were recultured for an additional 24 hr in medium containing 10% fetal bovine serum and the cell-free supernatants again harvested. To test Mϕ supernatants for IL-1 activity, they were added to cultures of B cells (2.5 × 10^4/well) and T cells (2.5–5 × 10^3/well) at a final dilution of 50%. After a 6-day incubation with PWM, the number of ISC was determined.
[b] Abbreviations as in Tables I and II.

Table IV. Requisite Role of IL-1 in the Generation of ISC in Humans[a,b]

Addition to NAC culture	PWM-Induced ISC (ISC per 10^6 cells $\times 10^{-3}$)	
	Expt. 1	Expt. 2
Nil	0	0
IL-1	0	0
Aged Mϕ	0.1	0.1
Aged Mϕ + IL-1	1.1	1.5

[a]NAC (5×10^4/well) were cultured in microwells with PWM. The cells were incubated either alone or supplemented with 48-hr preincubated Mϕ (5×10^4/well) and/or IL-1. After a 6-day incubation, the number of ISC was determined.
[b]Abbreviations as in Tables I and II.

antigens. In fact, they were comparable to fresh Mϕ in their capacity to support PWM-induced T-cell proliferation (Rosenberg and Lipsky, 1981). That their inability to support the generation of ISC was related to their diminished production of IL-1 was indicated by the finding that the addition of IL-1 to nonadherent cell cultures supported by aged Mϕ restored responsiveness. These results indicated that IL-1 played a necessary role in the differentiation of antibody-forming cells in humans but could not further delineate the function of IL-1 in this process.

In an attempt to confirm that IL-1 was required for human B-cell activation, experiments with a rabbit antiserum with activity against human IL-1 were undertaken (Lipsky *et al.*, 1983). This antiserum had been raised against human leukocytic pyrogen (LP), as previously described by Dinarello *et al.* (1977) and appeared to recognize and bind both leukocytic pyrogen and IL-1 (Rosenwasser *et al.*, 1979; Rosenwasser and Dinarello, 1981). It could therefore be used to examine the role of IL-1 in human B-cell activation. In the first set of experiments, Mϕ supernatants displaying IL-1 activity were absorbed with rabbit anti-LP followed by precipitation with Cowan I strain *Staphylococcus aureus* (Pansorbin). These experiments were done to determine whether the anti-LP antibody would remove the activity in human Mϕ supernatants that augmented the generation of ISC. As can be seen in Table V, Mϕ supernatants augmented the generation of ISC in cultures of B cells supplemented with small numbers of T cells. Treatment of these supernatants with Pansorbin alone or with control rabbit gammaglobulin and Pansorbin had no consistent effect on this augmentation. However, treatment of the supernatants with rabbit anti-LP plus Pansorbin consistently removed the activity from the Mϕ supernatants such that no augmentation of ISC generation was observed. These results indicated that the anti-LP had the capacity to remove the active principle from Mϕ supernatants responsible

Table V. Monocyte Factor-Mediated Augmentation of the Generation of ISC: Removal by Rabbit Anti-Leukocytic Pyrogen[a,b]

Addition to culture	PWM-Induced Ig-secreting cells (ISC per 10^6 B cells × 10^{-3})			
	Expt. 1	Expt. 2	Expt. 3	Expt. 4
Nil	12.8	10.0	5.6	2.8
Mφ sup	25.2	19.6	12.8	6.0
Control-absorbed Mφ sup	26.4	21.1	11.2	6.8
Anti-LP-absorbed Mφ sup	16.4	7.2	4.8	3.2

[a] Mφ supernatants were absorbed with anti-LP for 30 min at 4°C. They were then incubated for 30 min with Cowan I strain *Staphylococcus aureus* (Pansorbin) and centrifuged to remove Pansorbin and bound rabbit Ig. As controls, Mφ supernatants were absorbed with either rabbit gammaglobulin and Pansorbin or Pansorbin alone. After the absorption, each supernatant was added to cultures containing 2.5×10^4 B cells and 5×10^3 T cells at a final dilution of 50%. After a 6-day incubation with PWM, the number of ISC was determined.
[b] Anti-LP, anti-leukocytic pyrogen. Other abbreviations as in Table I.

for the augmentation of the generation of ISC, thereby supporting the conclusion that this activity could be accounted for by IL-1.

Additional experiments demonstrated that the anti-LP had no direct anti-cellular activity, reacting with neither B cells, T cells nor monocytes (Lipsky *et al.*, 1983). This was shown by preparing $F(ab^1)_2$ fragments of anti-LP and by examining their binding to peripheral blood mononuclear cells. No cellular reactivity was observed by indirect immunofluorescence using the fluorescence-activated cell sorter.

In the next series of experiments, the capacity of the anti-LP antibody to alter PWM-stimulated generation of ISC was examined. As can be seen in Table VI, anti-LP caused concentration-dependent inhibition of ISC generation. Additional experiments showed that the generation of ISC in response to *S. aureus* was also inhibited by anti-LP. Moreover, B-cell [^{3}H] thymidine incorporation in PWM-stimulated cultures supported by mitomycin C-treated T cells was also inhibited by anti-LP, but the degree of inhibition of B-cell proliferation caused by anti-LP was always less than the effect on ISC generation. Specificity for the action of anti-LP in these cultures was demonstrated by the finding that the addition of either crude Mφ supernatants or purified IL-1, but not T-cell supernatants, reversed the inhibition caused by anti-LP (Table VII). These results confirmed the conclusion that IL-1 plays a necessary role in the differentiation of ISC in humans, but again did not indicate the precise action of IL-1 in this system.

Table VI. Effect of Anti-Leukocytic Pyrogen on the Generation of ISC[a, b]

Addition to culture (μg/ml)	PWM-induced ISC (ISC per 10^6 cells × 10^{-3})	
	Expt. 1	Expt. 2
Nil	30.9	89.4
RγG		
1.0	29.1	71.7
10	22.8	69.9
100	18.0	67.8
RαLP		
1.0	18.6	64.2
10	6.0	44.1
100	1.8	9.0

[a] Peripheral blood mononuclear cells were incubated with PWM and assayed for the number of ISC after a 6-day incubation. Various concentrations of anti-LP (RαLP) or control rabbit gammaglobulin (RγG) were also added to culture as indicated.
[b] Abbreviations as in Table I.

C. Examination of the Role of IL-1 in Generation of T-Cell Help

The finding that T-cell supernatants (Table VII) did not reverse the inhibition of ISC generation caused by anti-LP suggested that the mechanism of anti-LP inhibition was not limitation of the production of necessary helper T-cell fac-

Table VII. Anti-Leukocytic Pyrogen-Inhibited Generation of ISC by Specifically Binding IL-1[a, b]

Addition to culture	PWM-induced generation of ISC (ISC per 10^6 cells × 10^{-3})			
	Expt. 1		Expt. 2	
	RγG	RαLP	RγG	RαLP
Nil	9.4	3.4	12.5	3.3
IL-1	9.2	13.4	15.0	11.9
T-cell sup	8.6	2.0	11.2	3.6

[a] Responding cells were incubated with PWM and either anti-LP (RαLP) or a control rabbit gammaglobulin (RγG), each at 10 μg/ml for 6 days at 37°C, after which the number of ISC was determined. In addition, where indicated, the cultures were supplemented with either purified IL-1 (a gift of L. Lachman) or supernatants from PWM-stimulated T cells.
[b] Abbreviations as in Table I.

Table VIII. Anti-Leukocytic Pyrogen-inhibited Generation of ISC in Cultures Supported by T Cells or T-Cell Supernatants[a, b]

Expt. #	Addition to B-cell cultures	*S. aureus*-induced ISC (ISC per 10^6 B cells $\times 10^{-3}$) Medium	RγG	RαLP
1	Medium	0	0	0
	T cells	171.2	167.6	56.0
	T-cell sup	41.2	37.6	0
2	Medium	0	0	0
	T cells	127.6	120.0	11.2
	T-cell sup	8.4	8.0	0
3	Medium	0	0	0
	T cells	22.0	24.0	0
	T-cell sup	9.2	8.8	0

[a] B cells (2.5×10^4/well) were cultured either alone or with $0.5–1 \times 10^5$ T cells or supernatant from PWM-stimulated T cells (final dilution: 50%). In addition, where indicated, the cultures also contained 25 μg/ml of $F(ab')_2$ anti-LP (RαLP) or control rabbit gammaglobulin (RγG). After a 6-day incubation with *Staphylococcus aureus*, the number of ISC was determined.

[b] Abbreviations as in Table I.

tors. In additional experiments, as shown in Table VIII, anti-LP was also found to inhibit the generation of ISC in B-cell cultures supported only by T-cell factors. If anti-LP were active solely by virtue of its capacity to interfere with the production of helper T-cell activity, inhibition in this circumstance would not have been anticipated. These results therefore suggested the hypothesis that IL-1 has a necessary role in the generation of ISC, not by promoting the production of helper T-cell factors, but rather by directly delivering a requisite signal to the B cell. In order to examine this question more fully, experiments were initially carried out in which the role of IL-1 in the generation of T-cell help was examined in greater detail.

For these experiments, supernatants were generated by stimulating sheep erythrocyte-rosetted, nylon–wool column-passed T cells with PWM, as indicated in Section II. The cells were exposed to PWM for 2 hr at 37°C and were then washed extensively before being incubated for 48 hr to permit elaboration of helper factors. This was done to minimize PWM contamination of the supernatants. Supernatants generated in this manner were found to have the capacity to support the differentiation of ISC in B-cell cultures rigorously deprived of T cells (Table IX). The T cells used to generate these supernatants were contaminated with 1–2% Mϕ. When these cells were cultured at the high cell densities necessary to generate active supernatants i.e., 10×10^6 T cells in 2 ml medium per culture tube, the total number of contaminating Mϕ i.e., $1–2 \times 10^5$ per tube, could well

Table IX. Generation of Active T-Cell Supernatants: Requirement for Mφ[a,b]

Addition to B-cell cultures	*S. aureus*-induced ISC (ISC per 10^6 B cells × 10^{-3})	
	Expt. 1	Expt. 2
0	0	0
Control T sup	19.2	10.4
Silica T sup	0	2.8
Control T cells	49.6	84.0
Silica T cells	60.8	102.4

[a]Silica T cells had been twice incubated with silica followed by density-gradient centrifugation. Control T cells were similarly incubated and centrifuged but not exposed to silica. Each T-cell population was then incubated with PWM, washed, and cultured to generate supernatants, or directly cocultured with B cells. 2.5×10^4 B cells were cultured alone or supplemented with 1×10^5 T cells or T-cell supernatant (final dilution: 50%). After a 6-day incubation with *Staphylococcus aureus*, the number of ISC was determined.
[b]Abbreviations as in Table I.

have been great enough to play an important role in supporting the activation of helper T cells. A more rigorous method of Mφ depletion was therefore necessary before one could examine the role of either Mφ or Mφ-secreted factors in the production of helper T-cell factors. In order to accomplish this, a technique of radical and specific Mφ depletion was used. This made use of the capacity of silica to function as a specific Mφ toxin (Thiele and Lipsky, 1982). As can be seen in Table IX, silica treatment of T cells markedly inhibited their subsequent capacity to generate helper factors necessary for B-cell differentiation into ISC. This inhibition did not appear to result from an effect on T-cell function *per se*, since silica-treated T cells were capable of supporting such responses when directly cocultured with the responding B-cell population, which itself contained adequate numbers of contaminating Mφ to support the generation of ISC. Moreover, experiments in which supernatants from control T cells were mixed with those from silica-treated T cells indicated that the latter did not contain suppressive factors, but rather lacked appropriate helper factors.

The capacity of silica-treated T cells to generate active T-cell helper factors was completely restored by coculturing them with Mφ (Table X). Of importance, neither crude Mφ supernatants containing IL-1 activity nor highly purified IL-1 were able to restore the capacity to produce helper factors to silica-treated T cells. These results suggested that intact Mφ, but not IL-1, were necessary for the generation of helper T-cell factors. It should be noted that, in these experiments, the control and silica-treated T cells were exposed to PWM and washed before being cocultured with Mϕ or IL-1. Thus, it is unlikely that the Mϕ were functioning merely to present the mitogenic stimulus to the T cells, although this may also be an important activity of Mϕ in this system. In additional experiments, PWM-pulsed Mϕ have been found able to present the mitogen to silica-treated T cells. The results presented in Table X, however, indicate that in addition to this function, Mϕ also appear to provide a signal necessary to activate helper T cells but that cannot be accounted for by IL-1. Additional experiments have indicated that direct cell contact between Mϕ and helper T cells facilitates the generation of helper T-cell factors. Thus, when the cells are cultured at the same total concentration per milliliter of culture medium, but under conditions in which the cell density is decreased and thus the opportunity for cell–cell contact is limited (flat-bottomed versus U-bottomed culture wells), the production of active helper T-cell factors is markedly reduced. These results support the conclusion that the generation of helper factors involves the necessity of a contactual interaction between Mϕ and T cells.

In order to examine in greater detail the role of IL-1 in the generation of helper T-cell factors, a number of other experiments were carried out. In the first set of experiments, the capacity of aged Mϕ that no longer produced IL-1 to restore the capacity of silica-treated T cells to generate T-cell replacing factor was examined. These Mϕ had been incubated for 48 hr *in vitro*; they no longer spontaneously produced IL-1. However, they were found to be comparable to fresh Mϕ, which spontaneously produced large amounts of IL-1, in their capacity to restore active helper factor production to silica-treated T cells. In additional

Table X. Role of Mϕ in the Generation of Active T-Cell Helper Factors[a,b]

Cells used to generate T-cell supernatants	*S. aureus*-induced ISC (ISC per 10^6 B cells × 10^{-3})		
	Expt. 1	Expt. 2	Expt. 3
No sup	0	0	0
Control T cells	14.8	13.6	9.2
Silica T cells	0	0	0
Silica T cells + Mϕ	12.8	8.4	5.6
Silica T cells + IL-1	0	0.4	0

[a]Control or silica-treated T cells were incubated with PWM, washed, and then cultured with intact monocytes (5–10%) or IL-1. After 48 hr, the supernatants were harvested and tested for their capacity to support *Staphylococcus aureus*-induced generation of ISC in cultures of T-cell-deprived B cells.

[b]Abbreviations as in Tables I and II.

experiments, T cells were preincubated for 48 hr in order to deplete the small number of residual Mϕ of their capacity to produce IL-1. These aged T cells were found comparable to fresh T cells in their capacity to produce active helper T-cells factors. Finally, the capacity of anti-LP to alter the production of helper T-cell factors was also examined. In these experiments, T cells were incubated with anti-LP during both their exposure to PWM and subsequent 48-hr incubation. Afterward, the anti-LP was removed by absorption with Pansorbin, and the supernatants were tested for their capacity to support the differentiation of B cells into ISC. In these experiments, the direct addition of 25 μg/ml of anti-LP to cultures of B cells supported by T cells inhibited the generation of ISC by more than 95%. The same concentration of anti-LP had no significant effect on the generation of helper T-cell factors. All these results support the conclusion that IL-1 has little function in the production of helper T-cell factors. It remains possible that a small amount of IL-1, perhaps directly transferred from Mϕ to T cell during cell–cell contact is necessary to facilitate the activation of helper T cells. If this is the case, however, the amount of IL-1 is below the level detectable in the system employed in these experiments. Moreover, the easily demonstrable inhibitory effect of the various techniques to limit IL-1 on the generation of ISC in mixed cell cultures is in marked contrast to the resistance of helper T-cell factor production to these same maneuvers. These results therefore suggest that the major role of IL-1 in the generation of ISC in humans may not be to facilitate the generation of helper T-cell factors, but rather to provide a necessary signal to B cells.

D. Direct Effect of IL-1 on B-Cell Activation

In order to examine this issue, experiments were carried out to determine whether IL-1 has a direct role in B-cell activation. Purified B cells were obtained and stimulated with PWM. For these experiments, more rigorous Mϕ depletion of the B cells with sequential glass adherence and silica exposure was carried out in order to decrease the number of contaminating Mϕ. As can be seen in Table XI, PWM stimulated the generation of no ISC in cultures of purified B cells. The addition of IL-1 alone did not increase the number of ISC. Modest responses were observed in some experiments when T-cell supernatants were added to these cultures. This response was presumably supported by the IL-1 produced by the small number of contaminating Mϕ, since, as pointed out by Table VIII, such responses could be totally inhibited by anti-LP. Markedly augmented responses were observed when both T-cell supernatants and IL-1 were added to the cultures. These results suggest that IL-1 and T-cell helper factors have a synergistic effect on B-cell activation and support the conclusion that IL-1 plays a role in triggering B cells to differentiate into ISC.

Table XI. Synergistic Effect of T-Cell Factors and IL-1 on B-Cell Activation[a, b]

Addition to B-cell culture	PWM-induced generation of ISC (ISC per 10^6 B cells $\times 10^{-3}$) Expt. 1	Expt. 2	Expt. 3
0	0	0	0
IL-1	0	0	0
T-cell sup	1.2	0.8	0
IL-1 + T-cell sup	20.8	7.2	6.0

[a] B cells (2.5×10^4/well) were cultured with PWM and the number of ISC determined after a 6-day incubation. Cultures were supplemented with IL-1 or T-cell supernatants (final dilution: 50%) or a mixture of the two as indicated.
[b] Abbreviations as in Table I.

E. Kinetics of the Effect of IL-1 and Helper T-Cell Factors on B-Cell Activation

In order to examine the relationship between the signals delivered by IL-1 and T-cell helper factors, kinetic experiments were carried out. Initially, the time in culture during which helper T-cell factor exerted its necessary action on B cells was examined. Experiments were set up in which B cells were stimulated with *S. aureus* and assayed for the generation of ISC after a 6-day incubation. T-cell supernatants were added either at the initiation of culture or at various times thereafter. As can be seen in Table XII, no ISC were generated in the absence of T-cell supernatants. The addition of T-cell supernatants at the initiation of culture effectively supported the generation of ISC. However, maximal responses were seen when T-cell supernatants were added after 24 hr of culture, and responses were still observed if these active T-cell supernatants were added after 48-hr stimulation. These results support the conclusion that helper T-cells factors are not required during the first 24–48 hr of human B-cell activation, but rather appear to play a necessary role subsequently in culture.

In an effort to determine the timing of the IL-1 signal on B-cell activation, experiments were set up in which B cells supported by small numbers of T cells were stimulated with PWM and assayed for the generation of ISC. As can be seen in Table XIII, either crude Mϕ supernatants or purified IL-1 augmented the generation of ISC when added at the initiation of culture. However, when the addition was delayed for 24 hr, no augmentation in responsiveness was observed. This finding suggested that IL-1 exerted its major effect on B cells early in the culture, before a requirement for helper T-cell factor was apparent. In order to confirm that IL-1 has a necessary role during the first few hours of culture,

Table XII. T-Cell Factor Support of the Generation of ISC[a,b]

Time of T-cell sup addition (hr)	*S. aureus*-induced ISC (ISC per 10^6 B cells × 10^{-3}) Expt. 1	Expt. 2	Expt. 3
No sup	0	0	0
Initiation	7.2	4.4	8.0
24	11.6	11.6	22.0
48	4.4	5.6	4.0
72	1.6	0.8	ND
96	0	0	ND

[a]B cells (2.5 × 10^4/well) were stimulated with *Staphylococcus aureus* and assayed for the number of ISC after a 6-day incubation. T-cell supernatant (final dilution: 50%) was added at the initiation of culture or at various times thereafter as indicated.
[b]ISC, immunoglobulin-secreting cells.

experiments using anti-LP were also carried out. Table XIV shows that anti-LP inhibited the generation of ISC only if added at the initiation of the culture. When addition of this antibody was delayed for 24 hr, no inhibition of the generation of ISC was observed. These results support the conclusion that IL-1 plays a necessary role during the first few hours of B-cell activation, whereas helper T-cell factors do not appear to be required until later.

Table XIII. Augmentation of the Generation of ISC by Mϕ Supernatants and IL-1[a,b]

Time of addition (hr)	PWM-stimulated Generation of ISC (ISC per 10^6 B cells × 10^{-3}): Expt. 1		Expt. 2	
	Medium	Mϕ sup	Medium	IL-1
Initiation	6.8	16.8	32.0	44.8
24	10.0	8.4	29.2	32.4
48	7.6	7.2	26.8	24.8
72	8.0	6.8	28.8	27.6

[a]A mixture of B cells (2.5 × 10^4/well) and T cells (2.5–5 × 10^3/well) was cultured with PWM and analyzed for the number of ISC after a 6-day incubation. Mϕ supernatant (final dilution: 50%) or purified IL-1 was added at the initiation of culture or at various times thereafter.
[b]Abbreviations as in Table I.

Table XIV. Anti-Leukocytic Pyrogen-Inhibited Generation of ISC: Required Presence during the First 24 hr of Culture[a, b]

Time of addition (hr)	PWM-induced generation of ISC (ISC per 10^6 cells × 10^{-3})					
	Expt. 1		Expt. 2		Expt. 3	
	RαLP	RγG	RαLP	RγG	RαLP	RγG
Initiation	5.6	16.4	2.8	19.4	4.2	25.8
24	22.4	16.2	13.2	13.6	33.0	39.8
48	19.0	14.6	14.4	11.6	46.8	33.8
72	20.2	22.2	15.4	12.2	37.6	32.4

[a]Peripheral blood mononuclear cells were stimulated with PWM and analyzed for the number of ISC after a 6-day incubation. Anti-LP (RαLP) or control rabbit gammaglobulin (RγG), each at 10 μg/ml, was added at the initiation of culture or at various times thereafter.
[b]Abbreviations as in Table I.

F. Role of Mitogen in Generation of ISC

Experiments were carried out to examine the role of the nonspecific polyclonal activator in B-cell activation and specifically the relationship between this signal and that delivered by IL-1. Peripheral blood mononuclear cells were incubated *in vitro* for 48 hr. Supernatants from these cultures were assayed and found to exhibit IL-1-like activity (Table XV). However, when these peripheral blood mononuclear cells were washed and subsequently cultured with PWM, no

Table XV. Effect of *in Vitro* Preincubation on the Generation of ISC[a, b]

Preincubation (hr)	Addition	PWM-induced ISC (ISC per 10^6 cells × 10^{-3})	
		Expt. 1	Expt. 2
Nil	Nil	10.4	2.7
48	Nil	0	0
48	IL-1	8.8	3.0

[a]Peripheral blood mononuclear cells were stimulated with PWM and assayed for the number of ISC after a 6-day incubation. In addition, an aliquot of the cells was incubated for 48 hr without mitogen, washed extensively, and then cultured for 6 days with PWM and with or without IL-1, after which the number of ISC was determined.
[b]Abbreviations as in Table I.

ISC were generated unless the cultures were also supplemented with additional purified IL-1. As previously noted, T cells preincubated for 48 hr in a similar fashion were capable of producing helper T-cell factor upon stimulation with PWM. Thus, it was likely that the diminished capacity of aged cells to respond to PWM with the differentiation of ISC resulted from B-cell deprivation of the signal transmitted by IL-1. Moreover, the results imply that B cells are only able to receive the IL-1 signal at or after the time of mitogenic stimulation. These experiments thus support the conclusion that IL-1 does not stimulate resting B cells; rather, it appears to have an action on B cells that have been triggered by a polyclonal activator.

IV. DISCUSSION

The experiments described in this chapter were undertaken to examine the role of IL-1 in human B-cell activation. The results indicate that IL-1 not only amplifies the generation of ISC, but also appears to deliver a requisite signal without which Ig synthesis does not occur. This was shown using two separate approaches. The first involved depleting Mϕ of their capacity to produce IL-1 by *in vitro* incubation. Such preincubations may not deplete these cells completely of their IL-1 content. Thus, for example, aged Mϕ may still contain intracellular IL-1 (Gery *et al.*, 1981), and more intense stimulation such as may occur with particulate materials or phorbol myristate acetate (PMA) may induce the release of small amounts of IL-1 from these aged cells. Nevertheless, they are markedly depleted in their capacity to secrete IL-1. In parallel with their diminished ability to produce IL-1, aged Mϕ manifest a significantly decreased ability to support the generation of ISC. That this deficiency was related to their diminished capacity to release IL-1 was demonstrated by the finding that the addition of purified IL-1 to culture restored the generation of ISC in cultures supported by aged Mϕ.

The role of IL-1 in the generation of ISC was also confirmed through studies that made use of a heterologous antibody raised against human leukocytic pyrogen that bound IL-1. The addition of this antibody to culture inhibited B-cell proliferation and the generation of ISC. A number of pieces of evidence supported the conclusion that inhibition of B-cell activation caused by anti-LP resulted from interference with the function of IL-1 and not from anticellular antibodies that might have been contaminating this antiserum. Thus, no anticellular reactivity was detected by indirect immunofluorescence using the fluorescence-activated cell sorter for analysis, and absorption of the antiserum with human peripheral blood mononuclear cells did not diminish its capacity to inhibit the generation of ISC. Specificity for the inhibition of B-cell activation was demonstrated by the finding that it could be completely reversed by the addition of Mϕ supernatants or highly purified IL-1, but not by T-cell supernatants. These results thus support the conclusion that IL-1 plays a necessary role in human B-cell activation.

Experiments were next undertaken to dissect the cellular site of action of IL-1 in the complex multicellular interactions resulting in the generation of ISC. Initial experiments suggested that IL-1 played little role in the generation of the helper T-cell factors necessary for the generation of ISC. Thus, while intact Mϕ were found necessary to support the stimulation of T-cell help, IL-1 appeared to have little or no role in helper T-cell activation. This was demonstrated by the finding that intact Mϕ, but not IL-1, could restore the capacity to produce helper factors to T cells that had been rigorously depleted of Mϕ by silica treatment. Moreover, aged Mϕ, which were markedly deficient in production of IL-1, were perfectly capable of restoring helper-factor production to silica-depleted T cells. Finally, the anti-LP antibody had little or no effect on generation of helper T-cell factors. All these results support the conclusion that the generation of helper T-cell factors in humans is dependent on the participation of intact Mϕ but that IL-1 appears to be minimally involved in helper T-cell activation. Although IL-1 may facilitate the generation of other T-cell lymphokines such as IL-2 and appears to be involved in the activation of T cells in a number of other model systems (Oppenheim and Gery, 1982), this Mϕ-derived product has little, if any, effect on the activation of human peripheral blood T cells by PWM (Rosenberg and Lipsky, 1981). In this regard, IL-1 plays at best only a minimal role in the production of helper factors by human T cells and also appears not to be involved in the induction of T-cell proliferation by PWM. This latter point is indicated, for example, by the finding that anti-LP has no effect on PWM-stimulated T-cell [^{3}H]thymidine incorporation even at concentrations 20-fold greater than those that will totally prevent the generation of ISC (Lipsky *et al.*, 1983). Similarly, Frost *et al.* (1978) were unable to show that Mϕ-secreted factors augmented proliferative responses of partially Mϕ-depleted human peripheral blood mononuclear cells, although such factors were able to augment responses to other T-cell mitogens such as phytohemagglutinin (PHA) and Concanavalin A (Con A). Thus, in humans PWM may stimulate a subpopulation of mature T cells, the activation of which does not require a signal from IL-1.

It should be noted, however, that current studies do not entirely rule out a role for IL-1 in the generation of helper T-cell factors. It is possible that IL-1 does play a role in these responses, but that only small amounts of IL-1 are necessary or that the relevant IL-1 may be directly transmitted from Mϕ to T cell during contactual interactions. The lack of effect on the production of helper T-cell factors, however, resulting from maneuvers designed to limit the amount of IL-1 in culture stands in marked contrast to the sensitivity of the generation of ISC in mixed cell cultures to the same manipulations. For example, anti-LP antibody inhibited the generation of ISC by more than 95% at concentrations that had no effect whatsoever on the generation of helper T-cell activities. Similarly, aged Mϕ, which were unable to support the generation of ISC, were perfectly capable of supporting the generation of helper T-cell factors. These results imply that the major action of IL-1 in the generation of ISC is not to facilitate the production of necessary helper T-cell factors, but possibly involves the delivery of a requisite signal directly to the responding B cell.

Current studies support the view that IL-1 conveys a necessary activation signal directly to the B cell. Thus, in cultures of purified B cells, IL-1 could be shown to participate synergistically with helper T-cell factors, while removal of IL-1 with anti-LP completely inhibited the generation of ISC. A number of studies in the mouse have also suggested that IL-1 is directly involved in B-cell activation. Thus, for example, Leibson *et al.* (1982) showed that supernatants from the Mϕ tumor line $P388D_1$ or from normal Mϕ taken from *Corynebacterium parvum*-immune mice augmented the generation of antibody-forming cells to the antigen SRBCs in murine spleen cell cultures depleted of T cells and macrophages. These investigators were unable, however, to show an absolute requirement for this Mϕ factor in the responses studied, demonstrating only an amplifying effect. Similarly, Hoffmann (1980) and Howard and Paul (1983) have suggested that IL-1 plays a direct role in triggering B-cell differentiation into antibody-forming cells. The studies discussed in this chapter demonstrate not only that IL-1 has a direct effect on the responding B cell, but also that IL-1 provides a necessary signal without which the differentiation into ISC does not occur.

The experiments also provide some insight into the role played by IL-1 in B-cell activation, as outlined in Fig. 1. The results suggest that IL-1 is essential during the first 24 hr of B-cell stimulation. Moreover, IL-1 has little demonstrable effect on resting B cells in the absence of a polyclonal B-cell activator. Preincubating B cells with IL-1 had little effect on their subsequent capacity to respond to a polyclonal B-cell activator in the absence of IL-1. However, in the presence of a B-cell activator, such as PWM, IL-1 was able to deliver a requisite signal preparing the B cell for the next step of differentiation. The experiments presented heretofore do not indicate whether B-cell activation involves sequential steps in which the mitogen induces IL-1 responsiveness or whether both mitogen and IL-1 must be present simultaneously to trigger B cells. Since resting B cells appear to be unresponsive to IL-1, it is possible that the polyclonal activator may be involved in inducing receptors for IL-1 on B cells. Alternatively, the mitogen may function as a ligand linking IL-1 to the appropriate B-cell receptor. Experiments in the mouse in which anti-immunoglobulin was used as the polyclonal B-cell activator tend to support the former conclusion (Howard and Paul, 1983). Either possibility is tenable at this point, however. Further insight will require biochemical analysis of the properties of putative IL-1 receptors on activated B cells.

Results of studies using murine B cells have suggested that IL-1 may play a role early in culture by preparing B cells to receive helper T-cell signals (Hoffman, 1980). In the studies reported here, a similar sequence of events may occur. Thus, the data support the view that IL-1 influences B-cell activation before

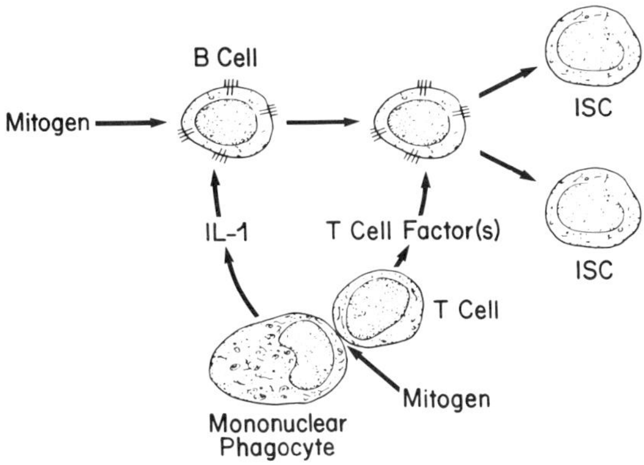

Figure 1. Schematic representation of the role of Mϕ and IL-1 in human B-cell activation.

T-cell signals are necessary. This conclusion is consonant with the work of Yoshizaki *et al.* (1982), who demonstrated that anti-Ig-stimulated human leukemic B cells will differentiate in the presence of a signal from T cells, but the T-cell factor does not appear to play a role until after the first 24 hr of incubation with anti-Ig. Similarly, the experiments reported here showed that T-cell signals do not appear to be involved in differentiation of human B cells into ISC until 24–48 hr of culture, well after the period of time when IL-1 has acted. These results thus support the view of Hoffmann (1980) that IL-1 plays a role early in B-cell activation, which may involve preparing B cells to receive appropriate T-cell signals necessary for their proliferation and subsequent development into ISC. The possibility that IL-1 is involved in the induction of receptors for T-cell helper factors may explain the observation that IL-1 activity is most apparent when T-cell help is suboptimal (Rosenberg and Lipsky, 1980). In the presence of large amounts of helper T-cell factors, only minimal induction of appropriate receptors on B cells may be necessary, whereas when T-cell help is limited, more receptors or greater receptor affinity may be necessary for optimal B-cell differentiation to ISC.

Howard and Paul (1983) have also suggested that IL-1 may play a role early in B-cell activation. In the murine system that these workers studied, however, IL-1 appeared to exert its influence before the differentiation signal conveyed by one T-cell factor (B-cell differentiation factor), but after initial activation by anti-immunoglobulin and another T-cell factor (B-cell growth factor). In the studies reported here, no T-cell influences were necessary before IL-1 in the induction of ISC. There are a number of possibilities to explain this discrepancy. First, in the experiments reported here, small numbers of T cells may have been contaminating the cultures that could be producing the requisite B-cell growth factor. This appears to be unlikely, however, because rigorous attempts to deplete T cells by a variety of techniques have not altered the responses or the sequence of events demonstrated in the current studies. Moreover, attempts to identify T cells before or after culture have indicated no significant contamination. An alternative and more attractive view is that the difference in the results relates to the differing nature of the B cells studied. Thus, Howard and Paul were studying the activation of small resting splenic B cells that appeared to be in the G_0 stage of the cell cycle at the initiation of the experiments. The human peripheral blood B cells that respond to PWM with differentiation into ISC, however, may not be comparable. Thus, PWM has been suggested to stimulate a distinct subpopulation of relatively large, low-density B cells that have ceased to express receptors for mouse erythrocytes and have a lower density of surface IgD (Dagg and Levitt, 1981; Kuritani and Cooper, 1982). This phenotype indicates that the PWM-responsive B-cell population is a distinct subset that may have been preactivated *in vivo.* Thus, the B cells that respond to PWM may well have already received the equivalent of anti-immunoglobulin and B-cell growth factor stimulation *in vivo*. Therefore, there may be no additional requirement for T-cell factors *in vitro* prior to their stimulation by a polyclonal activator and IL-1.

V. CONCLUSION

The data presented in this chapter indicate that IL-1 plays a necessary role in the activation of human B cells and their subsequent differentiation into immunoglobulin-secreting cells. The data support the view that IL-1 delivers a signal directly to the responding B cell. Moreover, the major effect of IL-1 is required early in the activation sequence and appears to involve the facilitation of the capacity to receive necessary helper T-cell signals. Only with appropriate sequential reception of these signals will differentiation of Ig-secreting cells occur. A better understanding of the precise nature of the receptors involved in this sequence of events and the biochemical consequences of signal transmission of these requisite factors should provide added insight into control of immunoglobulin production in humans.

Acknowledgments

The gifts of purified Interleukin-1 by Dr. L. Lachman and Dr. D. D. Wood, the kind donation of the anti-leukocytic pyrogen antibody by Dr. C. A. Dinarello and Dr. S. M. Wolff, the expert technical assistance of P. A. Thompson, and the skillful preparation of the manuscript by Ms. Debbie McInnis are gratefully acknowledged. This work was supported by grants AM-009989 and AM-00599 from the National Institutes of Health.

VI. REFERENCES

Dagg, M, K., and Levitt, D., 1981, *Cell. Immunol. Immunopathol.* **21**:39–49.
Dinarello, C. A., Renfer, L., and S. M. Wolff, 1977, *Proc. Natl. Acad. Sci. USA* **74**:4624–4627.
Frost, A. F., Monahan, T. M., and Abell, C. W., 1978, *Immunol. Commun.* **7**:251–260.
Gery, I., Davies, P., Derr, J., Krett, N., and Barranger, J. A., 1981, *Cell. Immunol.* **64**:293-303;
Ginsburg, W. W., Finkelman, F. D., and Lipsky, P. E., 1978, *J. Immunol.* **120**:33–39.
Hoffmann, M. K., 1980, *J. Immunol.* **125**:2076–2081.
Howard, M., and Paul, W. E., 1983, *Annu. Rev. Immunol.* **1**:307–333.
Koopman, W. J., Farrar, J. J., and Fuller-Bonar, J., 1978, *Cell. Immunol.* **35**:92–98.
Kuritani, T., and Cooper, M. D., 1982, *J. Exp. Med.* **155**:1561–1566.
Lachman, L. B., Page, S. O., and Metzgar, R. S., 1980, *J. Supramol. Struct.* **13**:457–466.
Leibson, H. J., Marrack, P., and Kappler, J., 1982, *J. Immunol.* **129**:1398–1402.
Lipsky, P. E., Thompson, P. A., Rosenwasser, L. J., and Dinarello, C. A., 1983, *J. Immunol.* **130**:2708–2714.
Oppenheim, J. J., and Gery, I., 1982, *Immunol. Today* **3**:113–119.
Rosenberg, S. A., and Lipsky, P. E., 1979, *J. Immunol.* **122**:926–931.
Rosenberg, S. A., and Lipsky, P. E., 1980, *J. Immunol.* **125**:232–237.
Rosenberg, S. A., and Lipsky, P. E., 1981, *J. Immunol.* **126**:1341–1345.
Rosenwasser, L. J., Dinarello, C. A., and Rosenthal, A. S., 1979, *J. Exp. Med.* **150**:709–714.
Rosenwasser, L. J., and Dinarello, C. A., 1981, *Cell Immunol.* **63**:134–142.
Thiele, D. L., and Lipsky, P. E., 1982, *J. Immunol.* **129**:1033–1040.
Unanue, E. R., 1972, *Adv. Immunol.* **15**:95–165.
Wood, D. D., 1979a, *J. Immunol.* **123**:2400–2407.
Wood, D. D., 1979b, *J. Immunol.* **123**:2395–2399.
Wood, D. D., and Cameron, P. M., 1975, *J. Immunol.* **114**:1094–1110.
Yoshizaki, K., Nakagawa, T., Kaieda, T., Muraguchi, A., Yamamura, Y., and Kishimoto, T., 1982, *J. Immunol.* **128**:1296–1301.

T-Cell Factors That Promote B-Cell Proliferation and Differentiation

Susan L. Swain and Richard W. Dutton

Department of Biology
University of California, San Diego
La Jolla, California 92093

I. INTRODUCTION

The goal of this chapter is to summarize and discuss the studies that have sought to understand just how helper T cells help B cells to proliferate and differeniate into antibody-secreting cells by the production of T-cell factors. The studies of Mitchison and others (Mitchison, 1969) showed that effective T-cell help was only delivered to B cells when both T cell and B cell recognized determinants on the same antigen molecule. This observation led to the hypothesis that T-cell help was delivered via an obligatory cell–cell interaction, and it was later shown that such interactions were major histocompatibility complex (MHC) restricted. Our own studies (Dutton *et al*, 1971) and those of others (Schimpl and Wecker, 1972) showed that in certain experimental models T cells could be replaced by factors contained in culture supernatants of activated T cells. For awhile, there were those who suggested that the latter mechanism represented a special case seen only with erythrocyte antigens or with previously activated B cell. It is now clear that both mechanisms of T-cell help exist. It is thought that some B cells become activated only via direct cell–cell interaction and that others can be affected directly by T-cell factors (Singer *et al.*, 1982). It has been shown that a major fraction of all resting B cells can be driven through activation, proliferation, and differentiation to immunoglobulin secretion solely with the aid of the appropriate soluble agents–antiimmunoglobulin and T-cell culture supernatants (Howard and Paul, 1983). All B cells can be made to respond to the B-cell mitogens, dextran sulfate, and lipopolysaccharide (LPS), in the presence of macrophage-derived factors (Wetzel and Kettman, 1981).

Singer and colleagues (1982) and others have provided strong evidence that it is only the Lyb-5^- subset of B cells that requires direct MHC-restricted T-cell–B-cell interactions and that the Lyb-5^+ and perhaps already activated Lyb-5^- B cells are responsive to factors alone. It seems most likely that both kinds of B cells are responsive to T-cell factors in the proliferation and differentiation events that occur after the initial stages of activation.

In the original studies with activated T-cell culture supernatants, the helper, or T-cell replacing factor (TRF), activity was thought of as a single factor. Subsequent studies have shown that the original TRF may consist of many components, and there is already good evidence that six separate factors, in addition to antigen, may be required to replace T cells. In early studies, lymphocyte populations from the spleens of unimmunized mice were T depleted and cultured with unfractionated culture supernatants of activated T cells and sheep red blood cells (SRBCs). The assay was the measurement of the number of cells secreting antibody to SRBC 4 days later in a direct hemolytic plaque assay. Even with this complex model we were able to show a requirement for two separate culture supernatants that acted synergistically (Swain *et al.*, 1981). One was an Interleukin-2 (IL-2)-containing supernatant and the other a supernatant from the long-term alloreactive T-cell line C.C3.11.75 (DL). We showed that purified IL-2 preparations were also active in this synergy assay and that the level of T-cell growth factor activity correlated closely with the activity of the same preparations in the synergy assay (Swain *et al.*, 1982). It is our current hypothesis that the activity needed in the IL-2-TRF synergy assay is IL-2 but that it is made active via its effect on contaminating non-B cells still present in the B-cell preparation. This issue is further discussed in Section F. The activity present in the C.C3.11.75 culture supernatants was termed (DL)TRF, but we now believe it to be a mix of at least two factors.

The original experimental system was clearly inadequate for further analysis; we have therefore adopted the use of a number of new models. What was needed were models in which (1) the three phases of the response—activation, proliferation, and secretion—could be measured separately; (2) a system in which the problem of contaminating non-B cells could be minimized or eliminated; and (3) methods to fractionate the complex culture supernatants into single or simpler mixtures of factors.

We have made progress in all three areas, which are outlined in this chapter. We have shown that the C.C3.11.75 culture supernatants contain at least two quite distinct activities: a B-cell growth factor (which we first called (DL)BCGF) (Swain and Dutton, 1982), and a secretion factor (DL)TRF. We have shown that the (DL)BCGF is different from the (EL4) BCGF described by Howard *et al.*

(1982) and that a factor very similar to the (DL)BCGF is also present in unseparated phorbol myristate acetate (PMA)-induced EL4 culture supernatants. We have suggested that these two BCGFs be called $BCGF_I$ and $BCGF_{II}$, respectively and that they act on different B-cell subsets or at different stages in the response (Swain *et al.*, 1983).

We were able to show that factors present in the C.C3.11.75 supernatants act directly on B cells, and not via some contaminating non-B cell. Finally, we have shown that IL-2 is not involved in the secretion stage of the response, of at least some B cells, and also that interferon is not active in this assay.

II. RESULTS AND DISCUSSION

A. Separate TRF and BCGF Activities in DL Culture Supernatants

The spleens of BALB/c mice taken 4–8 weeks after injection of the BCL_1 *in vivo* line consist predominantly of BCL_1 tumor cells. Cultures containing 5×10^4 of such cells from anti-Thy-1-treated mice contain very few contaminating non-B cells. These cells do not proliferate when cultured alone but are stimulated markedly by LPS (at 0.2–20 μg/ml) or by very low concentrations of the C.C3.11.75 culture supernatants (0.1–0.01%). The latter activity can be absorbed from the culture supernatants by fresh or glutaraldehyde-fixed BCL_1 cells, but not by a comparable number of normal B cells. The abosrbed supernatants still contain the TRF activity as assayed in the IL-2-TRF synergy assay. This finding shows that the BCGF and TRF activities are attributable to different factors and implies that the BCGF is either not involved or not limiting in the 4-day PFC (plaque forming cell) response to SRBC (Swain and Dutton, 1982).

B. Difference Between BCGF Activity in DL Culture Supernatants and EL4 BCGF

T-depleted B-cell populations from normal mice show a small but variable stimulation of proliferation in response to C.C3.11.75 culture supernatants (Swain *et al.*, 1982). This stimulation is not enhanced by the addition of anti-μ but is enhanced by the addition of dextran sulfate (DXS) at 50 μg/ml (Swain *et al.*, 1983); see Table I). We have shown that DXS alone does not stimulate a significant proliferation response but does produce increased levels of RNA characteristic of the G_0–G_1 transition (Table II). We conclude that (DL)BCGF acts on B cells activated by DXS. The observation that anti-μ does not synergize with (DL)BCGF despite the fact that it stimulates a portion of B cells to G_1 (Table II) suggested that (DL)BCGF was different from the EL4 BCGF described

Table I. Synergy between DXS and (DL)BCGF[a–c]

	Expt. 1	Expt. 2
None	305 (267–348)	460 (424–498)
(DL)BCGF		
1%	1,609 (1,506–1,719)	3,430 (3,336–3,526)
0.2%	1,037 (979–1,099)	2,278 (2,178–2,383)
0.04%	621 (506–763)	1.707 (1,563–1,865)
DXS (50 μg/ml)	2,438 (2,180–2,726)	1,443 (1,350–1,542)
DXS + (DL)BCGF		
1%	9,085 (7,741–11,047)	9,333 (9,014–9,663)
0.2%	9,711 (9,460–9,960)	6,052 (5,792–6,325)
0.04%	9,290 (8,613–10,021)	3.453 (3.219–3,705)

[a]BDF_1 mice with ATS treated (0.06 ml/, i.p.) 3 and 1 days before sacrifice. Spleen cells from these mice were treated with two MoAbs to Thy 1.2 and one MoAb to Ly 2.2 plus complement and then G10 passed; 5×10^4 cells/well were cultured in 0.1 ml with various factor additions.

[b]Data are expressed as mean counts per minute (cpm) for triplicate cultures (± SEM) of 72-hr cultures, pulsed with [^{125}I] IUdR for the final 6 hr.

[c]ATS, anti-thymocyte serum; (DL)BCGF, DL-B-cell growth factor; DXS, dextran sulfate; MoAbs, monoclonal antibodies.

by Howard *et al.* (1982) and that different subsets of B cells are responsive to the two BCGFs (Swain *et al.*, 1983). This finding was further substantiated by experiments that showed that the phenyl-Sepharose-purified EL4 BCGF had no activity on either DXS-stimulated normal B cells or BCL_1 cells (Swain *et al.*, 1983).

Table II. Cell-Cycle State of B Cells[a,b]

	G_0	G_1	S, M, G_2
Fresh B cells	96.5	2.1	1.4
BCL_1	8.9	88.1	3.0
Cultured B (48 hr)			
None	79.0	16.2	4.3
DXS (50 μg/ml)	52.4	31.4	15.9
Anti-μ (5 μg/ml)	20.8	54.0	24.4

[a]Cells were analyzed for cell-cycle state by comparing their ratio of DNA:RNA according to red and green fluorescence after staining with acridine orange. Fluorescence was analyzed on an orthocytofluorograph.

[b]B cells and BCL_1 were prepared as in proliferation assays (see footnotes to Tables I and III). Cultured B cells were cultured at 5×10^5/ml.

C. Presence of $BCGF_{II}$ Activity in EL4 Culture Supernatants

EL4 culture supernatants induced with 0.3 ng/ml PMA, however, do contain a factor active in the BCL_1 or DXS assays (Table III). This factor, apparently very similar to the (DL)BCGF, can be recovered from well-defined peaks on ACA 54 or ACA 34 columns in high yield and has an apparent molecular weight (M_r) in the neighborhood of 55,000 (Dutton *et al.*, 1984) in contrast to the phenyl-Sepharose-purified EL4 BCGF, which has an apparent M_r of 18,000. We have concluded that there are two quite distinct BCGF activities and have called them $BCGF_I$ and $BCGF_{II}$. Their properties are summarized in Table IV.

D. Comparisons with Human BCGFs

B-cell growth factors have also been described in the human system by Kishimoto and colleagues (Okada *et al.*, 1983). One of these factors, with a M_r of 55,000, is active on the human B-cell tumor line and, by these criteria, may be analogous to the 55,000-M_r $BCGF_{II}$ in the mouse.

Table III. EL4-Unseparated Supernatants Containing $BCGF_{II}$[a-c]

	BCL_1 proliferation		B + DXS
None	519 (495–545)	None	625 (501–779)
$EL4_{5\text{-}9\text{-}83}$		DL_H	
10%	7,026 (6,690–7,380)	5%	6,242 (6.060–6,430)
3%	3,473 (3,359–3,590)	1.25%	4,327 (3,561–5,259)
1%	1,802 (1,717–1,892)	0.31%	3,100 (2,993–3,211)
0.1%	817 (671–996)	0.08%	2,794 (2,773–2,814)
$EL4_{5\text{-}17\text{-}83}$		$EL4_{5\text{-}17\text{-}83}$	
10%	5,669 (5,269–6,763)	10%	2,980 (2,710–3,278)
3%	3,775 (3,519–4,050)	3%	3,110 (2,929–3,304)
1%	2,344 (2,315–2,373)	1%	1,058 (1,008–1,110)
0.1%	1,361 (1,304–1,422)		
LPS	7,410 (6,931–7,921)	LPS (50 μg/ml)	4,373 (4'256–4,493)

[a]EL4 at 5×10^5 cells/ml was induced with 0.3 ng/ml PMA and supernatant collected after 18 hr. BCL_1 cells were obtained from the spleens of tumor-bearing animals 5–8 weeks after inoculation with 10^6 cells. Spleen cells were treated with two MoAbs to Thy 1.2 and MoAb to Ly 2.2 plus complement. Such cells are 90–100% sIg^+ and 90–100% BCL_1 idiotype positive both at initiation of culture and after 3 days in culture with sources of $BCGF_{II}$. Triplicate cultures contain 5×10^4 cells.

[b]Proliferation of normal B to DXS (50 μg/ml) plus factor is as described in Table I footnote. All cultures were pulsed with [^{125}I]UdR for the last 6 hr and data represent mean counts per minute (cpm) of triplicate cultures (± SEM).

[c]BCGF, B-cell growth factor; DXS, dextran sulfate; LPS, lipopolysaccharide; MoAbs, monoclonal antibodies.

Table IV. Summary of Activities of Factor Preparations in B-Cell Proliferation Assays[a]

	BCL_1 proliferation	DXS-induced normal B proliferation	Anti-μ-induced normal B proliferation	BCGF type
Bulk supernatants				
EL4 (PMA-induced)	+++	+++	+++	I and II
DL (stimulator or IL-2-induced)	++++	++++	–	II
Purified BCGFs				
EL4 (M. H. phenyl-Sepharose 18,000)	–	–	++++	I
EL4 (ACA 54 45,000–65,000 fraction)	+++	+++	–	II
Other factors				
IL-2	–	–	–	None
IL-1	–	–	–	None

[a]BCGF, B-cell growth factor; DXS, dextran sulfate; IL-1, -2, Interleukin-1, -2; PMA, phorbol myristate acetate.

Human BCGFs have been reported to act synergistically in some experimental protocols (Okada *et al.*, 1983). Mouse $BCGF_I$ and $BCGF_{II}$ are weakly synergistic, in both the BCL_1 proliferation and DXS-induced normal B proliferation assays (S. L. Swain, unpublished results). Further experiments comparing mouse and human factors are needed to determine whether the two human BCGFs and two mouse BCGFs are analogous.

A hybridoma-secreting human BCGF has also been described by Fauci and colleagues (Butler *et al.*, 1983; Muraguchi *et al.*, 1983). This BCGF can be measured on normal B cells stimulated with anti-μ and thus appears to be analogous to mouse $BCGF_I$.

E. Direct Action of $BCGF_{II}$ on B Cells

In earlier experiments, we used a limiting dilution culture system in which highly enriched B cells from the spleens of normal mice were cultured at one cell/well. Such cells respond to a mixture of dextran sulfate and LPS by clonal growth and immunoglobulin (Ig) secretion (Wetzel and Kettman, 1981).

The response of suboptimally stimulated cells was shown to be markedly enhanced by the addition of a variety of T-cell line culture supernatants. Unfractionated C.C3.11.75 culture supernatants can increase the frequency of clonal

Table V. Proliferation of BCL_1 *in Vitro* Line Stimulated by ACA 34 Column Fractions (50,000–55,000 M_r) of an EL4 Culture Supernatant

Additions to the medium[a]	[^{125}]IUdR Uptake[b]
ACA 34 column fraction No.[c]	
None	230
20–29	340–600
30	580
34	1000
35	1500
36	3000
37	4300
38	3800
39	2900
40	1700
42	950
43–55	200–700

[a] 10^4 BCL_1 *in vitro* line cells were cultured in 0.1 ml RPMI 1640 in the absence of fetal calf serum.
[b] [^{125}]IUdR uptake was measured during the 6-hr period 20–26 hr after the start of incubation.
[c] Ten μl of the fractions was added to culture wells to give a final concentration of 10%; 50 ml of the EL4 24-hr culture supernatants was applied to an ACA 34 column (26-mm i.d., 778 mm long, flowrate 31 ml/hr); 8-ml fractions were collected.

growth severalfold, demonstrating unequivocally that components present in these supernatants can act directly on a single B cell (Wetzel *et al.*, 1982). Further experiments are in progress to determine which of the purified mouse factors—$BCGF_I$, $BCGF_{II}$, or (DL)TRF—are active in this system.

The fact that the $BCGF_{II}$ activity can be absorbed on BCL_1 also suggests that BCGF acts on B cells. The BCL_1 cells used for these experiments were prepared from the spleens of BCL_1 tumor-carrying mice and could contain contaminating non-BCL_1 cells. It was thus important that we were able to show that the proliferation of the cloned *in vitro* BCL_1 line was enhanced by column-purified EL4 $BCGF_{II}$ (Table V), confirming that $BCGF_{II}$ acts on B cells directly.

F. Measurement of TRF Activities

In our early studies, we assayed TRF activity by the response of purified B-cell populations to SRBC measured in the direct hemolytic plaque assay on day

4. This system obtained good responses when both IL-2-containing and DL supernatants were present together (Swain *et al.*, 1981). The DL culture supernatants contain variable amounts of other activities measurable in various assays, including BCGF, interferon (IFN), and sometimes small amounts of IL-1. It was therefore possible that the activity we had called (DL)TRF was attributable to the presence of some other factor, particularly IFN, or that other factors could also be active in the 4-day PFC response assay.

In our first attempts to investigate this question, we made various preparations of DL culture supernatants by different procedures and assayed both TRF and the virus-neutralizing activity of each preparation. The results we reported earlier (Swain *et al.*, 1982) indicated that there was no correlation between the two assays and that DL supernatants with undetectable amounts of IFN were very active in the TRF assay.

Next, we prepared culture supernatants from the cytotoxic T-cell line, CR15 (Klein *et al.*, 1982), which contained high titers of gamma-Interferon (γ-IFN), and tested them in the TRF assay. The supernatants showed modest levels of TRF activity, which were never as high as those in preparations of (DL)TRF with comparable amounts of IFN (Table VI).

The 4-day PFC response involves activation and requires a high degree of proliferation of the few SRBC specific B cells present in each culture, as well as

Table VI. Effect of IFN in IL-2-TRF Synergy Assay[a-c]

	Expt. 1	Expt. 2
None	11 (5–25)	36 (23–56)
(DL)TRF		
2%	938 (917–960)	1,172 (1,135–1,211)
0.4%	361 (306–425)	518 (472–596)
0.8%	280 (216–364)	434 (295–640)
(Cr15) IFN		
10%	96 (92–100)	251 (189–334)
2%	74 (23–163)	241 (233–249)
0.4%	131 (93–185)	99 (72–135)
0.08%		28 (16–48)

[a]BDF_1 B cells were prepared as indicated in the footnote Table I. B cells at 6×10^5/well were cultured with 20% IL-2 containing supernatant and 0.1% SRBC. (DL)TRF had 768 units of IFN and (Cr15) γ-IFN had 1536 units of IFN. Direct PFCs were determined on day 4.

[b]Data are expressed as PFCs per culture and represent the geometric mean (± SEM) of triplicate microcultures.

[c]IFN, interferon; IL-2, Interleukin-2; PFC, plague-forming cell; SRBC, sheep red blood cell; TRF, T-cell replacing factor.

the differentiation to Ig-secretion step, in which TRF is said to be involved. It would thus be expected to score factors that affected the earlier steps, provided that some level of TRF activity was present.

We therefore assayed these same culture supernatants in a BCL_1-secretion assay. The number of BCL_1 cells is not expected to be limiting in this assay, and the B cells are already activated, hence the possibility that factors for activation and proliferation will not be required. We and our colleagues (Puré *et al.*, 1981) had earlier shown that DL supernatants increased the number of BCL_1 cells detectable in an Ig-secretion assay. We used this same model to determine whether IL-2 or γ-IFN had a role in stimulating secretion.

Table VII shows that DL culture supernatant (containing IFN) was strongly active in this assay. IL-2-containing culture supernatants displayed no activity when added alone, nor did they enhance the response to the DL culture supernatants. We therefore concluded that the requirement for IL-2 in the 4-day PFC response to SRBC was most likely for some earlier step. γ-IFN-containing culture supernatants from the CR15 and FS7.20.18 line of Marrack and Kappler were also inactive, suggesting that whatever role γ-IFN may have in the other

Table VII. Activities of Factor Preparations in Inducing BCL_1 Secretion[a–c]

Expt. No.		PFCs/culture
1	None	45
	(DL)TRF	3990
	(DL)*TRF	3200
	FS7.20.18	50
2	None	36
	(DL)*TRF	532
	Cr15	20
	(DL)*TRF + Cr15	480
3	None	23
	IL-2	43
	(DL)TRF	248
	(DL)TRF + IL-2	266

[a]Factors were tested at 10% for their ability to cause BCL_1 to differentiate to PFCs. 2.5×10^4 BCS_1 were cultured in duplicate, and results are the mean PFCs/culture for the duplicate wells.

[b](DL)TRF was a batch with 768 units/ml of IFN; (DL)*TRF had <3 units/ml of IFN and no BCGF activity (I or II). FS7.20.18 had 768 units of IFN, and Cr15 had 1536 units of IFN. IL-2 from BW.Mls cell line was the same IL-2 that synergizes with TRF (see Table VI).

[c]BCGF, B-cell growth factor; IFN, interferon; IL-2, Interleukin-2; TRF, T-cell replacing factor.

model system, it is not involved in the secretion step, at least for BCL_1 cells. The BCL_1 cell is a tumor cell, however, and it is possible that the secretion assay used here may not truly reflect the physiological processes that take place in the normal B-cell response to antigen. It is also possible that the assay reflects the activity of only one subpopulation of B cells. Further assays with a variety of B-cell lines having different properties are planned to help resolve this issue.

It is of interest that this activity, in contrast to $(DL)BCGF_{II}$, is not absorbed by the BCL_1 tumor cells. Thus no evidence that IFN acts as a B-cell differentiation factor is seen in these studies. We propose that its enhancing effects in the antigen-specific system might be due to some indirect effect leading to enhancement of some other step in the B-cell life cycle.

III. SUMMARY AND CONCLUSIONS

We have developed new protocols for the separate assay of proliferation and differentiation in the B-cell response to antigen. With these assays, we have shown that there are two different B-cell growth factors—$BCGF_I$ and $BCGF_{II}$—that appear to act on different subpopulations of B cells. $BCGF_{II}$ has been shown to act directly on B cells and can be absorbed by BCL_1 cells. $BCGF_{II}$ is present in culture supernatants of EL4 and has an apparent molecular weight in the neighborhood of 55,000. These BCGFs can be distinguished from IL-2 TRF, γ-IFN, and other lymphokines by a variety of procedures. Another activity present in the culture supernatants of the C.C3.11.75 long-term alloreactive T-cell line enhances the secretion of immunoglobulin by the BCL_1 tumor cell line. It appears to be a component of the activity previously assayed by the 4-day PFC response to SRBC and designated (DL)TRF. IL-2 and γ-IFN are inactive in this assay, suggesting they may well play an indirect role, or a role in earlier stages of the B-cell response, in those B-cell differentiation assays in which they score.

ACKNOWLEDGMENTS

We wish to thank Dr. Jim Watson, for purified IL-2, Dr. Maureen Howard, for purified (EL4)BCGF, Dr. John Kappler and Dr. Philippa Marrack, for FS7.20.18, Dr. John Klein and Dr. Michael Bevan, for the Cr15 line, and John Klein again, for doing the IFN determinations. This work is supported by grants AI-08795 and CA-09174 from the National Institutes of Health, grant IM-1P from the American Cancer Society, and the American Heart Association's Established Investigatorship to Dr. Susan Swain.

IV. REFERENCES

Butler, J. L., Muraguchi, A., Lane, H. C., and Fauci, A. S., 1983, *J. Exp. Med.* **157**:60.

Dutton, R. W., Falkoff, R., Hirst, J. A., Hoffmann, M., Kappler, J. W., Kettman, J. R., Lesley, J. F., And Vann, D., 1971, *Progress Immunology* **1**:355.

Dutton, R. W., Wetzel, G. D., and Swain, S. L., 1984, *J. Immunol.* **132**:2451.

Howard, M., and Paul, W. E., 1983, *Annu. Rev. Immunol.* **1**:307.

Howard, M., Farrar, J., Hilfiker, M., Johnson, B., Takatsu, K., Hamaoka, T., and Paul, W. E., 1982, *J. Exp. Med.* **155**:914.

Klein, J. R., Raulet, D. H., Pasternack, M. S., and Bevan, M. J., 1982, *J. Exp. Med.* **155**:1198.

Mitchison, N. A., 1969, in: *Immunological Tolerance* (M. Landy, and W. Braum, eds), p. 149, Academic Press, New York.

Muraguchi, A., Butler, J. L., Kehrl, J. H., and Fauci, A. S., 183, *J. Exp. Med.* **157**:530.

Okada, M., Sakaguchi, N., Yoshimura, N., Hara, H., Shimazu, K., Hoshida, N., Yoshizaki, K., Kishimoto, S., Yamamura, Y., and Kishimoto, T., 1983, *J. Exp. Med.* **157**:583.

Puré, E., Isakson, P. C., Takatsu, K., Hamaka, T., Swain, S. L., Dutton, R. W., Dennert, G., Uhr, J. W., and Vitetta, E. S., 1981, *J. Immunol.* **127**:1953.

Schimpl, A. L., and Wecker, E., 1972, *Nature* **237**:15.

Singer, A., Asano, Y., Shigeta, M., Hathcock, K. S., Ahmed, A., Fathman, G., and Hodes, R. J., 1982, *Immunol. Rev.* **64**:137.

Swain, S. L., and Dutton, R. W., 1982, *J. Exp. Med.* **156**:1821.

Swain, S. L., Dennert, G., Warner, J. F., and Dutton, R. W. 1981, *Proc. Natl. Acad. Sci. USA* 78:2517.

Swain, S. L., Wetzel, G. D., Soubiran, P., and Dutton, R. W., 1982, *Immunol. Rev.* **64**:11.

Swain, S. L., Howard, M., Kappler, J. W., Marrack, P., Watson, J., Booth, R., Wetzel, G. D., and Dutton, R. W., 1983, *J. Exp. Med.* **158**:822.

Wetzel, G. D., and Kettman, J. R., 1981, *J. Immunol.* **126**:723.

Wetzel, G. D., Swain, S. L., and Dutton, R. W., 1982, *J. Exp. Med.* **156**:306.

T-Cell-Replacing Factor and Its Acceptor Site on B Cells: Molecular Properties and Immunogenetic Aspects

Toshiyuki Hamaoka

Institute for Cancer Research
Osaka Universtiy Medical School
Fukushimaku, Osaka, 553, Japan

I. INTRODUCTION

It has been generally postulated that B-cell proliferation and differentiation into immunoglobulin (Ig)-producing cells are regulated by several soluble factors derived from macrophages and T cells. This has been demonstrated in both antigen-specific responses (Dutton *et al.*, 1971; Schimpl and Wecker, 1972; Hamaoka *et al.*, 1973; Harwell *et al.*, 1976, 1980; Delovitch and McDevitt, 1977; Takatsu *et al.*, 1980b; Andersson and Melchers, 1981; Takatsu and Hamaoka, 1982; Swain *et al.*, 1982; Howard *et al.*, 1982) and nonspecific responses induced by anti-Ig as a stimulator analogous to the antigen (Kishimoto and Ishizaka, 1975; Parker *et al.*, 1979; Pure *et al.*, 1981; Isakson *et al.*, 1982; Yoshizaki *et al.*, 1982; Nakanishi *et al.*, 1983). However, the biochemical identification and characterization of such soluble factors and the determination of a cascade reaction of those factors in B-cell proliferation and differentiation have been difficult due to the mixture of activities closely related in those functions. One approach to solving this problem has been to use soluble products from monoclonal T-cell hybridomas, which release selected lymphokine activity.

Our laboratory has been interested in identifying a soluble factor involved in the B-cell differentiation process, since the analysis of this process will provide us with the fundamental information for the final stage of T–B-cell interactions for antibody production and present an intriguing model for elucidation of the gene-control mechanisms involved in B-cell differentiation. The T-cell-derived lymphokines that stimulate activated B cells to differentiate into antibody-forming cells have been generally designated as T-cell-replacing factor (TRF).

This chapter reviews the recent progress of our analysis of the molecular properties of TRF derived from a T-cell hybridoma, B151K12. In addition, an attempt is made to further elucidate the immunogenetic aspects of the TRF acceptor site on B lymphocytes, since the identification and characterization of TRF as inducer molecule and its acceptor site as responder molecule are both important issues for further understanding the final step of B-cell differentiation.

II. ESTABLISHMENT OF A T-CELL HYBRIDOMA SPONTANEOUSLY PRODUCING TRF

In studying the molecular properties of TRF, we have established a T-cell hybrid clone, B151K12, which has the ability to produce TRF without any mitogenic stimulation. This TRF induces differentiation of B cells into specific antibody-producing cells. With the fusion of the AKR-derived thymoma cell line BW5147 and *Mycobacterium*-primed and boosted BALB/c T cells, a total of 513 clones of proliferating hybrid cells were obtained. The TRF activity in cultured fluid supernatant (CFS) was measured, and the most potent TRF producers without any further antigenic stimulations were selected. For the TRF assay, various strains of mice were immunized intraperitoreally (i.p.) with 100 μg DNP–KLH in 4 mg aluminum hydroxide gel (Alum) along with 1×10^9 *Bordetella pertussis* vaccine and were given booster doses of 5 μg of the same antigen in saline 8–10 weeks later. Spleen cells were prepared from the mice 10 days after the booster injection and were treated with anti-brain-associated Thy-1 antibody plus selected rabbit complement (C) or with monoclonal anti-Thy-1.2 (F7D5) antibody and complement to deplete T cells. A half-volume each of the dialyzed CFS containing TRF or various testing lymphokines, and 5×10^6/ml of hapten-primed B cells (T-cell depleted) were mixed together. To these cell suspensions, hapten–protein conjugates were added to a final concentration of 40 ng/ml; 0.2 ml of the cell suspensions were distributed into each well of a tissue culture plate (Microplate II) and cultured for 5 days. Anti-hapten IgG PFC (plaque-forming cell) responses were assayed by the method described previously (Takatsu *et al.*, 1980b).

The TRF in CFS produced by a monoclonal T-cell hybridoma, B151K12, exhibited stimulatory activity toward B cells in a totally antigen nonspecific manner (Takatsu *et al.*, 1980a). The T-cell-replacing character of the CFS from the clone B151K12 was ascertained on the basis of its triggering of the anti-hapten IgG PFC responses of T-cell-depleted hapten-primed spleen cells upon stimulation with the hapten–heterologous carrier, DNP-ovalbumin (DNP-OVA). More definitively. DNP-(D-glutamine: D-lysine copolymer), to which the T cells are not definitely expected to respond, was also able to trigger DNP-primed B cells in the presence of the CFS of B151K12 (Takatsu *et al.*, 1980b).

Studies by Watson *et al.* (1979) and Watson and Mochizuki (1980), Parker (1980) Parker *et al.* (1979) and Harwell *et al.* (1980) have demonstrated that many conventional sources of helper T-cell-replacing activity are mixtures of Interleukin-2 (IL-2), TRF, and perhaps IL-1. In order to determine the property of the CFS of B151K12, the CFS was measured for its IL-2 activity on the basis of ability to maintain the growth of an IL-2-dependent T-cell clone, CTLL.B6, and for its IL-1 activity by the thymocyte costimulator assay (Paetkau *et al.*, 1976). Various sources of IL-2 and IL-1 were used as positive controls in this assay. Unlike the culture supernatant derived from antigen-reactive helper T cells stimulated with antigen, the B151K12 supernatants lack any obvious IL-1, IL-2, and killer helper-factor activity (Hamaoka *et al.*, 1981a). Moreover, B151K12 supernatant does not contain any measureable interferon activity.

Most conventional TRF assays respond to IL-2 and often to IL-1 (Hoffman *et al.*, 1978). However, Harwell *et al.* (1980) reported that rabbit anti-mouse thymocyte serum (ATS)-pretreatment of spleen cell donors combined with *in vitro* depletion with anti-Thy-1 antibody produced a spleen population that concanavalin A (Con A)-stimulated T-cell culture supernatant, but not IL-2 from their FS6-14.13 line, would reconstitute for a primary plaque-forming cell response to sheep red blood cells (SRBCs). It seemed likely that these spleen cells were now dependent on an additional activity or activities present in the Con A supernatant. Furthermore, studies by Parker (1980) suggested that B cells responded by proliferation to anti-Ig plus IL-2 and that some component or other factor(s) in Con A supernatant was necessary for their further differentiation to antibody-producing cells.

In order to rigorously exclude the possibility that the B-cell-triggering activity of the CFS of B151K12 was due to stimulation of the residual T-cells contamination in the B-cell population, spleen cells from DNP-KLH-primed mice pretreated with rabbit anti-thymocyte-specific antiserum 2 days before sacriface were further treated with monoclonal anti-Thy 1.2 plus complement. Recovered splenic B cells were tested for their ability to respond to the various lymphokines derived from T-cell hybridomas listed in Table I, after partial purification as shown in Figs. 1 and 2. As summarized in Table II, the addition of A55-24-derived IL-2 or FS6-derived B-cell growth factor (BCGF-1 or BSFp-1) or BCGF-1 plus IL-2 were all not sufficient to reconstitute the plaque-forming cell response. Moreover, the addition of Ultrogel AcA54-semipurified IL-1 derived from the lipopolysaccharide (LPS)-pulsed J774.1 macrophage cell line did not induce any PFC response under these conditions. In contrast, the addition of CFS of B151K12 alone gave rise to a significant number of plaque-forming cells after 5 days of culture.

Table I. Lymphokine-Producing T-cell Hybridomas[a]

Hybridoma	Lymphokine activities BCGF[b]	IL-2[c]	TRF[d]
FS6-14.13	++	++	–
A55-24	–	+	–
B151K12	–	–	++

[a]BCGF, B-cell growth factor; IL-2, Interleukin-2. TRF, T-cell replacing factor.

[b]The BCGF assay employed involved the culture of 5×10^4 purified B cells/well with anti-IgM antibodies at a final concentration of 2 μg/ml in the presence of varying dilutions of CFS. Culture were incubated for 3 days with a final 16-hr pulse of [^{3}H]thymidine, and the [^{3}H]thymidine incorporated into cells was measured.

[c]The IL-2 activity was measured by the increase in proliferation of IL-2-dependent T-cell clone (CTLL.B6; our newly established C57BL/6 anti-C3H/He cytotoxic T-cell line) in the presence of CFS.

[d]TRF activity was assessed using rigorously T-cell-depleted DNP-primed B cells, viz, spleen cells from DNP-KLH-primed and -boosted mice having received i.p. injection of anti-thymocyte serum (ATS) 2 days prior to the experiments and then treated with anti-Thy-1 antiserum plus rabbit complement. These DNP-primed B cells were stimulated *in vitro* with DNP–OVA in the presence of varying dilutions of CFS from B151K12 cells before and after fractionation. After 5 days, anti-DNP IgG PFC responses were enumerated. In some experiments, TRF activity was measured using BALB/c chronic leukemia B cells (BCL1), as described by Pure *et al.* (1981).

In collaboration with us, Vitetta and colleagues (Pure *et al.*, 1981) attempted to demonstrate the TRF activity of the CFS of B151K12 in the polyclonal activation of murine B lymphocytes. Supernatants from the B151K12 cell lines alone induced polyclonal IgM secretion by adult B cells as well as murine chronic leukemia BCL1 B cells maintained *in vivo*. We extended this type of approach using anti-Thy-1 antibody plus C-treated and Percoll-purified BCL1 cells. BCL1 cells were cultured with CFS from various T-cell hybridomas without any antigenic stimulation for 3 days, and the number of IgM PFC was enumerated by using protein A-bound SRBC as detector cells. The CFS from the B151K12 cell line alone induced polyclonal IgM secretion by Percoll-purified neoplastic B cells. By contrast, BCGF-1 and IL-2 from FS6-14.13 and A55-24 again did not induce any polyclonal IgM secretion. The addition of either *Escherichia coli*-expressed murine γ-interferon (γ-IFN) or J774.1-derived IL-1 also did not induce any significant PFC response under these conditions. The addition of purified IL-3

Table II. Induction of B-Cell Differentiation by Various Lymphokines[a]

Responder B cells	Lymphokines	PFC response/well[h]
	–	32 (1.02)
DNP-KLH-	IL-1[b]	40 (1.11)
primed cells	IL-2[c]	58 (1.12)
(1.0 × 10^6/well)	BCGF[d]	71 (1.21)
	IL-2 + BCGF	62 (1.10)
	B151-TRF[e]	482 (1.08)
	–	10 (1.01)
	IL-1	10 (1.12)
	IL-2	12 (1.08)
BCL1	BCGF	14 (1.21)
cells	IL-2 + BCGF	14 (1.14)
(1.0 × 10^5/well)	B151-TRF	504 (1.07)
	γ-IFN[f]	17 (1.14)
	IL-3[g]	12 (1.11)

[a] Abbreviations as in Table I.
[b] IL-1 is the semipurified fraction by Ultrogel AcA 54 gel-filtration of CFS of lipopolysaccharide (LPS)-pulsed J 774.1 macrophage tumor-cell line added at a 10%-equivalent concentration of the original CFS.
[c] IL-2 is derived from A55-24 CFS shown in Fig. 2; the predominant peak of IL-2 activity in pI range of 5.3 was added at a 5%-equivalent concentration of the original CFS.
[d] BCGF is derived from FS6-14.13 CFS shown in Fig. 1 and is added to the well at a 10%-equivalent concentration of the original CFS according the report of Howard *et al.* (1982).
[e] B151-TRF represents the CFS of B151K12 in this experiment added to a well at 50% v/v.
[f] γ-IFN is the *Escherichia coli*-expressed murine γ-interferon (lot 1641/46, 1 mg/ml 1 × 10^9 u/ml) kindly supplied by D. Goeddel (Genentech, Inc.) and added 4.5 × 10^6 u/well.
[g] IL-3 is the purified preparation generously supplied by J. N. Ihle and added 100 ng/well.
[h] These denote the anti-DNP IgG and BCL1 IgM PFC responses after 5- and 3-day cultures, respectively. PFC responses were assayed by the methods described previously (Takatsu *et al.*, 1980b; Pure *et al.*, 1981). The values represent geometric means and standard errors.

alone again did not exhibit any significant B-cell-triggering activity (Table II). Thus, B151K12 hybridoma produced obvious TRF activity in the culture supernatant without any further stimulation, and the TRF derived from B151K12 T-cell hybridoma constitutes a distinct lymphokine activity that induces B-cell differentiation via its direct action on the B cells.

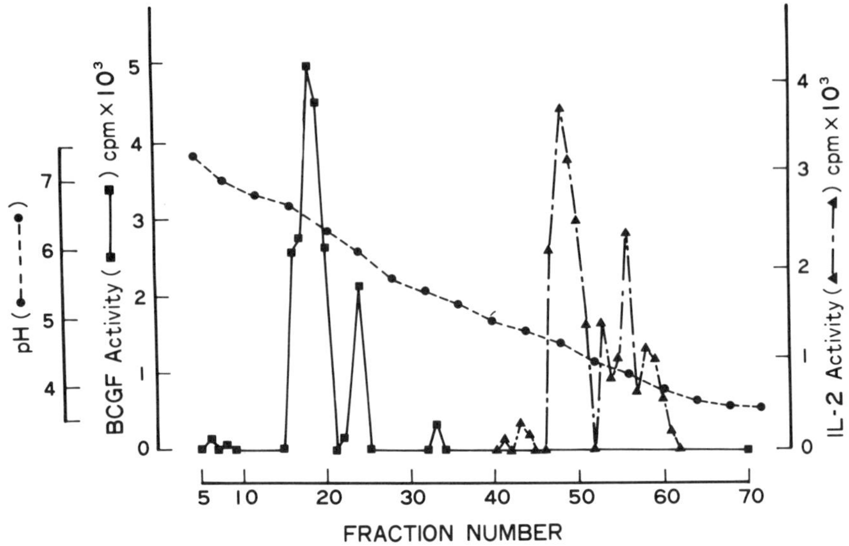

Figure 1. Chromatofocusing of CFS from Con A-stimulated FS6-14.13. Fraction Nos. 15–19 were pooled and used as the BCGF source in Table II. BCGF, B-cell growth factor; CFS, culture fluid supernatant; Con A, Concanavalin A; cpm, counts per minute; IL-2, Interleukin-2.

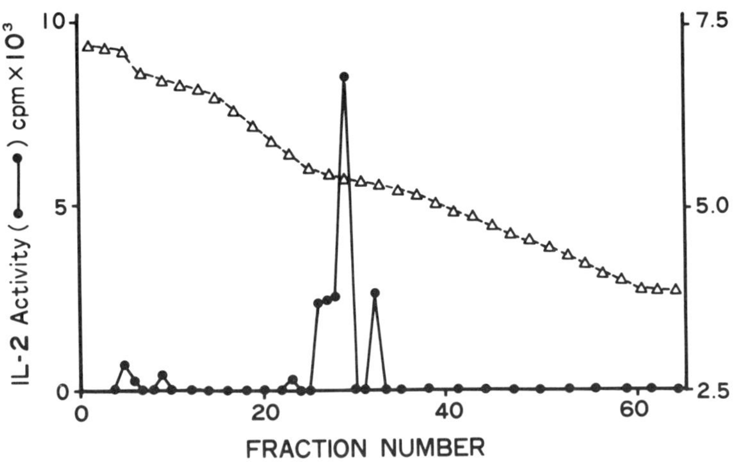

Figure 2. Chromatofocusing of IL-2 from A55-24 CFS. A55-24 is our newly established T-cell hybridoma. It is formed by fusion of *Mycobacterium*-primed T cells with BW5147 and produces only IL-2 without any antigenic stimulation. Fraction Nos. 26–29 were pooled and used as the IL-2 source in Table II. Abbreviations as in Fig. 1.

III. PHYSICOCHEMICAL PROPERTIES OF TRF

The cultured fluid supernatant of B151K12 was salted out with $(NH_4)_2 SO_4$ in the range of 50–80% saturation. Most of the TRF activity was recovered in this fraction. After extensive dialysis, samples were applied to either a chromatofocusing column (pH range: 7.0–4.0) or an Ultrogel AcA 54 gel-filtration column. TRF activity in each fraction was assayed using BCL1 cells. As shown in Fig. 3, the TRF activity was mainly eluted at fractions between the isoelectric points (pI) of 4.9–5.1 by chromatofocusing. By gel filtration, the TRF activity was mainly recovered at fractions in the range of 45,000-60,000 M_r, as shown in Fig. 4. However, some of the TRF activity seemed to associate with other fractions, such as the globulin fraction of fetal calf serum (FCS) carried over from the B151K12 culture medium. These results suggest that the TRF molecule tends

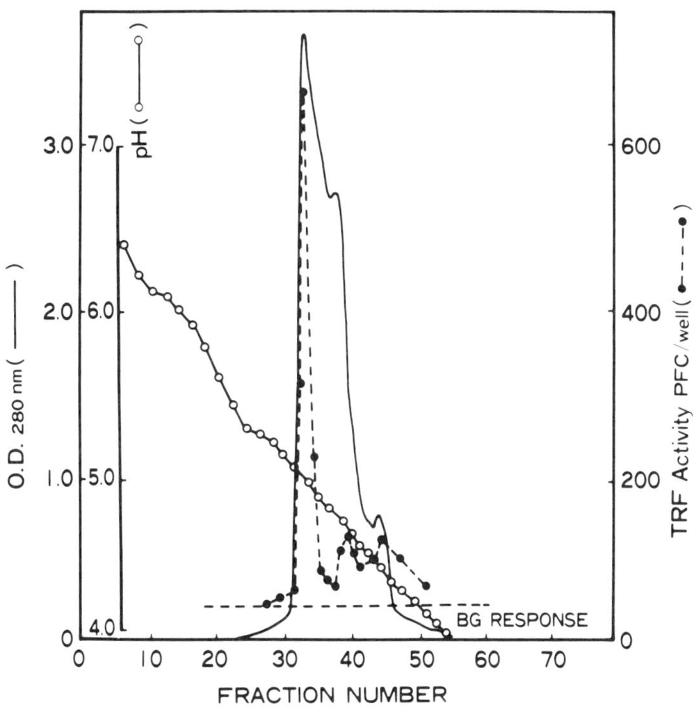

Figure 3. Chromatofocusing analysis of CFS from B151K12. After removal of Polybuffer, each fraction was assayed for TRF activity by adding to the culture of BCL1 cells a 50% (v/v)-equivalent dose to original CFS. BG response represents the PFC response without addition of B151K12 CFS fractions. BG, background, TRF, T-cell replacing factor.

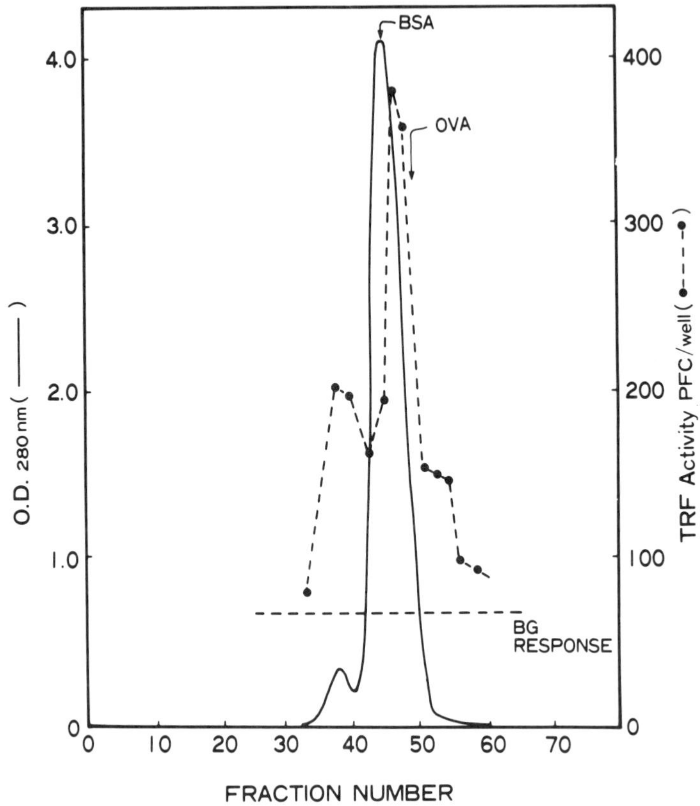

Figure 4. Gel-filtration profile of B151K12 CFS on Ultrogel AcA 54 column. B151K12 CFS was precipitated with ammonium sulfate (50–80%) and subjected to gel filtration on a 2.5 × 100-cm column in phosphate buffer, pH 7.0 at flow-rate of 9 ml/hr. TRF activity was assayed as in Fig. 3.

to bind nonspecifically to the proteins contained in the culture medium, possibly due to its hydrophobicity.

Although by this fractionation procedure the TRF activity could be enriched to a certain extent, clear separation of TRF molecule from other proteins such as bovine serum albumin (BSA) was utterly impractical due to the similarity in physicochemical properties of TRF-active fraction and BSA. In order to further establish an effective condition to separate TRF molecule from BSA, a possible difference in the hydrophobicity of these respective molecules was applied and the CFS of B151K12 was submitted to analysis by reverse-phase high-performance liquid chromatography (RP-HPLC) under the newly devised condition demonstrated in Fig. 5. Under this particular condition, the TRF activity was eluted in

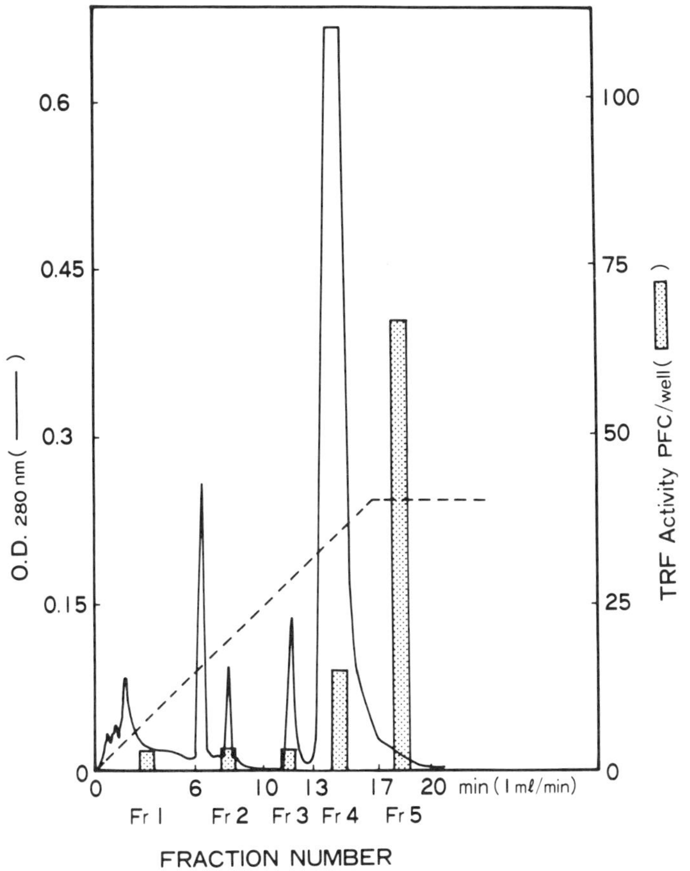

Figure 5. Reverse-phase HPLC fractionation of B151K12 TRF; 500 μl of 10 times concentrated B151K12 CFS was injected into a 4 × 50mm Nucleosil C18 (10 μm) column. Dotted line represents a linear gradient from 0 to 80% of solvent B in solvent A for 16 min. Solvent A denotes a pH 3 buffer solution of 0.1 M NaH_2PO_4 and H_3PO_4, and solvent B comprises the constituents of solvent A, isopropanol, and ethylene glycol with a ratio of 1:3:1. The flow rate was 1 ml/min. A total of five pooled fractions were collected and submitted to the TRF assay. The samples were concentrated 7 times by Diaflow membrane CF24, and dialyzed against RPMI 1640 medium before assay. Measurement of TRF activity was essentially the same as in Figure 3.

a fraction clearly distinct from BSA peak, and an extraordinarily sharp peak of the TRF activity was obtained. RP-HPLC analysis demonstrated that the TRF molecule is more hydrophobic than BSA. After having purified the TRF-active fraction up to this point, the physiochemical properties of TRF were analyzed; the properties of B151K12 TRF as monitored by its activity are summarized in Table III. In particular, it is worth noting that the TRF molecule is free of Ia

Table III. Properties of B151K12-TRF

Reacting cells	Activated B cells and chronic leukemia B cells (BCL1), but not T cells
Function	Terminal differentiation to antibody-forming cells
Activity absorbed on	Activated B cells and certain neoplastic B cells, but not on T cells
Molecular weight	45,000–60,000 by Ultrogel AcA 54 gelfiltration
pI	4.9–5.1 by chromato-focusing
Ia	Negative
Reactivity with	Binding to lima bean agglutinin and *Dolichos biflorus* agglutinin; no binding to soybean agglutinin
Heat stability	Stable (56°C, 1 hr)
pH stability	Stable between pH 2.0–11.0 in Britton Robinson buffer overnight
Proteolytic enzyme stability	Inactivated by trypsin (5 U), α-chymotrypsin (5U), papain (5 U), and protease VIA (1.5 U)
0.1% Sodium Dodecyl Sulfate	Stable
4M guanidine HCl	Stable
4M urea:	Stable
Other properties	No binding to blue Sepharose Stable by lyophilization

molecule, as revealed by its nonbinding property to the anti-Ia immunoadsorbent column. The glycoprotein nature of the TRF molecule was indicated by its efficient binding to the lectin column such as lima bean agglutinin (LBA) and *Dolichos biflorus* agglutinin (DBA), which specifically bind to the terminal sugar residue of GalNAC. The bound TRF activity to these columns was effectively eluted by 0.05-0.2 M GalNAC solution, as shown in Table IV. TRF could also be effectively eluted from those columns with 1.5 M NaCl solution.

Although these physiochemical properties of the TRF activity seemed to be convenient to some extent for the purification of the TRF molecule, contamination by the fetal calf serum (FCS) component in culture fluid supernatant decreased the efficiency of further purification of TRF due to limitations in the

Table IV. Partial Purification of B151K12-TRF by LBA-Sepharose and DBA-Gel[a]

TRF		IgM PFC/Culture	OD280	Specific activity
(−)		10 (1.02)	−	
B151K12-TRF	unfractionated	2821 (1.15)	19.0	1
B151K12-TRF absorbed on LBA-Sepharose	Eluted with 0.2 M GalNAC	1190 (1.24)	0.073	110
	Eluted with 1.5 M NaCl	2134 (1.03)	0.128	113
(−)		12 (1.01)	−	
B151K12-TRF	unfractionated	2468 (1.21)	14.9	1
B151K12-TRF absorbed on DBA-Gel	Eluted with 0.05 M GalNAC	235 (1.11)	0.06	235
	Eluted with 1.5 M NaCl	521 (1.12)	0.01	314

[a]LBA, lima bean agglutinin; DBA, *Dolichos biflorus* agglutinin.

capacity of the HPLC column for protein. In order to increase the efficiency of HPLC column separation, culture was established to protein-free media, in which the B151K12 hybridoma can secrete TRF almost to the same extent as in FCS-containing medium. It was found that a 48-hr culture supernatant of B151K12 in FCS-free RPMI1640 medium contained approximately half the TRF activity of that in 5% FCS-containing medium. Thus, from protein-free culture, the relative TRF activity recovered in the medium was approximately 500 times higher than from FCS-containing medium as calculated on a protein basis, and we could fractionate the TRF molecule by RP-HPLC, using a large volume of TRF-containing medium at one time. Figure 6 illustrates one example of RP-HPLC fractionation of TRF using 500 ml of protein-free culture fluid supernatant. By this procedure, the TRF activity was obtained in fractions 13–15. These TRF-enriched fractions were pooled, concentrated and radiolabeled with ^{125}I-Bolton–Hunter reagent under conditions which maintained full TRF activity. The pooled radiolabeled TRF-enriched fractions were used to further characterize the TRF molecule and its corresponding acceptor molecule on B cells.

IV. IMMUMOGENETIC PROPERTIES OF THE TRF-ACCEPTOR SITE ON B CELLS

For the ultimate identification of the TRF molecule out of various contaminating substances and analysis of its structure and function, the identification of TRF-binding acceptor site on B cells is another fundamental issue. In other words,

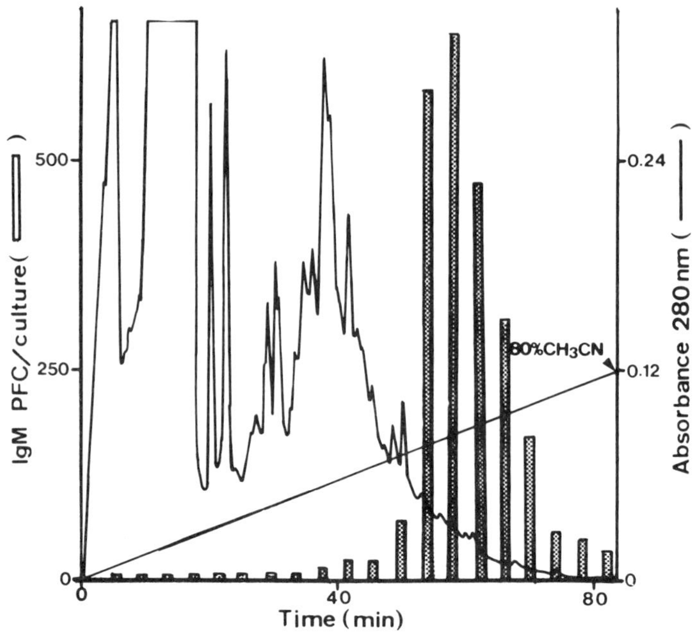

Figure 6. Preparation of TRF-enriched fraction from B151K12-TRF. Reverse-phase HPLC fractionation was conducted by charging 100 ml of 5 × concentrated CFS from a protein-free culture of the B151K12 hybridoma into a 10 × 300 mm YMCAP-324 column (Yamamura Chemical Laboratory Co., Ltd.) after passage through a Sep-Pack C column. The fractions were eluted by linear gradient from 0–80% of CH_3CN in 0.1% trifluoroacetic acid for 100 min with flow rate of 1 ml/min. Aliquots of a fraction comprising 4 ml each were submitted to the TRF assay after the samples were processed as described in Fig. 5.

the demonstration of the specific binding of the TRF molecule to the acceptor molecule may be one of the most definitive criteria for defining and identifying the TRF molecule and its function. Thus the TRF-acceptor molecule may provide a specific detecting reagent for the TRF molecule. In this context, we have been interested in the identification and characterization of TRF-acceptor site on B cells. Along this line, an intriguing genetic defect in the TRF responsiveness of B cells found in the mutant mice of DBA/2Ha strain enabled us to approach this issue. In this particular mutant strain, the expression of the TRF-acceptor site on B cells is defective, and this permitted us to prepare rather easily the specific antibody to the TRF-acceptor molecule.

A. X-Chromosome-Linked Recessive Gene Control in the Defective Expression of the TRF-Acceptor Site on B Cells Found in DBA/2Ha Mutant Mice

As we demonstrated previously, B cells not only from syngeneic mice, but from other allogeneic mice as well, responded to B151K12-TRF, indicating that

TRF triggers B cells beyond the major histocompatibility barrier. Importantly, antigen-primed B cells from X-linked B-cell defective CBA/N mice responded well to B151K12-TRF, whereas B cells from the mutant mice of DBA/2Ha strain failed to show any significant PFC response even after antigen priming (Tominaga *et al.*, 1980). By taking advantage of the low-response character of DBA/2Ha B cells, the B-cell responsiveness to B151K12-TRF was genetically analyzed by using B cells from an F1 hybrid of the low-responder strain DBA/2Ha and high-responder BALB/c. The results showed that the B cells from (DBA/2Ha × BALB/c) DCF1 male mice were incapable of responding to the B151K12-TRF, whereas DCF1 female mice responded quite well to the TRF, indicating that major differences in the ability of DBA/2Ha and BALB/c mice to respond to the factor are not controlled by an autosomal gene. Rather, these results suggest that a major component involved in the response of B cells to the TRF is X-chromosome linked. To further substantiate the X-linked gene control of TRF responsiveness, B cells from the backcross progenies of DCF1 female mice by DBA/2Ha male mice or F2 progenies were examined for their ability to respond to the TRF. The data further indicated that the responsiveness to the TRF is controlled by the gene linked to the X chromosone of the high-responder parent (Takatsu *et al.*, 1981c).

In order to test the possibility that a particular acceptor site for TRF on DBA/2Ha B cells is absent, experiments were conducted to measure the ability of B cells from high TRF-responder BALB/c mice and low TRF-responder DBA/2Ha mice to absorb TRF activity. Residual TRF activities after absorption of CFS from B151K12 with those B cells were determined. Also as demonstrated previously (Tominaga *et al.*, 1980), B cells from BALB/c mice were able to absorb the TRF activity. In contrast, B cells from DBA/2Ha mice could not absorb the TRF activity, indicating that low responsiveness of DBA/2Ha B cells to TRF is reflected by the absence of a particular acceptor site for TRF.

B. Production of Antiserum Against the Putative TRF-Acceptor Site on B Cells and Its Blocking of TRF Action on B Cells

Recently, antisera specific for various differentiation markers on B cells have been raised and submitted to functional analysis. An antiserum against a subset of B cells receiving immunogenic stimuli from some thymus-independent antigens (markers denoted Lyb 3 and Lyb 5), which CBA/N mice do not bear on their surface, was raised by the immunization of a low-responder strain with B cells from a high-responder strain (Huber *et al.*, 1977; Ahmed *et al.*, 1977).

In an analogous manner, in order to ascertain further whether the low-response characteristic of DBA/2Ha B cells to TRF is due the absence or low expression of TRF acceptor site on B cells, attempts were made (1) to raise an antiserum in DCF1 hybrid male mice (TRF low responders and putatively TRF-acceptor site-negative) by immunization with BALB/c B cells (TRF high responder), and (2) to test whether such an antiserum would suppress manifestation of TRF activity on B cells. In this situation, the possibility of generating an antibody to a histocompatibility difference is theoretically negligible. In order to detect the antibody activity, DNP-primed B cells from BALB/c mice were mixed with the B151K12-TRF and stimulated with DNP conjugates in continuous presence of DCF1 male anti-BALB/c B-cell antiserum. As a control, serum from TRF-high-responder DCF1 female mice immunized with BALB/c B cells according to precisely the same protocol as for the DCF1 male mice, was also added to the culture. It was found that the DCF1 male anti-BALB/c B-cell antiserum strikingly inhibited the B-cell responses mediated by the B151K12-TRF. In contrast, the DCF1 female anti-BALB/c antiserum showed no inhibitory activity under these experimental conditions. Furthermore, the suppressive activity of the DCF1 male anti-BALB/c B-cell antiserum was successfully removed by absorption using DNP-primed B cells from TRF-high responder BALB/c and C57BL/6 mice, but not from TRF-low-responder DBA/2Ha mice (Tominaga *et al.*, 1980).

The possibility that DCF1 male anti-BALB/c B-cell antiserum might still contain some unidentified nonspecific inhibitors of B-cell responses *in vitro* was ruled out by the fact that the continuous presence of DCF1 male anti-BALB/c B-cell antiserum in the culture suppressed anti-DNP PFC responses mediated by TRF, whereas presence of the antiserum did not suppress cognate T–B-cell interactions (Tominaga *et al.*, 1980). In order to further substantiate the B-cell specificity of the antibody, DNP-primed B cells were first treated with the biotinylated F(ab′)2 fragment of DCF1 male anti-BALB/c B-cell antibody followed by treatment with avidin–ricin-A-chain conjugates and were then cultured with DNP–OVA in the presence of B151K12-TRF. The responsiveness of B cells to TRF thus treated with biotinylated antibody in combination with avidin–ricin-A-chain conjugates was strikingly abolished, whereas this treatment did not affect B-cell activity responsive to cognate interaction with helper T cells. Treatment of B cells either with biotinylated antibody alone or with avidin–ricin A chain alone did not affect responsiveness to TRF under this condition (Takatsu *et al.*, 1982a; Hashimoto *et al.*, 1984). These results indicate that antigen-primed B cells responsive to the TRF molecule are distinct from those responsive to direct interaction with helper T cells and further substantiate the specificity of this antibody for a subpopulation of the TRF-responsive B cells.

The addition of this antiserum to the culture of BCL1 tumor cells in the presence of TRF also clearly inhibited the PFC responses induced by the TRF. Thus, taken collectively, these data imply that this antiserum contains antibodies specific for the putative TRF-acceptor site on a certain subpopulation of B lymphocytes.

C. TRF-Substituting Activity of the Anti-TRF-Acceptor Site Antibody in Triggering B Cells

The antibody-mediated blocking of TRF-induced triggering of B cells described above does not rule out the possibility that the DCF1 male anti-BALB/c B-cell antiserum may contain antibodies against some unknown X-chromosomal product(s) present in parental B cells and that these antibodies may sterically block the putative TRF-acceptor site, which may be incidentally located adjacent to such X-chromosome product(s) on the B-cell surface. If that is the case, the blocking activity of the antiserum per se does not necessarily mean that the antiserum contains specific antibodies against the putative TRF-acceptor site. If the DCF1 male anti-BALB/c B-cell antiserum contains specific antibodies against the TRF-acceptor site, it can be predicted that the antiserum will mimic the function of the effector molecule, i.e., TRF, by binding to the acceptor site and will trigger B cells under appropriate conditions, just as in the case of a hormone receptor and its specific antibody (Kahn *et al.*, 1979; Schechter *et al.*, 1979). We examined whether this antiserum contains antibodies capable of replacing the T-cell function in the triggering of B-cell differentiation.

Various strains of 6-week-old mice were immunized intravenously with suboptimal doses of 1×10^6 SRBCs in combination with DCF1 male anti-BALB/c B-cell antiserum in a volume of 5 μl. After 4 days, the mice were sacrificed, and the number of IgM PFC to SRBC in the spleens was determined. The results

Table V. Characteristics of (DBA/2Ha × BALB/c)F1 Male Anti-BALB/c B-Cell Antiserum

Ig class	IgG1 and IgG2a
Reactive with	B cells but not T cells
Absorbed by	Antigen-primed B cells from TRF-high responder, but not with those from low responder Some neoplastic B cells
C-dependent cytotoxicity	Negative
Blocking activity in TRF-induced PFC response	Yes
TRF-substituting activity	Yes
Blocking activity in lymphokine-induced CTL response from thymocytes	No

showed that antiserum raised in TRF-nonresponder DCF1 male mice against TRF-responder parental BALB/c B cells induced augmented primary IgM anti-SRBC antibody responses when intravenously injected in combination with suboptimal doses of antigen into TRF-high-response animals. Although injection of the antiserum alone induces a small but significant polyclonal PFC response, the antiserum acts synergistically with antigen to produce enhanced antigen-specific PFC responses (Hamaoka *et al.*, 1981b; Takatsu, *et al.*, 1981a).

Thus, the DCF1 male anti-BALB/c B-cell antiserum contains antibodies capable of substituting for TRF activity. Moreover, the fact that the antiserum reacted selectively with B cells but not with T cells as shown by fluorescence-activated cell sorter (FACS) analysis, and that the stimulating activity of the indicates that the reactivity of the antiserum is B-cell specific. The antibody activity was associated with IgG1 and IgG2a. These properties of the DCF1 male anti-BALB/c B-cell antiserum are summarized in Table V.

D. Relationship between the TRF-Acceptor Site Detected by (DBA/2Ha × BALB/c) F1 Male Anti-BALB/c B-Cell Antiserum and Other Known B-Cell Differentiation Markers

It has been reported that CBA/N mice also demonstrate X-linked immune defect and lack a subpopulation of B cells expressing Lyb-3 and Lyb-5 determinant. B cells that express the Lyb-5 determinant are a late-appearing subpopulation in normal mice that have been reported to respond to TRF (Singer *et al.*, 1981).

An alloantiserum, designated anti-Lyb 3 and anti-Lyb 5, that reacts exclusively with this subset of B cells in all mouse strains other than CBA/N was rasised by immunizing defective mice with Lyb-3$^+$ cells (Huber *et al.*, 1977; Ahmed *et al.*, 1977). In particular, it was demonstrated that this anti-Lyb-3 antiserum acts synergistically with antigen to produce enhanced antigen-specific PFC responses in various strains of mice, but not in CBA/N. It was thought worthwile to test whether the TRF acceptor site detected by the antiserum present in DCF1 male anti-BALB/c B-cell antiserum is identical to, or closely associated with, the Lyb-3 or Lyb-5 molecule(s). We examined the effect of this antiserum on primary anti-sheep red blood cell (SRBC) responses in CBA/N and DBA/2Ha mice. Enhancement of anti-SRBC responses was observed not only in BALB/c, but in CBA/N mice as well. In contrast, intravenous injections of DCF1 male anti-BALB/c B-cell antiserum failed to augment the anti-SRBC PFC response in DBA/2Ha mice (Takatsu *et al.*, 1982b), indicating that the augmenting effect was clearly due to a specific reaction of this antiserum with a component that is absent in DBA/2Ha mice. The fact that *in vitro* stimulation of DNP-primed CBA/N B cells with a DNP conjugate as antigen, in combination with antiserum, produced a greater than 10-fold increase in DNP-specific PFCs indicated that enhancement of the antibody response in CBA/N mice is clearly due to a specific

Table VI. Conversion of Nonresponder Status of CBA/N B Cells to Responder to TRF by Antigen Priming

Responder B cells[a]	TNP–Ficoll (4 ng/ml)	B151TRF	Anti-TNP IgG PFC/culture
CBA/N	–	–	0
CBA/N	–	+	0
CBA/N	+	–	0
CBA/N	+	+	258 (1.12)

[a]Responder B cells were spleen cells from CBA/N mice immunized with 100 μg DNP–KLH i.p. in alum 4 months previously and boosted i.p. with 5 μg of the same antigen in saline 10 days before sacrifice. Responder cells were treated with monoclonal anti-Thy 1 plus C.

interaction of this antiserum with a component that is present in CBA/N mice and different from both Lyb 3 and Lyb 5 (Tominaga *et al.*, 1982).

Despite our demonstration that the TRF-acceptor site and Lyb-3 and Lyb-5 molecules are serologically different, it appears that the TRF-acceptor-site-positive B-cell subset is functionally identical to the Lyb-3$^+$ -and Lyb-5$^+$ B-cell population. In order to analyze this point further, the responsiveness of CBA/N B cells to TNP–Ficoll from DNP-KLH-primed and -boosted mice was tested *in vitro* in the presence of TRF. The results demonstrated that the B-cell response of CBA/N mice to TNP–Ficoll was markedly augmented by the presence of TRF, whereas virtually no significant anti-TNP PFC responses were elicited from the same B cells by stimulation with either TNP–Ficoll or TRF alone (Table VI). Under these experimental conditions, however, the stimulation of nonprimed B cells from CBA/N with TNP–Ficoll plus TRF did not induce any significant anti-TNP PFC responses (data not shown). More definitively, Ono and Singer, in collaboration with our laboratory (1984), recently demonstrated that the CBA/N B cells acquired responsiveness to TRF after priming with SRBC, thus corroborating the TRF responsiveness of DNP-KLH-primed B cells of CBA/N mice DNP-KLH. Most importantly, however, this TRF responsiveness was not affected by treatment with anti-Lyb-5 antiserum plus complement, indicating that Lyb-5 marker and TRF-acceptor molecule are distinct from each other and that the Lyb-5$^-$ B-cell population in CBA/N mice could be rendered responsive to TRF after appropriate antigenic priming.

V. PHYSICOCHEMICAL CHARACTERIZATION OF THE TRF-ACCEPTOR MOLECULE

(DBA/2Ha × BALB/c)F1 male anti-BALB/c B-cell antiserum was obtained by taking advantage of X-linked recessive gene control of the expression of TRF acceptor site on B cells as described in Section IV, and it was demonstrated that this antiserum contains antibodies specific for the putative TRF acceptor site. Moreover, the serological properties of TRF-acceptor site on B cells identified by this antiserum were apparently different from the Lyb-3 and Lyb-5 markers on B cells.

Using this combination of immunization to obtain antibody as a specific reagent, we proceeded to the physiochemical analysis of TRF-acceptor molecule on the B-cell membrane. We used BCL1 B cells as a source of the TRF-acceptor-site-positive B-cell population, since BCL1 cells can bind TRF as determined by this specific TRF-absorbing activity; it can also specifically bind DCF1 male anti-BALB/c B-cell antibody, as demonstrated by FACS analysis, using biotinylated antibody and fluorescence isothiocyanate (FITC)-labeled avidin molecule.

A. Preparation of Soluble BCL_1 Membrane Protein Fraction Containing the TRF-Acceptor Molecule

In order to obtain TRF-acceptor molecule from BCL1 membrane, we strove to solubilize membranes under conditions in which the acceptor molecule retains its full TRF-binding activity. BCL1 cells or MOPC 104E myeloma cells, used as controls, were disrupted with a Polytron TP-10 (Brinkmann) at dial setting 7 for 1 min in 5 vol 0.3 M sucrose; the membrane fraction was collected by ultracentrifugation according to the method of Tsushima and Friesen (1973). The membrane fraction obtained was solubilized by 2% Lubrol-PX (polyoxyethylene dodecyl ether) for 30 min on ice, and the protein fraction was precipitated by 80% saturated $(NH_4)_2SO_4$. The protein fraction thus obtained was extensively dialyzed against phosphate buffer and was tested for TRF-binding activity by determining its ability to block the TRF-induced BCL1 IgM PFC response.

The membrane protein fraction from BCL1 cells, but not from MOPC 104E cells, strikingly inhibited the TRF-induced PFC response, clearly indicating that this membrane protein fraction contains the TRF-acceptor site with its potent TRF-binding activity (see results summarized in Table VII). However, although the data are not shown here, the membrane protein fraction obtained from NP40- and Triton X100-solubilized membrane fraction showed no TRF-binding activity.

After confirming that TRF-acceptor activity in the Lubrol-PX solubilized membrane fraction of BCL1 was fully retained after treatment with sodium dodecyl sulfate (SDS), the TRF-acceptor molecule with TRF-binding activity was directly demonstrated by SDS-polyacrylamide gel electrophoresis (SDS-PAGE). The electrophoretically separated membrane protein bands containing the TRF-acceptor molecule were transferred to a nitrocellulose membrane, which was then quenched by 3% gelatin and dipped into semipurified $[^{125}I]$-TRF solution (380,000 cpm/10 ml) obtained as described in Section III. After incubation

Table VII. Inhibition of TRF-Induced PFC Response of BCL1 Cells by Lubrol PX-Solubilized Membrane Protein Fraction from BCL1 Cells

Responder B cells[a]	TRF	Membrane protein fraction added ng/ml[b]		IgM PFC/culture	% inhibition
BCL1	–	–		2	
BCL1	+	–		197 (1.06)	0
BCL1	+	MOPC 104E	500	196 (1.09)	0
BCL1	+	MOPC 104E	100	235 (1.12)	0
BCL1	+	MOPC 104E	20	190 (1.16)	3
BCL1	+	BCL1	500	12 (1.24)	94
BCL1	+	BCL1	100	61 (1.30)	69
BCL1	+	BCL1	20	177 (1.04)	10

[a]Responder cells (2×10^5/well) were obtained from the spleens of BCL1-bearing mice.
[b]The protein concentration of the membrane fraction was determined by the Lowry method. The membrane was solubilized with 2% (v/v) Lubrol PX in 25 mM Tris-HCl buffer, pH 7.6, and the 80% saturated ammonium-precipitated protein fraction was extensively dialyzed in Spectopor tube O/N against 10 mM Tris-HCl, pH, 7.4 buffer containing 2 mM $CaCl_2$ and 2 mM $MgCl_2$ in the presence of Bio-beads SM-2.

at 37°C for 3 days, the membrane was thoroughly washed and used for autoradiography. As shown in Fig. 7, [^{125}I]-TRF specifically bound to the 120,000 M_r molecule of BCL1 membrane protein but not to any protein band of MOPC 104E. Likewise, nitrocellulose membrane blots of those membrane proteins, separated by SDS-PAGE, were stained with DCF1 male anti-BALB/c B-cell antiserum in conjunction with horseradish peroxidase-labeled anti-mouse immunoglobulin antiserum. Although the photograph is not shown here, the antiserum contains antibodies that detect at least 10 bands of membrane proteins including the 120,000 M_r molecule. This result is not surprising, since there is a high probaspecificity to the TRF-acceptor-site-positive B-cell population was established by the functional assay. On the basis of these results, we attempted to establish a monoclonal antibody specific for the TRF-acceptor site, which might enable us to identify the TRF-acceptor molecule much more definitively.

B. Establishment of a Monoclonal Antibody Specific for the TRF-Acceptor Molecule

In order to obtain a monoclonal antibody specific for the TRF acceptor site on the B-cell surface, we screened several hundred B-cell hybridomas secreting antibody reactive with TRF-acceptor molecule-positive BCL1 cells. Spleen cells from DCF1 male mice hyperimmunized with BALB/c B cells were fused with P31X63-Ag8.U1 (P3U1) cells (HGPRT$^-$ myeloma) using polyethlene glycol 1000.

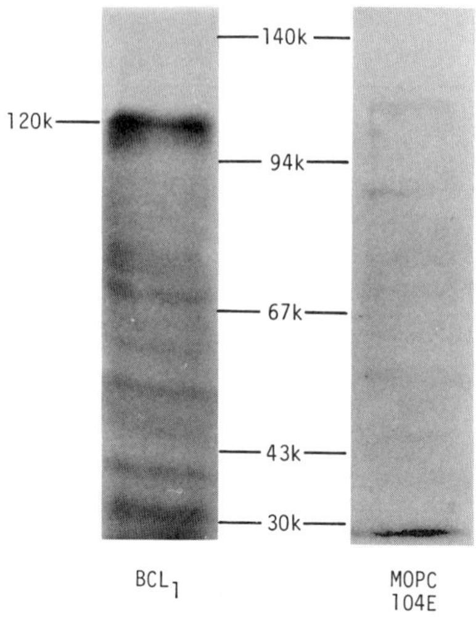

Figure 7. Detection of TRF acceptor molecule by binding to a ^{125}I-labeled TRF fraction. BCL1- and MOPC 104E-membrane protein fractions solubilized with 2% Lubrol PX were submitted to SDS-PAGE (8% gel), and transferred onto a nitrocellulose membrane. After quenching with 3% gelatin, the membrane was dipped in I^{125}-labeled, semipurified TRF solution (380,000 cpm/10ml), and the TRF binding protein was detected by autoradiography.

Detection of the hybridoma clones that produce antibody specific for the TRF-acceptor site was accomplished by reacting the BCL1 cells with hybridoma supernatant and measuring the binding of [^{125}I] protein A from *Staphylococcus aureus* Cowan I to the BCL1 cells. In some experiments, the supernatant of individual hybridoma was biotinylated, and reaction of hybridoma antibody to BCL1 was detected by the binding of [^{125}I] avidin. Likewise, in the FACS analysis for detection of the specific binding of biotinylated antibody to BCL1, FITC-labeled avidin molecule was used as the staining reagent. After screening and selecting antibody-producing hybridoma clones with potent binding activity to BCL1 cells but not to other syngeneic TRF-acceptor-negative cell lines, such as BALB/c-derived T-cell lymphoma (BAL.9), Abelson virus-transformed pre-B-cell line (AT8-2), and myeloma (P3U1), these monoclonal antibodies were further submitted to the functional assay described above for DCF1 male anti-BALB/c B-cell antiserum; measuring both blocking activity for TRF-mediated B-cell responses and triggering activity for anti-SRBC responses *in vivo*.

As summarized in Tables VIII and IX, the monoclonal antibody derived from one of the selected hybridomas [designated as anti-B-cell activation receptor (BAR)-1 antibody] exhibited the most potent activity, as measured by these two assays, suggesting its specificity for the TRF-acceptor site. In order to ascertain further the specificity of the anti-BAR-1 monoclonal antibody for the TRF-acceptor site, inhibition of TRF-binding to BCL1 cells by this monoclonal antibody was tested. BCL1 cells pretreated with or without monoclonal anti-BAR-1 antibody were used to absorb cells of B151K12-TRF; residual TRF activity in the supernatant after absorption with thus antibody-pretreated BCL1 cells was measured. Pretreatment of BCL1 cells with the DCF1 male anti-BALB/c B-cell

Table VIII. Blocking Effect of Anti-BAR-1 Monoclonal Antibodies on TRF-Induced B-Cell Differentiation

		BCL1 cells		DNP-primed B cells	
B151-TRF	Hyb-CFS or Antiserum[a]	IgM PFC /Culture	% Suppression	Anti-DNP IgG PFC/culture	% Suppression
–	–	53 (1.03)	–	23 (1.12)	–
+	–	1301 (1.01)	0	430 (1.08)	0
+	P3U1	1296 (1.06)	1	411 (1.11)	5
+	Anti-BAR-1	368 (1.26)	75	192 (1.21)	59
+	DCF1 anti-BALB/c	521 (1.18)	62	181 (1.16)	62

[a]Antibodies added to the culture were 5% anti-BAR-1 hybridoma CFS containing approximately 100 ng/ml monoclonal antibody or 0.5% DCF1 anti-BALB/c B-cell antiserum at final concentration.

antiserum as a positive control or with anti-BAR-1 antibody [as the experimental group] significantly inhibited the TRF-absorbing capability of BCL1 cells (see Table X). More intriguing, as consistent with the analysis that used DCF1 male anti-BALB/c B-cell antiserum (data not shown), the presence of B151K12-TRF evidently inhibited antibody binding to BCL1 cells as shown by staining with biotinylated anti-BAR-1 monoclonal antibody and FITC-avidin. This is evident by the FACS analysis shown in Fig. 8. Thus, on the basis of these data taken

Table IX. Triggering Effect of DCF1 Male Anti-BALB/c B-Cell Antiserum or Anti-BAR-1 Monoclonal Antibody on Anti-SRBC Responses *In Vivo*

Antibody injected[a]	Antigen	Anti-SRBC IgM PFC/spleen
–	–	205 (1.10)
–	SRBC	420 (1.02)
DCF1 male Normal serum	SRBC	820 (1.04)
DCF1 male Anti-BALB/c	SRBC	8700 (1.08)
anti-BAR-1	–	290 (1.25)
anti-BAR-1	SRBC	4550 (1.05)

[a]Doses of antibody injected were 0.5 ml of 100 times diluted DCF1 male anti-BALB/c antiserum or 0.5 ml of 10 times diluted anti-BAR-1 hybridoma CFS.

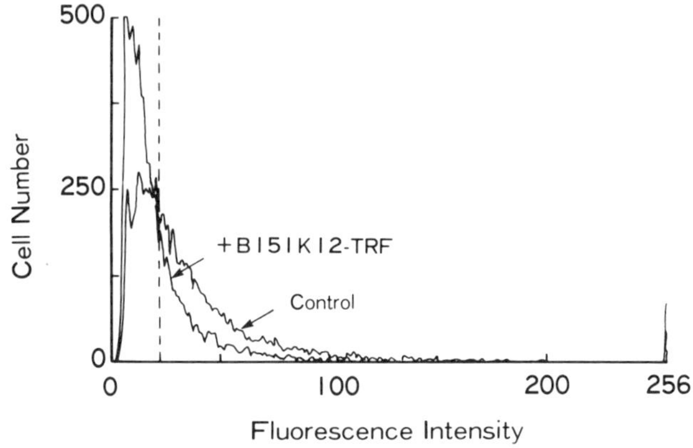

Figure 8. Inhibition of binding of anti-BAR-1 monoclonal antibody to BCL1 cells by the presence of B151K12-TRF. BCL1 cells were stained with biotinylated anti-BAR-1 antibody and FITC-labeled avidin in the presence or absence of the TRF-enriched fraction.

collectively, it can be concluded that the anti-BAR-1 monoclonal antibody seems to be specific for the TRF-acceptor site on B cells.

SDS-PAGE analysis of the above BCL1 Luburol PX-solubilized membrane protein fraction under nonreducing conditions in conjunction with protein transfer to nitrocellulose paper, demonstrated that this anti-BAR-1 monoclonal anti-

Table X. Blocking Effect of DCF1 Male Anti-BALB/c B-Cell Antiserum or Anti-BAR-1 Monoclonal Antibody on TRF-Absorbing Activity of BCL1 Cells

TRF absorbed with[a]		Residual TRF activity	
Cells	Antibody pretreatment	IgM PFC/well	%
None	None	440 (1.12)	100
BCL1	None	192 (1.03)	43
BCL1	DCF1 male normal	205 (1.10)	46
BCL1	DCF1 male anti-BALB/c	438 (1.02)	*99*
BCL1	P3U1	182 (1.04)	41
BCL1	Anti-BAR-1	410 (1.08)	*93*

[a]BCL1 cells used for absorption of TRF were pretreated with the above-listed antibodies for 1 hr on ice under the conditions described in Table VIII and then washed. The concentration of antibodies exposed to BCL1 cells was four times more than in Table VIII.

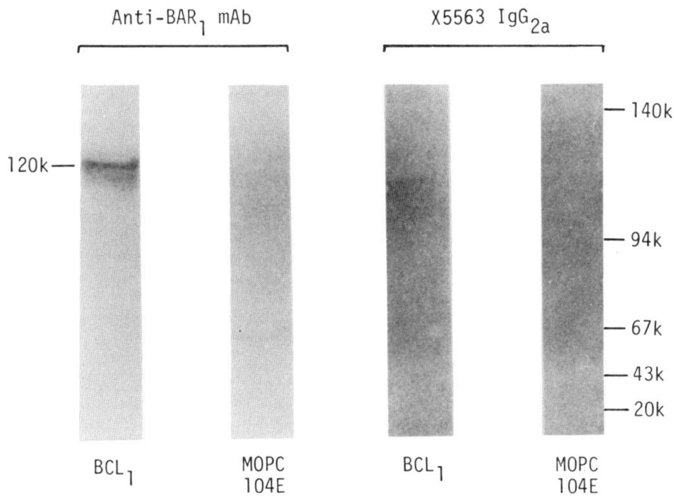

Figure 9. Detection of an anti-BAR-1 monoclonal antibody-reactive membrane protein in BCL1 cells. Solubilized membrane protein fractions of BCL1 and MOPC 104E were submitted to SDS-PAGE and transferred to nitrocellulose membranes. After reacting with anti-BAR-1 monoclonal antibody or X5563 IgG 2a as control, the membranes were stained with horse radish peroxidase-labeled anti-mouse immunoglobulin antibody.

body specifically reacted with a band of 120,000 M_r (Fig. 9), which seemed to correspond to a band detected by the [^{125}I]-TRF binding assay (Fig. 7). Moreover, although the photograph is not shown, this monoclonal antibody also reacted with a 60,000-M_r molecule when the BCL_1 membrane protein fraction was reduced with 20 mM 1,4-dithiothreitol.

C. Separation and Characterization of the TRF-Acceptor Molecule

In order to ascertain whether the 120,000-M_r protein molecule detected by the anti-BAR-1 monoclonal antibody represents the authentic TRF acceptor molecule, an affinity column was prepared by coupling purified anti-BAR-1 monoclonal antibody to CNBr-activated Sepharose beads, and tested for specific absorption of the TRF acceptor activity. As a control column, X5563 IgG2a myeloma protein was used in the place of nomoclonal antibody. The TRF acceptor activity contained in the Lubrol-PX-solubilized BCL1 membrane protein fraction was specifically absorbed by the anti-BAR-1 antibody column but not by the X5563-column; absorbed TRF-acceptor activity was successfully eluted by 0.1 M glycine-HC1 buffer pH 2.0. These results are summarized in Table XI.

Table XI. Specificity of Anti-BAR-1 Monoclonal Antibody to the TRF Acceptor Molecule as Demonstrated by Specific Binding to and Elution from Anti-BAR-1–Sepharose

B151-TRF	BCL1 membrane protein fraction added to the culture as inhibitor of TRF assay (ng/ml)	BCL1 response (IgM PFC/culture)	% Inhibition
–	–	10	–
+	–	450(1.09)	0
	Crude membrane protein		
+	274	324(1.16)	28
+	54	339(1.06)	25
+	11	414(1.08)	8
	Anti-BAR-1 column effluent		
+	274	407(1.06)	10
+	54	406(1.10)	10
+	11	459(1.06)	0
	Anti-BAR-1 column eluate[a]		
+	274	104(1.02)	67
+	54	240(1.08)	47
+	11	291(1.07)	36
	X5563 IgG2a column effluent		
+	274	310(1.08)	32
+	54	340(1.03)	25
+	11	425(1.05)	6
	X5563 IgG2a eluate[a]		
+	274	411(1.04)	9
+	54	467(1.04)	0
+	11	463(1.03)	0

[a]BCL1 membrane protein fraction was eluted from the antibody column by 0.1M glycine-HCl buffer pH 2.0 and neutralized with 0.5M tris-(hydroxymethyl) aminomethane.

To further characterize the molecular properties of the protein with TRF acceptor activity, the fraction eluted from the anti-BAR-1 column was radioiodinated using IODO-BEADS (Pierce Chemical Company), and submitted to SDS-PAGE analysis in conjunction with autoradiography. One of the representative results is shown in Fig. 10. The protein molecule eluted from the anti-BAR-1

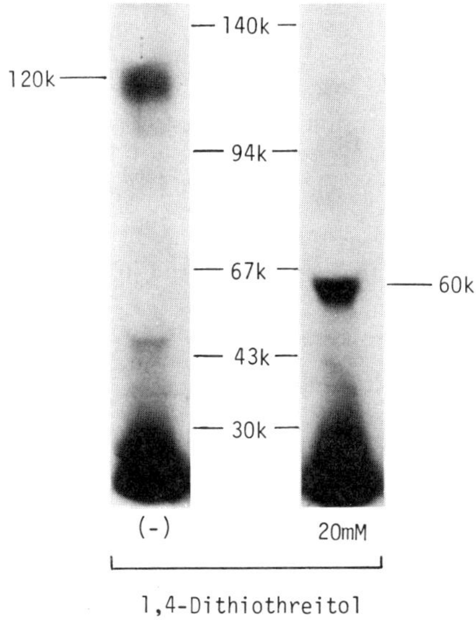

Figure 10. Molecular characterization of the TRF acceptor by autoradiography. TRF acceptor molecule, affinity-purified with anti-BAR-1 monoclonal antibody, was labeled with ^{125}I and submitted to SDS-PAGE analysis under nonreducing and reducing conditions.

column yielded a 120,000 M_r band, the size of which was reduced by half after reduction with 20 mM 1, 4-dithiothreitol.

Thus, anti-BAR-1 monoclonal antibody is specific for the TRF acceptor molecule on the surface of B cells, and the TRF acceptor molecule represents a disulfide-linked homodimer of a 60,000 M_r polypeptide. The purified TRF acceptor molecule will be a definitive binding probe for the ultimate identification and functional characterization of the TRF molecule.

VI. DISCUSSION

Accumulating bodies of evidence indicate that soluble factors produced by activated T cells are involved in B-cell proliferation and differentiation. However, the precise molecular nature of these factors have remained elusive. In the present study, the physicochemical properties of a B-cell differentiation factor, generally designated as TRF, derived from a hybridoma T-cell clone B151K12 were analyzed, and the immunogenetic properties of the acceptor site to this factor were described in detail. However, it is generally postulated that even in the lymphokine activity, which governs a very limited step of terminal B-cell differentiation, there appear to be several kinds of factors involved. For example, Paul and colleagues, in collaboration with our laboratory (Nakanishi *et al.*, 1983), have presented the evidence indicating that two kinds of B-cell differentiation factor are required for, or synergistically act on, the development of Ig-producing cells in addition to BCGF. One of them is B151K12-TRF and the other pI 4.5 fraction derived from EL4 CFS. Vitetta and associates (Pure *et al.*, 1983) also demonstrated the existence of a B-cell differentiation factor (BCDF) determining the isotype specificity of the B cells triggered, such as $BCDF_\mu$ and $BCDF_\gamma$, which induces preferentially IgM and IgG antibody-forming cells.

Even though there seem to be various factors govering terminal B-cell differentiation, we chose to define the molecular properties of TRF (B151K12-TRF), as well as characterize the acceptor molecule for this TRF. Such determinations may provide invaluable information about the molecular relatedness of this TRF to other B-cell differentiation factors and may also provide a firm molecular basis for future structural analyses of the genes or gene family that encodes these biologically important molecules. Another aspect of our interest in analyzing the terminal B-cell differentiation is that this provides an intriguing model for studies of the intracellular biochemical events and gene-regulation mechanisms responsible for differentiation processes in mammalian cells, since to the best of our knowledge no definitive *in vitro* model has developed for such analyses.

Despite the establishment of a simple model of B-cell differentiation as discussed herein, it is clear that we are still far from a complete understanding of the molecular mechanism by which a TRF governs the terminal stage of the B-cell differentiation. A number of conclusions can be drawn, however, about a B-cell differentiation factor present in the culture supernatant of B151K12 T-cell hybridomas and its corresponding acceptor site on B cells.

The factor from B151K12 exhibits an obvious T-cell-replacing activity and acts directly on B cells. It does not display any other known lymphokine activity. In particular, under the experimental conditions in which the addition of various lymphokines such as IL-1, IL-2, BCGF-1, IL-3, and γ-IFN did not induce any B-cell differentiation, purified B151K12 factor displayed obvious TRF activity. Regarding the TRF-acceptor site on B cells, expression of the specific acceptor site is controlled by an X-linked gene, and the acceptor molecule was identified as a 120,000-M_r membrane-associated protein. Moreover, our preliminary result showed that the ^{125}I-labeled purified acceptor molecule bound specifically to Con A-Sepharose. This indicates that the molecule has a sugar side chain with a mannose core that is typical of an *N*-glycosylated protein. This acceptor molecule receives a signal from TRF by binding the TRF molecule and transmits an activation signal involved in terminal B-cell differentiation.

The following questions concern the immunological aspects of the TRF molecule and its acceptor site on B cells.

1) Does the TRF molecule comprise a single polypeptide chain structure, and is the sugar moiety (GalNAC) on the TRF molecule required for its function? Our recent experiment demonstrated that the [^{125}I]-labeled TRF fraction

described in Fig. 6 significantly bound to LBA- and DBA-Sepharose and likewise, addition of GalNAC to the TRF assay specifically inhibited the BCL1-response, indicating that the GalNAC moiety of the TRF molecule plays a crucial role for TRF binding and transmission of the signal to the TRF acceptor molecule. We are currently striving to further purify the TRF molecule based on these physicochemical properties and to ultimately identify the TRF molecule by its specific binding to the purified TRF acceptor molecule. We are also attempting to produce a monoclonal antibody specific for the TRF molecule for use in its final purification and in the determination of its structure. Another approach to determine the functional aspect of TRF structure is the utilization of mRNA from B151K12 hybridoma cells and pursuing molecular cloning and sequencing of the gene encoding this TRF. These issues are now in progress in our laboratory.

2) At what stage does the TRF acceptor site molecule emerge on the surface of B cells in the process of B-cell maturation from progenitor cells? Concerning this point, we addressed ourselves to the question of whether B cells bearing such TRF acceptor site develop early in ontogeny of B-cell generation or late, after receiving nominal antigenic stimulus. If the TRF-acceptor molecule appears early in ontogeny of B-cell generation, the neonatal treatment with anti-TRF-acceptor antibody would eliminate such a TRF acceptor$^+$ B-cell subpopulation.

It has been reported that passive administration of anti-immunoglobulin, anti-allotypic, or anti-idiotypic antiserum in the neonatal stage (within 24 hr) could eliminate the relevant B-cell population, resulting in impaired antibody synthesis (Lawton *et al.*, 1972; Warner, 1974; Metcalf *et al.*, 1981). To examine the possibility that treatment at birth with antiserum against the TRF-acceptor site could induce such a B-cell elimination, we injected 5 μl DCF1 male anti-BALB/c B-cell antiserum i.p. into neonatal BALB/c mice within 24 hr after birth. As a control, a group of mice from the same litter was treated with DCF1 male normal mouse serum. After 5 weeks, all the mice were immunized with 100 μg DNP-KLH included in 4 mg aluminum hydroxide gel and 1×10^9 pertussis vaccine and were used as donors of DNP-primed B cells.

In order to determine the effect of treatment with antibody against the TRF-acceptor site on the development of B cells responsible for TRF-mediated antibody response, DNP-KLH-primed splenic B cells (treated with anti-Thy 1.2 plus C) from either the antibody-treated or control mice were cultured with graded amounts of TRF derived from B151K12 at the stimulation with DNP-OVA. A significant anti-DNP IgG PFC response was observed when DNP-KLH-primed splenic B cells from control mice were stimulated with DNP-OVA in the presence of B151K12-TRF, whereas a remarkably lower anti-DNP IgG PFC response (one-fourth to one-fifth that of control) was induced by the B151K12-TRF in DNP-primed splenic B cells from the anti-TRF-acceptor site antibody-treated mice (Takatsu *et al.*, 1982a). Under these conditions, however, the activity of the B-cell type that interacts with T cells in cognate fashion was not affected significantly. Thus, the injection of anti-TRF-acceptor site antibody into neonatal BALB/c mice selectively suppressed the development of TRF-responsive B-cell activity. Importantly, to obtain such effect the antiserum had to be injected within 48 hr after birth.

In the generation of TRF-acceptor site-positive subpopulations of B cells, it can be postulated that a portion of the immature B cells differentiates into a B-cell subpopulation with the acceptor site in the early stages of differentiation, which is susceptible to neonatal treatment with antibody. Neonatal treatment with antibody may block this differentiation process or inactivate the acceptor-positive B-cell subpopulation. An important deduction that can be drawn from this result is that the emergence of the TRF-acceptor molecule does not necessarily require nominal antigenic stimulus via Ig-receptor on B cells, since the above system measured the specific anti-DNP PFC response of B cells primed with DNP–KLH 5 weeks after having been treated neonatally with anti-TRF-acceptor site antibody, and eliminating the antibody-reactive B-cell subpopulation. This deduction is rather contradictory to the general notion postulating that the TRF-acceptor site on B cells may emerge after receiving signals via Ig-receptor and other lymphokine stimuli such as BCGF-1. Although the above supposition does not exclude the possibility that the number of TRF-acceptor site on B cells may increase and that B cells functionally mature to respond to TRF after receiving these signals, it rather implies that the TRF-acceptor molecule or its related primordial molecule reactive with this anti-acceptor antibody emerges before receiving such lymphokine and nominal antigenic signals. However, the definitive answer concerning kinetics and timing of appearance of the acceptor molecule are extraordinarily intriguing issues. The anti-BAR-1 monoclonal antibody described herein will definitely provide us with the specific reagent for this approach. Moreover, it is worthwhile to add finally that, by our recent analysis, this antibody successfully detects 120,000 Mr TRF acceptor molecule in the solubilized membrane protein fraction of antigen-non-primed spleen cells from BALB/c and CBA/N but not from DBA/2Ha mice.

VII. CONCLUSION

This review provides evidence indicating that a B-cell differentiation factor (generally designated as TRF) derived from a T-cell hybridoma is a distinct lymphokine molecule that governs the terminal B-cell differentiation into antibody-forming cells and that is clearly distinguishable from other T-cell-derived lymphokines such as IL-2, BCGF-1, IL-3, and γ-IFN. The TRF-active fraction was apparently separable from BSA by means of reverse-phase HPLC and by lectin columns specific for GalNAC. For the future utilization of the

TRF-acceptor molecule as a probe to ultimately identify the TRF molecule and to analyze the interaction of TRF with the acceptor, the solubilized protein fraction was obtained from the membrane of TRF-responsive chronic leukemic B cells (BCL1). This protein fraction exhibited specific inhibition of the TRF-mediated B-cell differentiation, indicating that this protein fraction contains the TRF-acceptor molecule. By taking advantage of the fact that the expression of TRF-acceptor site on B cells is controlled by an X-linked recessive gene and defective in DBA/2Ha mutant mice, a monoclonal antibody specific for the TRF acceptor site was obtained from a hybridoma established from spleen cells of TRF-low responder (DBA/2Ha × BALB/c)F1 male mice immunized with TRF-high-responder parental BALB/c B cells. The monoclonal anti-BAR-1 antibody thus obtained inhibited TRF binding onto the BCL1 cells; reciprocally, treatment of BCL1 with TRF clearly interfered with the binding of anti-BAR-1 antibody to BCL1 cells. Moreover, this anti-BAR-1 monoclonal antibody specifically bound the TRF acceptor molecule in solubilized BCL1 membranes, and membrane proteins affinity-purified, by using this antibody revealed a glycoprotein of 120,000 M_r, consisting of a disulfide-linked homodimer of a 60,000-M_r glycoprotein. This 120,000-M_r molecule also specifically bound ^{125}I-labeled TRF semipurified by RP-HPLC, thus providing direct evidence that this molecule represents the authentic TRF acceptor.

Further analysis of the precise structure of the TRF acceptor and its interaction with the TRF molecule will provide invaluable information for understanding the molecular mechanism of terminal B-cell differentiation mediated by helper T cells, which occurs via this site. In addition, determining the structure of the genes encoding TRF and its acceptor molecule would be helpful in elucidating the mechanism of genetic control of T–B cell interactions. This has been another intriguing issue ever since the discovery of MHC-linked genetic control of T–B cell interactions (Katz *et al.*, 1973).

Acknowledgments

I would like to express my deep appreciation to Ms. Kazuko Ishimura for her infinite patience and outstanding secretarial assistance. Many thanks are expressed to my colleagues at the Institute: Yoshinobu Hara, Yohsuke Takahama, Norio Ishii, Shin-ichi Hayashi, Gen Yamada, and Noburn Hashimoto, who have shared their data with me. Special thanks are given to Ellen S. Vitetta (Texas Southwestern Medical School) and John W. Kappler (Department of Medicine, National Jewish Hospital) for providing the *in vivo* line of BCL1 cells and the FS6-14.13 hybridoma T-cell clone. I am also deeply indebted to David Goeddel (Genentech, Inc.) and James N. Ihle (National Cancer Institute–Frederik Cancer

Research) for providing the *Escherichia coli*-expressed murine γ-interferon and purified Interleukin-3 used in this study. Support was provided in part by a grant-in-aid from the Japanese Ministry of Education, Culture and Science and from the Japanese Ministry of Health and Welfare.

VIII. REFERENCES

Ahmed, A., Scher, I., Sharrow, S. O., Smith, A. H., Sachs, D. H., and Sell, K. W., 1977, *J. Exp. Med.* **145**:101.

Andersson, J., and Melchers, F., 1981, *Proc. Natl. Acad. Sci. USA* **78**:2497.

Delovitch, T. L., and McDevitt, H. O., 1977, *J. Exp. Med.* **146**:1019.

Dutton, R. W., Falkoff, R., Hirst, J. A., Hoffman, M., Kappler, J. W., Kettman, J. R., Lesley, J. F., and Vann, D., 1971, *Prog. Immunol.* **1**:355.

Hamaoka, T., Katz, D. H., and Benacerraf, B., 1973, *J. Exp. Med.* **136**:538.

Hamaoka, T., Takatsu, K., Okuno, K., and Tsuchida, T., 1981a, *J. Immunol.* **126**:659.

Hamaoka, T., Takatsu, K., Tominage, A., Sano, Y., Tomita, S., and Hashimoto, N., 1981b, in: *Mechanism of Lymphocyte Activation* (K. Resch and H. Kirchner, eds.), p. 480, Elsevier–North-Holland, New York.

Harwell, L., Kappler, J., and Marrack, P., 1976, *J. Immunol.* **116**:1379.

Harwell, L., Skidmore, B., Marrack, P., and Kappler, J., 1980, *J. Exp. Med.* **152**:893.

Hashimoto, N., Takatsu, K., Masuho, Y., Kishida, K., Hara, T., and Hamaoka, T., 1984, *J. Immunol.* **132**:129.

Hoffman, M. K., Koenig, S., Mitter, R. S., Oettigen, A. F., Ralph, P., and Hammerling, U., 1978, *J. Immunol.* **122**:497.

Howard, M., Farrar, J., Hilfiker, M., Johnson, B., Takatsu, K., Hamaoka, T., and Paul, W. E., 1982, *J. Exp. Med.* **155**:94.

Huber, B., Gershon, R., and Cantor, H., 1977, *J. Exp. Med.* **145**:10.

Isakson, P., Pure, E., Vitetta, E. S., and Krammer, P. H., 1982, *J. Exp. Med.* **155**:734.

Kahn, C. R., Baird, K. L., Jarett, D. B., and Flier, J. S., 1979, *Proc. Natl. Acad. Sci. USA* **75**:4209.

Katz, D. H., Hamaoka, T., Dorf, M. E., Maurer, P. H., and Benaceraf, B., 1973, *J. Exp. Med.* **138**:734.

Kishimoto, T., and Ishizaka, K., 1975, *J. Immunol.* **114**:1177.

Lawton, A. R., Asofsky, R., Hylton, M. B., and Cooper, M. D., 1972, *J. Exp. Med.* **135**:277.

Metcalf, E. S., Scher, I., Mond, J. J., Wilburn, S., Chapman, K., and Finkelman, F. D., 1981, in: *B Lymphocytes in the Immune Responses: Functional, Developmental and Interactive Properties* (N. R. Klinman, D. R. Mosier, I. Sher, and E. S. Vitetta, eds.), p. 211, Elsevier–North Holland, New York.

Nakanishi, K., Howard, M., Muraguchi, A., Farrar, J., Takatsu, K., Hamaoka, T., and Paul, W. E., 1983, *J. Immunol.* **130**:2219.

Ono, S., Yaffe, L., Takatsu, K., Hamaoka, T., and Singer, A., 1984, (submitted).

Paetkau, V., Millis, G., Gerhart, S., and Montione, V., 1976, *J. Immunol.* **117**:1320.

Parker, D. C., 1980, *Immunol. Rev.* **52**:115.

Parker, D. C., Fothergill, J. J., and Wadsworth, D., 1979, *J. Immunol.* **123**:931.

Pure, E., Isakson, P., Takatsu, K., Hamaoka, T., Swain, S. L., Dutton, R. W., Uhr, J., Dennert, G., and Vitetta, E. S., 1981, *J. Immunol.* **127**:1953.

Pure, E., Isakson, P. C., Kappler, J. W., Marrack, P., Krammer, P. H., and Vitetta, E., 1983, *J. Exp. Med.* **157**:600.

Schechter, Y., Hernaez, L., Schlessinger, J., and Cuatrecasas, P., 1979, *Nature* **278**:835.

Schimpl, A., and Wecker, E., 1972, *Nature (New Biol.)* **237**:15.

Singer, A., Morrissey, P. J., Hathcock, K. S., Ahmed, A., Sher, I., and Hodes, R. J., 1981, *J. Exp. Med.* **145**:501.

Swain, S. J., Wetzel, G. D., Souliran, P., and Dutton, R. W., 1982, *Immunol. Rev.* **63**:111.
Takatsu, K., and Hamaoka, T., 1982, *Immunol. Rev.* **64**:25.
Takatsu, K., Tanaka, K., Tominaga, A., Kumahara, Y., and Hamaoka, T., 1980a, *J. Immunol.* **125**:2646.
Takatsu, K., Tominaga, A., and Hamaoka, T., 1981c, *Immunol. Lett.* **3**:137.
Takatsu, K., Tominaga, A., and Hamaoka, T., 1981c, *Immunol Lett.* **3**:137.
Takatsu, K., Sano, Y., Tomita, S., Hashimoto, N., and Hamaoka, T., 1981a, *Nature* **292**:360.
Takatsu, K., Tanaka, K., Tominaga, A., and Hamaoka, T., 1981b, in: *B Lymphocytes in the Immune Response: Functional, Developmental, and Interactive Properties* (N. R. Klinman, D. R. Mosier, I. Sher, and E. S. Vitetta, eds.), p. 331, Elsevier–North-Holland, New York.
Takatsu, K., Hashimoto, Y., Hashimoto, N., Sano, Y., and Hamaoka, T., 1982a, in: *UCLA Symposia on Molecular and Cellular Biology*, Vol. XXIV: *B and T cell Tumors* (E. S. Vitetta, and C. F. Fox eds.), p. 161, Academic Press, New York.
Takatsu, K., Sano, Y., Hashimoto, N., Tomita, S., and Hamaoka, T., 1982b, *J. Immunol.* **128**:2575.
Tominaga, A., Takatsu, K., and Hamaoka, T., 1980, *J. Immunol.* **124**:2423.
Tominaga, A., Takatsu, K., and Hamaoka, T., 1982, *J. Immunol.* **128**:2581.
Tsushima, T., and Friesen, H. G., 1973, *J. Clin. Endocrinol. Metab.* **37**:334.
Warner, N. L., 1974, *Adv. Immunol.* **19**:67.
Watson, J., and Mochizuki, D., 1980, *Immunol. Rev.* **51**:257.
Watson, J., Gillis, S., Marbrook, J., Mochizuki, D., and Smith, K. A., 1979, *J. Exp. Med.* **150**:849.
Yoshizaki, K., Nakagawa, T., Kaieda, T., Muraguchi, A., Yamamura, Y., Kishimoto, S., and Kishimoto, T., 1982, *J. Immunol.* **128**:1296.

In Vivo Administratration of Interleukin-2

Martin A. Cheever and Philip D. Greenberg

Division of Oncology
University of Washington School of Medicine
and the Fred Hutchinson Cancer Research Center
Seattle, Washington 98195

I. INTRODUCTION

Interleukin-2 (IL-2), also known as T-cell growth factor (TCGF), induces the replication of antigen-activated T cells *in vitro*. However, little is known concerning its function *in vivo* as a pharmacologic agent. The purpose of this chapter is to review evidence from animal models that IL-2 administered *in vivo* can induce T-cell growth *in vivo* and thereby augment specific T-cell immunity. In addition, an attempt is made to identify clinical immunodeficiency states in which the administration of IL-2 might be therapeutic; some of the potential toxicities of IL-2 and effects on immunity that might limit its use as a systemic reagent are discussed.

In vitro studies have provided much information about the biology and function of IL-2 as a T-cell proliferative signal; this work forms the theoretical basis for predicting its potential uses *in vivo*. *In vitro* cell-mediated immune reactions result from a complex series of interactions among antigen, antigen-reactive cells, and secreted factors (reviewed in Oppenheim and Gery, 1982). Macrophages process antigen and present it to T lymphocytes, in addition to producing an essential lymphocyte-activating factor, Interleukin-1 (IL-1) (Smith *et al.*, 1980). The specific binding of antigen to T cells bearing clonally distributed antigen receptors provides the first signal for T-cell proliferation and results in the expression of membrane receptors for IL-2 (Smith *et al.*, 1979; Bonnard *et al.*, 1979; Robb *et al.*, 1981). A subset of T cells, functionally defined as amplifier T cells, synthesizes and secretes IL-2, but only after specific activation by antigen and stimulation by the macrophage-produced IL-1. The binding of IL-2 to its receptor on antigen-activated T cells provides the second signal for T-cell proliferation and induces replication (Wagner and Röllinghoff, 1978). Antigen-specific daughter cells are generated that also express IL-2 receptors, but that will now continue to proliferate *in vitro* even in the absence of antigen, as long as adequate amounts of exogenous IL-2 are provided (Gillis and Smith, 1977; Nabholz *et al.*, 1978; Rosenberg *et al.*, 1978). Thus, although the specificity and magnitude of a T-cell response *in vitro* is initially determined by the antigen and number of antigen-reactive T cells present, theoretically unlimited expansion of activated antigen-specific T cells can be accomplished *in vitro* by continuous addition of exogenous IL-2 to cell cultures.

In vitro studies suggest that the magnitude of T-cell immunity reflects the resultant proliferation of activated T cells and is thus controlled at the level of production of and response to IL-2. *In vivo*, several studies have demonstrated that IL-2 administration can augment specific T-cell reactivity and therefore provide indirect evidence that IL-2 can induce T-cell growth *in vivo*. In those studies, semipurified preparations of IL-2 administered to mice after antigen inoculations were shown to augment the cytotoxic T-cell response to haptenated-self and alloantigens and to induce helper T cells for an antibody response to heterologous erythrocytes (Wagner *et al.*, 1980a, b; Stötter *et al.*, 1980). More recently, highly purified IL-2 has been shown to augment the effect of IL-2-dependent long-term cultured T lymphocytes for tumor therapy (Cheever *et al.*, 1982a,b) and to augment cytotoxic T-cell responses to alloantigens (Hefeneider *et al.*, 1983; Rosenberg *et al.*, 1983). Although these results demonstrated that the administration of IL-2 *in vivo* can enhance specific T-cell immunity *in vivo*, the results need not necessarily reflect T-cell growth in response to exogenous IL-2. Although *in vitro* studies suggest that IL-2 functions predominantly as an inducer of T-cell replication, either IL-2 (Kern *et al.*, 1981) and/or other lymphokines present in preparations of semipurified IL-2 such as those used in the above studies (Wagner *et al.*, 1982b) appear to be necessary for induction of T-cell differentiation. Thus, the augmentation of T-cell immunity identified *in vivo* following the administration of exogenous IL-2 might represent either T-cell differentiation or proliferation.

II. GROWTH OF CULTURED T CELLS *IN VIVO* INDUCED BY ADMINISTRATION OF IL-2 *IN VIVO*

Establishment of effective therapeutic regimens using IL-2 requires the development of animal models in which the effects of IL-2 administration on T-cell growth can be quantified. For initial studies, we have begun to examine the effects of IL-2 in a model in which the *in vivo* growth and survival of T lymphocytes previously cultured long-term *in vitro* in response to IL-2 can be measured (Cheever *et al.*, 1984). Such long-term-cultured T lymphocytes are exquisitely dependent *in vitro* upon exogenous IL-2 for proliferation and survival, express high-affinity IL-2 receptors, and rapidly absorb and deplete IL-2 from culture media. Thus, the adoptive transfer of these cells potentially creates a situation *in vivo* in which T cells dependent on exogenous IL-2 for survival are present in a relatively IL-2-deficient environment.

In order to identify and quantify the growth of donor T cells *in vivo*, the model has required the use of donor and host mice congenic for the T-cell marker Thy 1. Donor T cells were derived from spleens of C57BL/6 mice, which are Thy 1.2 and denoted B6, and the recipients were B6.PL(74NS) mice, denoted B6/Thy 1.1. B6/Thy-1.1 mice have been established as a strain congenic to B6 at the Thy-1 locus, the only difference being the introduction of the gene for the Thy-1.1 antigen and deletion of the gene for the Thy-1.2 antigen. As predicted, since C57BL/6 mice are low responders to Thy antigens (Zaleski *et al.*, 1981), no immune response to disparities at the Thy-1 allele was detectable following transfer of donor T cells into cyclophosphamide-pretreated congenic hosts. Moreover, the transfer of specific T-cell immunity as measured in functional assays was equally effective regardless of whether the donor of immune T cells was syngeneic or congenic (Greenberg and Cheever, 1983).

Donor spleen cells, obtained from B6 mice immunized *in vivo* with FBL-3 (a syngeneic Friend virus-induced leukemia), were activated by culture *in vitro* for 7 days with irradiated FBL-3; the activated T cells were then nonspecifically expanded in number by culture to day 19 with partially purified IL-2 from supernatants of concanavalin A (Con A)-stimulated spleen cells. These long-term-cultured T lymphocytes retained specific cytolytic reactivity to FBL-3 in a standard 4-hr chromium release assay (Cheever *et al.*, 1981). Host mice were pretreated on day 0 with cyclophosphamide (CY) to augment the transfer of donor T cells, and the donor cell inoculum was mixed *in vitro* with irradiated FBL-3 immediately before injection to provide specific antigenic stimulation to immune donor T cells *in vivo*. The number of donor T cells persisting within host ascites, spleen, and mesenteric lymph nodes was determined at selected points in time using fluorescein-tagged monoclonal antibody to Thy 1.2.

When no exogenous IL-2 was provided, long-term-cultured donor T cells were observed to die rapidly *in vivo*, with less than 1% remaining in host ascites and spleen by day 8 (Fig. 1) (Cheever *et al.*, 1984). However, administration of partially purified IL-2 daily by intraperitoneal (i.p.) inoculation resulted in a marked increase in both the percentage of ascitic cells of donor origin and the total number of donor T cells within host ascites (Table I). The increase was dependent on the dose of IL-2 inoculated with the highest dose of IL-2 tested, producing a 17-fold increase in donor T cells between days 4 and 6. This represents approximately four doublings in 48 hr. The changes in donor T-cell number observed

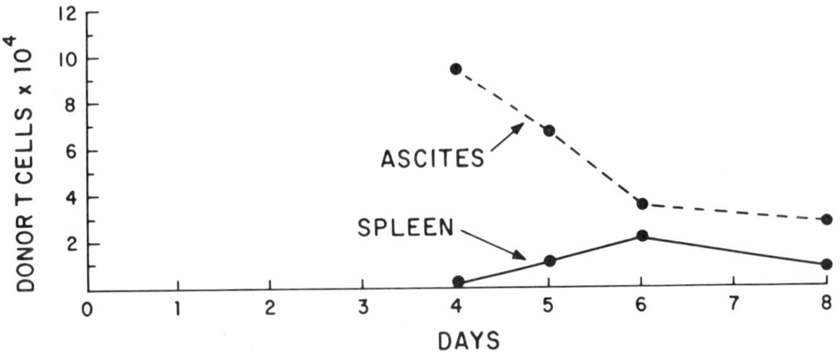

Figure 1. Survival of long-term cultured T lymphocytes following transfer *in vivo*. B6/Thy-1.1 mice were injected i.p. on day 0 with 5 × 10^6 long-term cultured T lymphocytes (i.e., spleen cells from B6 mice immunized *in vivo* with FBL-3, and subsequently activated by culture for 5 days with irradiated FBL-3 and numerically expanded by culture through day 19 with IL-2). All mice were pretreated with cyclophosphamide (CY) at a dose of 180 mg/kg and donor cells were mixed with 2 × 10^7 irradiated FBL-3 cells immediately prior to injection *in vivo*. On the days noted, host mice were sacrificed and cells from ascites and spleen were labeled with fluoresceinated antibody to Thy 1.2. Viable donor T cells were enumerated by phase/fluorescence microscopy.

within each host site examined reflected the net outcome of cell growth, cell death, and traffic to or from other sites and therefore provided only an indirect measurement of donor T-cell growth. However, the observation that donor T cells had increased in number at all sites examined strongly supports the conclusion that IL-2 administered *in vivo* induces the growth of long-term-cultured T cells *in vivo*.

The IL-2 administered *in vivo* in the preceding experiments had been only partially purified and thus may have contained other lymphokines and/or monokines in addition to IL-2 (Lafferty *et al.*, 1978). Therefore, in order to determine whether IL-2 alone is sufficient to induce *in vivo* T-cell growth, the IL-2 preparation was further purified. A murine T-cell lymphoma was stimulated by phytohemagglutinin (PHA) and phorbol myristate acetate (PMA), and the supernatant was purified by ammonium sulfate precipitation, DEAE ion-exchange chromatography, and reverse-phase high-pressure liquid chromatography (RP-HPLC). The purified material had no detectable lymphokine activity other than that ascribed to IL-2, produced a single spot of 14,000 M_r on two-dimensional polyacrylamide gels, and had a specific activity of approximately 1.4 million U/μg (Cheever *et al.*, 1984). The IL-2 was lyophilized in the presence of mouse serum protein in order to ensure stability during handling and storing prior to use *in vivo*.

Mice were injected with long-term cultured T cells and were inoculated with graded doses of purified IL-2 (Fig. 2). The purified IL-2 increased the number of

Table I. Partially Purified IL-2 Administered *in Vivo* Increases the Percent and Number of Donor Long-Term Cultured T Lymphocytes *in Vivo*[a]

		Ascites			Spleen		
Day	IL-2 dose units/day	Total cells × 10^4	Percent donor T cells	Total donor T cells × 10^4	Total cells × 10^4	Percent donor T cells	Total donor T cells × 10^4
4	–	186	3.7	6.9	593	0.011	0.065
	80	75	11.1	8.3	680	0.014	0.095
	320	51	25.0	12.8	380	0.023	0.087
6	–	168	2.9	4.9	2825	0.042	1.19
	80	420	8.3	34.9	2100	0.215	4.51
	320	1032	19.3	199.2	3350	0.585	19.60

[a]On day 0, B6/Thy 1.1 mice were injected i.p. with 5×10^6 long-term cultured T lymphocytes (i.e., spleen cells from B6 mice immunized *in vivo* with FBL-3 and subsequently activated by culture for 5 days with irradiated FBL-3 and numerically expanded by culture through day 19 with IL-2) either alone or with subsequent daily i.p. inoculation with 80 or 320 units of partially purified IL-2. All mice were pretreated with CY, 180 mg/kg, and donor cells were mixed with 2×10^7 irradiated FBL-3 cells immediately prior to injection. On days 4 and 6, donor T cells within host ascites and spleen were identified with fluoresceinated antibody to Thy 1.2 and enumerated.

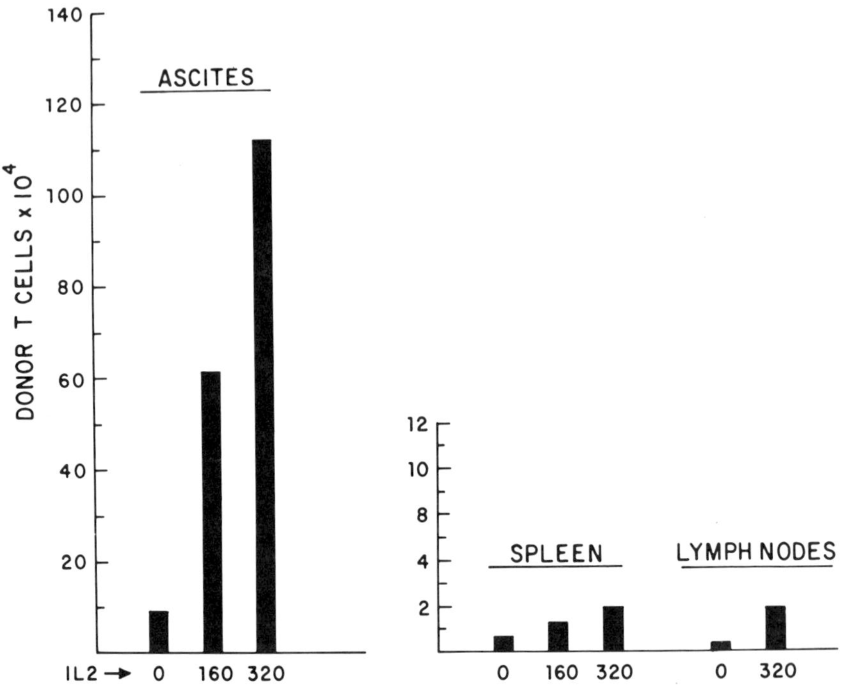

Figure 2. Purified IL-2 administered *in vivo* increases the survival of long-term culture T lymphocytes *in vivo*. B6/Thy-1.1 mice were injected on day 0 with 5×10^6 long-term cultured T lymphocytes (see Fig. 1 for definition) alone or with subsequent daily i.p. injections of graded doses of purified IL-2. All mice were pretreated with CY and donor T cells were injected *in vivo* mixed with irradiated FBL-3. On day 5, donor T cells within host ascites, spleen and mesenteric lymph nodes were enumerated by phase/fluorescence microscopy.

donor T cells in host ascites, spleen, and mesenteric lymph nodes in proportion to the dose inoculated. Thus, exogenous IL-2 alone is sufficient to induce the *in vivo* growth of donor long-term-cultured T lymphocytes.

The demonstration that cultured T cells grow *in vivo* in response to exogenous IL-2 strongly suggests that IL-2 will have application as a therapeutic agent. However, it is necessary to establish that IL-2 induced T-cell growth *in vivo* results in augmented T-cell function *in vivo*. We had previously addressed the issue of IL-2 function *in vivo* in models for the therapy of leukemia in which disseminated antigenic leukemia can be eradicated specifically by the adoptive transfer of T cells immune to the leukemia (Fefer *et al.*, 1976; Cheever *et al.*, 1982b; Greenberg and Cheever, 1983). Briefly, adult B6 mice are injected i.p. on day 0 with a lethal inoculum of FBL-3, a transplantable Friend virus-induced leukemia. By day 5, leukemic cells have disseminated and are detectable in both blood and spleen. All mice receiving FBL-3 on day 0 and no treatment die by day 14 (Fig.

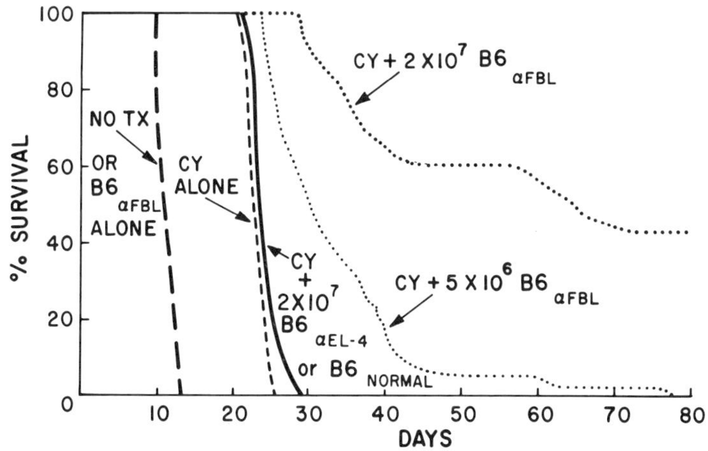

Figure 3. Adoptive chemoimmunotherapy of FBL-3. C57Bl/6 mice, denoted as B6, were inoculated i.p. on day 0 with 5×10^6 FBL-3 tumor cells. On day 5, tumor-bearing mice received therapy with CY at 180 mg/kg plus either 5×10^6 or 2×10^7 spleen cells from B6 mice immunized previously with irradiated FBL-3 denoted as $B6_{\alpha FBL}$. Alternatively, mice received therapy with immune cells alone ($B6_{\alpha FBL}$ ALONE), cyclophosphamide alone (CY ALONE), CY plus cells from mice immune to the EL-4 tumor (CY + $B6_{\alpha EL\text{-}4}$), or spleen cells from normal nonimmune B6 mice (CY + $B6_{NORMAL}$). The cumulative results of four experiments are presented with 32 mice per treatment group.

3). Treatment with a single injection of CY i.p. (180 mg/kg) approximately doubles median survival time, but all mice eventually die with tumor. Treatment on day 5 with immune cells alone has no apparent *in vivo* antitumor effect. However, as an adjunct to the CY, immune cells have a significant dose-dependent effect in prolonging survival and curing mice. In this circumstance, CY both reduces the tumor burden by a direct tumoricidal effect (Greenberg *et al.*, 1980) and eliminates suppressor cells that interfere with the expression of adoptively transferred immunity (North, 1982).

The *in vivo* efficacy of long-term-cultured T lymphocytes has been established in this adoptive chemoimmunotherapy model (Cheever *et al.*, 1981, 1982a, b) and confirmed by others in a similar model (Eberlein *et al.*, 1982). Spleen cells from *in vivo*-primed B6 mice, which were activated *in vivo* by culture with tumor and numerically expanded *in vitro* by culture with IL-2 for 19 days, retained specific cytolytic activity *in vitro* and mediated a specific antitumor effect in the treatment of disseminated leukemia (Fig. 4). Moreover, the efficacy of donor long-term-cultured T lymphocytes *in vivo* was dependent on the dose of donor T cells inoculated, with larger doses of cells further prolonging survival and curing a higher percentage of mice. Thus, any technique that induces numerical expansion of donor T cells *in vivo* would be expected to augment the therapeutic activity. To test this, mice treated with long-term-cultured T cells were given daily i.p. inoculations of IL-2 (Fig. 5). Exogenous IL-2 had no detect-

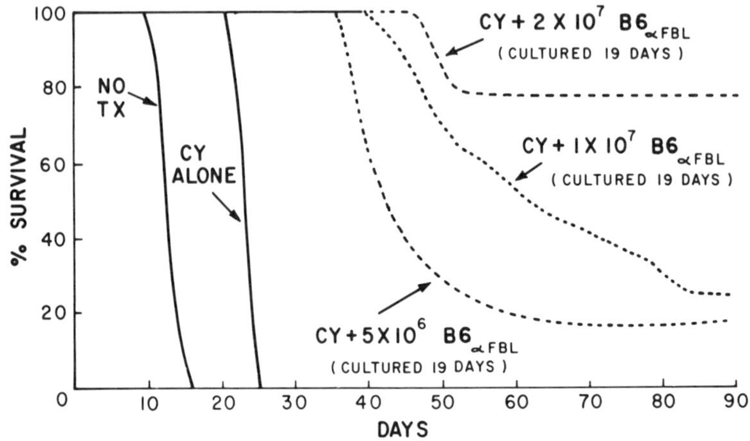

Figure 4. Efficacy of long-term cultured T lymphocytes in the adoptive chemoimmunotherapy of FBL-3. C57Bl/6 mice (B6) inoculated i.p. on day 0 with 5×10^6 FBL-3 received either no therapy (NO TX), treatment on day 5 with CY at 180 mg/kg (CY ALONE), or treatment with CY plus variable dose of long-term cultured T lymphocytes from mice sequentially immunized *in vivo* to FBL-3, activated by secondary sensitization *in vitro* and numerically expanded by culture through day 19 with Interleukin-2 [B6αFBL (cultured 19 days)]. The cumulative results of two experiments are represented with 16 mice per treatment group.

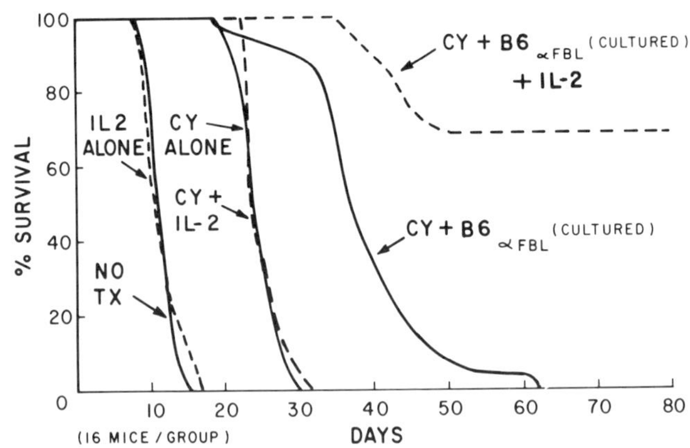

Figure 5. Partially purified IL-2 augments the function of IL-2-dependent long-term cultured T lymphocytes in chemoimmunotherapy. C57Bl/6 mice (B6), inoculated i.p. on day 0 with FBL-3 received either no therapy (NO TX), therapy on days 5–9 with Interleukin-2 i.p. at a dose of 80 units/day (IL-2 ALONE), treatment on day 5 with CY at a dose of 180 mg/kg (CY ALONE), treatment on day 5 with CY plus treatment on days 5–9 with IL-2 (CY + IL-2), treatment on day 5 with CY and 5×10^6 long-term cultured T lymphocytes [CY + B6αFBL (cultured)], or treatment on day 5 with CY and 5×10^6 long-term cultured T lymphocytes plus IL-2 on days 5–9 [CY + B6αFBL (cultured) + IL-2]. The cumulative results of two experiments are represented with 16 mice per treatment group.

able intrinsic antitumor effect, but did significantly augment the efficacy of tumor-specific long-term-cultured T lymphocytes in tumor therapy (Cheever *et al.*, 1982a, b). It is likely that the increased efficacy of the transferred T cells *in vivo* resulted directly from growth of donor T cells, since IL-2 did not augment the therapeutic effect of long-term-cultured T cells, which were rendered incapable of proliferation by irradiation. Thus, an IL-2 regimen that induced *in vivo* growth of cultured T cells was also found to enhance their functional efficacy *in vivo*.

III. FAILURE OF IL-2 TO INCREASE THE GROWTH OF NONCULTURED T CELLS *IN VIVO*

The use of cultured T cells *in vivo* serves as an excellent indicator system to evaluate the ability of IL-2 to function *in vivo*. As the technology for identification, selection, *in vitro* growth, and cloning of human T cells improves, the use of IL-2 *in vivo* as an adjunct to the adoptive transfer of specifically reactive T lymphocytes might prove effective therapy for neoplastic or infectious diseases. However, approaches involving manipulation of cells *in vitro* will always be cumbersome; IL-2 could have more general therapeutic value if regimens could be devised in which administration of IL-2 alone augmented autochthonous immunity. The development of appropriate regimens will require knowledge as to when during the evolution of a normal *in vivo* immune reaction IL-2 is produced in excess and when or under what circumstances a lack of IL-2 production limits the magnitude of immune reactivity.

We have begun to study these issues by examining the growth and response to exogenous IL-2 of noncultured immune donor T cells that have been transferred into nonimmune congenic host mice (Cheever *et al.*, 1984). Immune cells were transferred into naive hosts in order to permit eventual differentiation of the effect of exogenous IL-2 on immune T cells (i.e., donor) and nonimmune T cells (i.e., host). B6/Thy-1.1 mice were injected i.p. on day 0 with spleen cells from B6 mice previously immunized with irradiated FBL-3; donor T cells in host ascites and spleen were enumerated on selected days (Fig. 6). As in the previously described experiments, host mice were pretreated with CY, and noncultured donor T cells were mixed with irradiated FBL-3 immediately before injection. The results demonstrated that the number of donor T cells within the host ascites and spleen increased approximately 16-fold between days 4 and 8.

The *in vivo* survival of noncultured splenic T cells injected *in vivo* without exogenous IL 2 was thus markedly different than the survival of long-term-cultured T cells without IL-2. Long-term-cultured T lymphocytes inoculated *in vivo* without IL-2 progressively decreased in number over time; by contrast, after a short lag period, noncultured T cells grew rapidly. Long-term-cultured T lymphocytes are exquisitely dependent *in vitro* on exogenous IL-2 for survival. The *in*

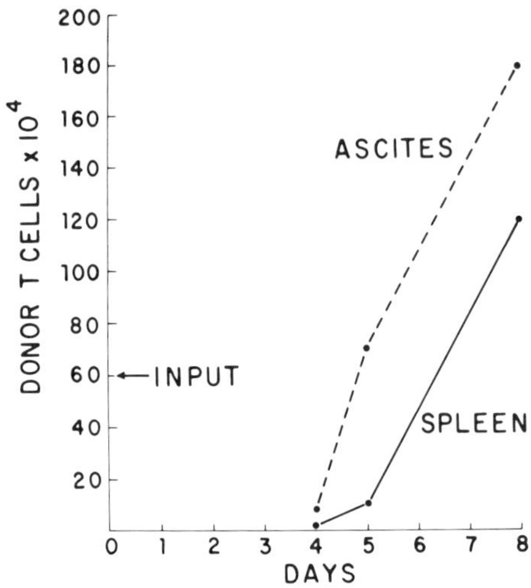

Figure 6. *In vivo* growth of non-cultured donor T cells injected without exogenous IL-2. On day 0, B6/Thy-1.1 mice were pretreated with CY, 180 mg/kg, and were injected i.p. with 2×10^7 irradiated FBL-3 cells mixed with 5×10^6 noncultured spleen cells from B6 mice previously immunized with FBL-3. On selected days, donor T cells within host ascites and spleen were enumerated by phase/fluorescence microscopy.

vivo demise of adoptively transferred long-term-cultured T lymphocytes without supplementary exogenous IL-2 implies that such cells remain IL-2 dependent *in vivo* and that endogenous IL-2 is unavailable and/or insufficient to maintain their viability. The *in vivo* growth of donor T cells from noncultured spleens injected without exogenous IL-2 implies that IL-2-producing donor amplifier T cells responding to tumor antigen are producing adequate amounts of IL-2 *in vivo* to sustain donor T-cell proliferation. Previous studies have demonstrated the presence of Lyt-1^+2^- amplifier T cells in the spleens of mice immune to FBL-3 tumor (Greenberg *et al.*, 1981). However, studies will be necessary to determine the relative contribution of antigen-specific donor T-cell-derived IL-2 production to the observed growth of transferred donor T cells.

During the period in which noncultured donor T cells proliferate rapidly *in vivo*, one would predict that administration of exogenous IL-2 would have little effect, either in inducing donor T-cell growth or in augmenting T-cell function. Although only one IL-2 regimen has thus far been evaluated as an adjunct to the transfer of noncultured immune spleen cells, experimental results support this hypothesis. On day 0, B6/Thy-1.1 mice pretreated with CY were injected with irradiated FBL-3 mixed with noncultured spleen cells from mice immune to FBL-3. Daily i.p. inoculation of partially purified IL-2 at a dose of 80 U/day had no demonstrable effect on the number of donor T cells detectable in ascites or spleen on day 5 (Cheever *et al.*, 1984) (Fig. 7). Similarly, this regimen of exogenous IL-2 failed to augment the functional efficacy of noncultured immune cells in adoptive therapy experiments (Cheever *et al.*, 1982a) (Fig. 8). Thus, unlike long-term-cultured T lymphocytes, which require exogenous IL-2 for survival, noncultured immune spleen cells appear to produce adequate endogenous IL-2 to maintain viability and to proliferate *in vivo*.

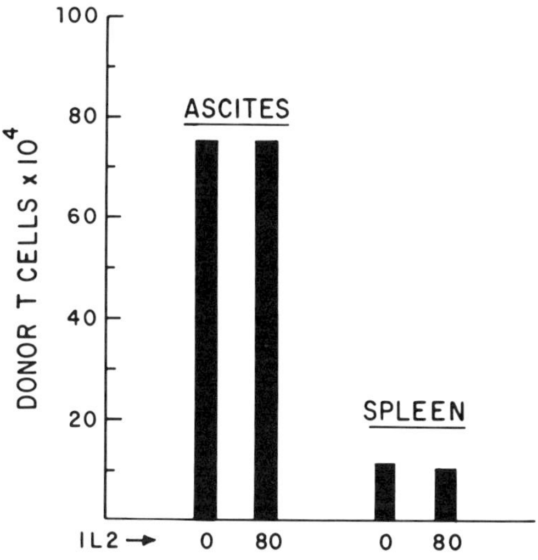

Figure 7. IL-2 administered *in vivo* fails to increase the number of *non-cultured* donor T cells *in vivo*. B6/Thy-1.1 mice were injected i.p. on day 0 with 5×10^6 noncultured spleen cells (1.2×10^6 T cells) from B6 mice immune to FBL-3 either alone or with subsequent daily i.p. inoculation with partially purified IL-2 at a dose of 80 units/day. All mice were pretreated with CY, and donor cells were injected with 2×10^7 irradiated FBL-3 cells. On day 5, donor T cells in host ascites and spleen were enumerated.

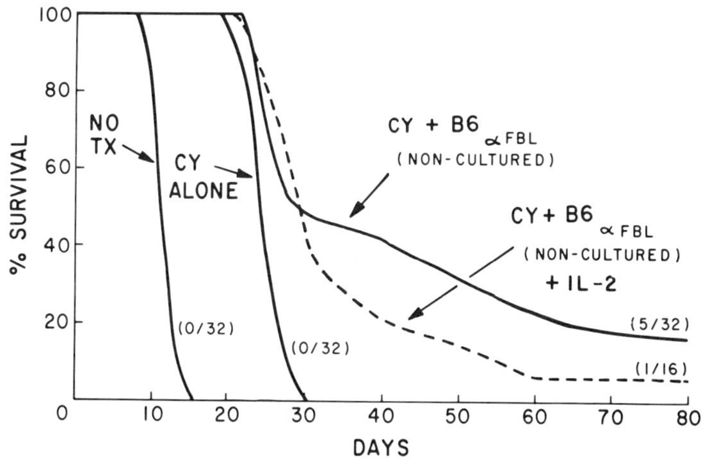

Figure 8. Failure of IL-2 administered *in vivo* on days 5–9 to enhance the function of non-cultured immune cells in chemoimmunotherapy. C57B1/6 mice, denoted B6 mice, inoculated i.p. on day 0 with 5×10^6 FBL-3 received either no therapy (NO TX), treatment on day 5 with CY (CY ALONE), treatment on day 5 with CY and 5×10^6 noncultured cells from mice immune to FBL-3 [CY + B6αFBL (noncultured)] or treatment on day 5 with CY and $5 \times 10_6$ noncultured immune cells plus IL-2 on days 5–9 at a dose of 80 units/day [CY + B6αFBL (noncultured) + IL-2]. The cumulative results of two experiments are represented with 16 mice per group.

The observation that exogenous IL-2 failed to increase the number (i.e., the growth rate) of noncultured T cells *in vivo* implies that the production of IL-2 *in vivo* during the period tested provided the maximal achievable stimulation with this lymphokine. Thus, *in vivo* IL-2 production was equal to or in excess of IL-2 utilization and/or degradation. It is possible that, at a later point in time after cell transfer, the production of donor T-cell-derived IL-2 may become insufficient to maintain the viability and/or maximal proliferation of donor T cells. At that time, the administration of exogenous IL-2 *in vivo* might be effective. Since the production of IL-2 *in vivo* during ongoing immune reactions has been difficult to quantitate, in part as a result of its short *in vivo* half-life (Paetkau *et al.*, 1982; Donohue and Rosenberg, 1983) and the presence of serum inhibitors to its function (Hardt *et al.*, 1981), models similar to that presented may prove useful for obtaining further evidence as to when during the evolution of an immune response IL-2 production is in relative excess or relative deficiency.

The long-term-cultured T lymphocytes used in the preceding experiments and shown to proliferate *in vivo* in response to exogenous IL-2 had been previously cultured with exogenous IL-2 (i.e., the T-cell population used had been selected to be IL- dependent by virtue of previous growth *in vitro* in response to exogenous IL-2). This T-cell population was used for initial studies, since it was presumed that cells expressing IL-2 receptors and adapted to *in vitro* growth with exogenous IL-2 would provide the most sensitive assay for *in vivo* IL-2 activity. The failure of exogenous IL-2 to augment the growth or function of noncultured immune cells *in vivo* raised the question of whether prior adaptation to growth with exogenous IL-2 *in vitro* is necessary to render T cells responsive to exogenous IL-2 *in vivo*. Thus, immune spleen cells activated by 5-day culture with irradiated FBL-3 and not cultured with exogenous IL-2 were studied.

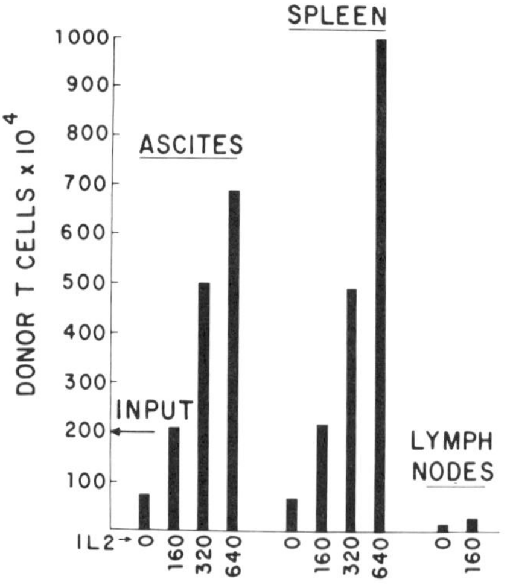

Figure 9. IL-2 administered *in vivo* induces the *in vivo* growth of donor T cells previously cultured short-term without exogenous IL-2. On day 0, B6/Thy-1.1 mice were injected with 2×10^6 spleen cells from B6 mice previously immunized *in vivo* with FBL-3 and subsequently activated by culture for 5 days with irradiated FBL-3. Host mice received either cultured cells alone or with subsequent daily i.p. inoculation with graded doses of purified IL-2. In addition, all mice were pretreated with CY and donor T cells were injected with irradiated FBL-3. On day 6 *in vivo*, donor T cells within host ascites, spleen, and mesenteric lymph nodes were enumerated.

Mice were injected on day 0 with short-term-culture-activated spleen cells followed by daily inoculations of purified IL-2 (Fig. 9). In mice receiving cells and no exogenous IL-2, 70% of the total number of donor T cells infused were recoverable on day 6 in ascites and spleen. By contrast, the total number of donor T cells at the same sites in mice receiving daily i.p. inoculation of 160, 320, or 640 units of purified IL-2 increased approximately 200%, 500%, and 800%, respectively. Therefore, the administration of exogenous IL-2 induced the *in vivo* growth of donor T cells activated by short-term culture with antigen but not previously exposed to exogenous IL-2. These results affirm that prior adaptation to growth with exogenous IL-2 *in vitro* will not be required for *in vivo* responsiveness.

IV. PHARMACOKINETICS OF IL-2 ADMINISTRATION

In vivo studies with adoptively transferred cultured T cells provide compelling evidence that IL-2 can function *in vivo* as a pharmacological modifier of T-cell responses. However, development of effective IL-2 regimens will require more information about the production, consumption, and localization of IL-2 *in vivo* during normal T-cell responses as well as the pharmacology of IL-2 following *in vivo* administration.

A major obstacle to dissecting the role of IL-2 *in vivo* has been the difficulty in measuring IL-2 in serum or other biological fluids during an ongoing immune reaction. Lymph node cells participating in an *in vivo* immune reaction can be removed, placed into culture, and shown to produce measurable quantities of IL-2 *in vitro* (Gautam *et al.*, 1983). However, the amount of IL-2 produced and released systemically during immune reactions has not been quantifiable because (1) it has a short serum half-life (Paetkau *et al.*, 1982; Donohue and Rosenberg, 1983); (2) inhibitors to its function exist in normal sera (Hardt *et al.*, 1981; Wagner *et al.*, 1982a); and (3) there is no reproducible radioimmunoassay or an enzyme-linked immunoadsorbent assay (ELISA) with which to measure its molecular presence in biological fluids. Thus, measurements of IL-2 to date have been largely functional (i.e., the ability of a biological sample to induce proliferation of IL-2-dependent T-cell lines *in vitro*). Unfortunately, measurement of the amount of IL-2 present in such samples with functional assays lacks sufficient precision for detailed pharmacokinetic studies since the proliferative response measured does not reflect the total amount of IL-2 produced, but rather indicates the net excess amount of IL-2 that has been produced and neither degraded nor blocked by inhibitors to IL-2 function.

Despite these obstacles, some useful kinetic data have been obtained from functional studies. IL-2 administered intravenously has been shown to have a half-life of several minutes (Paetkau *et al.*, 1982). This short half-life is not attributable to adsorption onto cells expressing IL-2 receptors, but rather to renal tubular catabolism of filtered IL-2 (Donohue and Rosenberg, 1983). The serum half-life can be prolonged by inoculating the IL-2 subcutaneously or intraperitoneally rather than intravenously (Donohue and Rosenberg, 1983). However, the optimal dose, route, or timing of IL-2 to induce T-cell growth *in vivo* has not been defined.

In our studies on the growth of long-term-cultured T cells, i.p. inoculation of IL-2 daily for 5 days induced dose-dependent proliferation of the transferred T cells with the highest dose tested, 320 U/day, inducing a doubling of donor T-cell number approximately every 12 hr (Table I). The potential efficacy and toxicity of IL-2 inoculated at higher doses or at different intervals still requires testing. For example, the therapeutic use of IL-2 may require frequent *in vivo* administration, similar to that required to maintain the growth and viability of T cells *in vitro*. Alternatively, as IL-2 induces the *in vivo* replication of cells bearing high-affinity IL-2 receptors, ever-increasing doses of IL-2 may be required to prevent T-cell death.

In the studies on *in vivo* T-cell growth described above, both donor T cells and IL-2 were inoculated intraperitoneally. Since the majority of donor T cells were subsequently found in ascites, it is reasonable to assume that donor T-cell growth occurred for the most part within the ascitic fluid. Although IL-2 inoculated i.p. did result in increases in donor T cells in host spleen and lymph nodes, such increases might reflect traffic to those sites rather than proliferation following egress from the ascites. This hypothesis is consistent with the observation by others that inhibitors to IL-2 function are present in mouse sera and potentially limit or localize the functional activity of IL-2 to the vicinity of IL-2 production or, in this circumstance, the site of inoculation. Whether exogenously administered IL-2 can induce T-cell growth at sites distant to IL-2 inoculation has not yet been evaluated.

V. INHIBITORS OF IL-2 FUNCTION

Serum inhibitors of IL-2 function may pose obstacles to therapy with exogenous IL-2. These inhibitors of T-cell proliferation, which have not yet been characterized, may be produced or regulated by T cells, since such factors are detected in the sera of normal mice but not in the sera of either T-cell-deficient athymic nude mice or mice treated with doses of cyclophosphamide toxic to lymphocytes (Hardt *et al.*, 1981; Wagner *et al.*, 1982a). Whether these serum inhibitors are specific for IL-2-induced proliferation is unknown. However, inhibition of IL-2-dependent T-cell growth *in vitro* by normal sera can be partially overcome by adding exogenous IL-2. It is possible that serum inhibitors may represent immunoregulatory molecules that function to control the magnitude of T-cell proliferation, such as circulating IL-2 receptors that have been shed from cell surfaces. However, studies of the relationship between endogenous IL-2 production and *in vivo* T-cell proliferation in inducing inhibitors to IL-2 function have yielded inconsistent results. Sera of mice undergoing a graft-versus-host reaction across H-2 disparities expressed increased inhibition of IL-2 function (Hardt *et al.*, 1981), whereas sera from mice undergoing an *in vivo* anti-Mls reaction, a potent inducer of IL-2 production *in vitro*, exhibited decreased inhibition (Gautam *et al.*, 1983). Unfortunately, the results of assaying the amount of IL-2 inhibitor in these experiments may be confounded by the potential presence of functionally active IL-2 in the serum in addition to the IL-2 inhibitors. Thus, analysis of the role and importance of serum IL-2 inhibitors will require methods designed to purify and characterize the inhibitory factor(s).

VI. POTENTIAL BIOLOGICAL EFFECTS AND TOXICITIES OF IL-2 THAT MIGHT LIMIT ITS ABILITY TO AUGMENT SPECIFIC T-CELL IMMUNITY

Similar to the action of polypeptide hormones, the activity of IL-2 appears to be limited to cells bearing specific high-affinity membrane receptors to the molecule (Robb *et al.*, 1981; Robb, 1982). By virtue of the restricted distribution of such IL-2-receptor-bearing cells to the lymphoid system, the toxicities as well as benefits of purified IL-2 should result from consequences of alterations in lymphocyte number and function. However, since the normal immune response involves multiple immunoregulatory circuits and cascades of interrelated responses, subsets of T cells of varied function reactive to the same antigen and responding to IL-2 may mediate disparate or conflicting functions, such as cytotoxicity and suppression. There is, in fact, little reason to expect that the administration of IL-2 *in vivo* will augment immune reactivity in a predicted positive direction to yield only the desired effect. For example, inappropriate timing or quantities of IL-2 might lead to excessive effector function or inappropriate suppressor function or might disturb the normal mechanism(s) for developing and maintaining tolerance and precipitate either autoimmunity or immune paralysis. Such issues must be resolved by extensive testing of IL-2 in appropriate animal models.

Exogenously administered IL-2 might also have significant effects on host immunological memory. T lymphocytes can be divided into a long-lived compartment containing memory T cells with a very low proliferative rate, and a short-lived compartment containing T cells with a high proliferative rate and a rapid turnover (reviewed in de Sousa, 1981). T cells activated by antigen and subsequently driven to proliferate *in vitro* by exogenous IL-2 die rapidly after withdrawal of IL-2. There is as yet no evidence that memory T cells capable of surviving for long periods without IL-2 are either generated or persist during IL 2-induced proliferation *in vitro*. If *in vivo* administration of high-dose exogenous IL-2 expands T-cell reactivity by increasing the number of short-lived T cells, but does not induce or permit the generation of memory T cells *in vivo*, then short-term augmentation of T-cell reactivity might occur at the expense of clonal deletion of the specific antigen-reactive cells. Depending on the particular immunogen, this might potentially result in either the loss of desirable reactivity to a potentially harmful environmental agent or the beneficial acquisition of tolerance to a self-determinant.

In vitro studies have shown that IL-2 can induce proliferation not only of T cells specifically activated by antigen, but also of other lymphocytes such as mitogen-activated T cells, natural killer (NK) cells, and an unclassified cytotoxic cell descriptively termed a lymphokine-activated killer (LAK) cell (Bonnard *et al.*, 1979; Dennert *et al.*, 1981; Grimm *et al.*, 1982; Vose and Bonnard, 1983). Although all such cells may potentially provide benefit against infectious agents or malignancies, their induction and growth *in vivo* may interfere significantly with the ability of IL-2 in augmenting a desired specific immune reaction.

Even if IL-2 regimens can be developed that uniquely induce *in vivo* growth of T cells of a desired antigen specificity, proliferating T cells are known to produce a myriad of lymphokines (reviewed in Krammer *et al.*, 1982), such as colony-stimulating factor, macrophage inhibition factor, macrophage activating factor, B-cell growth factor, T-cell replacing factor, immune interferon, T-cell differentiation factor, and even IL-2 itself—all of which, if produced in an uncontrolled or nonphysiological fashion—might lead to undesired consequences for normal T- and B-cell function, as well as inflammation and hematopoiesis. Thus, a great deal of study needs to be done with a large variety of assays and models to elucidate the ramifications of infusing pharmacological doses of IL-2.

VII. IDENTIFICATION OF IMMUNODEFICIENT STATES POTENTIALLY RESPONSIVE TO IL-2 ADMINISTRATION

Antigen-specific cell-mediated immunity is dependent in part on proliferation of antigen-reactive T cells in response to IL-2. Thus, deficient T-cell immunity can result either from a lack of cells able to elaborate IL-2 or a lack of cells able to respond to IL-2. Effective therapeutic use of IL-2 to overcome immunodeficiency will require identification of clinical and experimental settings in which the only or overriding problem is deficient IL-2 production. Thus, the role of IL-2 is being examined in many disease states. As examples, the immunodeficient states associated with autoimmune disease, aging, and chronic graft-versus-host disease have been reported to involve defects of both production and response to

IL-2 (Altman *et al.*, 1981; Gillis *et al.*, 1981; Mori *et al.*, 1983). Thus, although too little is known of the physiological and pharmacological role(s) of IL-2 *in vivo* to predict with confidence the utility of IL-2 administration in any clinical setting, it seems unlikely that IL-2 will prove effective in overcoming these immunodeficient states. In contrast, acquired immunodeficiency syndrome (AIDS) has been targeted for early therapy trials with IL-2. This syndrome represents an immunoregulatory disorder, in which there is a profound and possibly selective decrease of the OKT4-bearing helper T cells (Fauci *et al.*, 1983). If the remaining subsets of effector OKT8-bearing suppressor/cytotoxic T cells can be activated normally *in vivo* by specific antigen stimulation and can be induced to proliferate *in vivo* by the administration of IL-2, the immunodeficiency occurring in this syndrome might be alleviated. A preliminary report of a phase I study of IL-2 therapy in AIDS has described several minor clinical responses (Mertelsmann *et al.*, 1983). With the forseeable improvement in the efficacy of IL-2 regimens, such responses may become more significant.

Several common clinical settings have been identified in which the major problem apppears to be lack of IL-2 production, including patients receiving adrenal glucocorticosteroids, anticancer chemotherapy, or radiation therapy. Glucocorticosteroids *in vivo* are potent regulators of T-cell immunity, with glucocorticosteroid excess producing lymphopenia, lymphoid atrophy, and immunodeficiency (Smith, 1982). Although the precise mechanism for these *in vivo* changes remains to be elucidated, *in vitro* studies have shown that glucocorticosteroids prevent production of IL-2 and that the resultant inhibition of clonal expansion of activated T cells can largely be overcome *in vitro* by providing exogenous IL-2 (Gillis *et al.*, 1979a, b; Smith, 1982).

Chemotherapy and radiation therapy have also been shown to depress *in vivo* T-cell immunity. Spleen cells from mice treated with a moderate dose of cyclophosphamide contain cytotoxic T-lymphocyte precursors but fail to respond vigorously to antigenic stimulation due to inadequate IL-2 production. Thus, reactivity can be restored *in vitro* by either exogenous IL-2 or the addition of Lyt-$1^{+}2^{-}$ T lymphocytes capable of producing IL-2 (Merluzzi *et al.*, 1980, 1981a, b). Similarly, following sublethal total-body irradiation, cytotoxic T-lymphocyte precursors recover more quickly than do IL-2-producing cells, and radiation-induced inhibition of cytotoxic T-lymphocyte generation can be restored *in vitro* by the addition of cells capable of producing IL-2 (Kanagawa *et al.*, 1983).

It is unknown to what extent the lymphopenia and immunodeficiency induced by glucocorticosteroids, chemotherapy, and radiation therapy can be prevented or mitigated by concurrent administration of IL-2 *in vivo* or the degree to which immunological reconstitution following treatment with these agents can be hastened by subsequent administration of IL-2. However, the recent demonstration that an infusion of IL-2 into CY-pretreated mice stimulates the generation of cytotoxic T cells (Merluzzi *et al.*, 1983) implies that IL-2 may prove of significant benefit in these settings.

VIII. CONCLUSIONS

IL-2 will soon be available in large quantity for potential therapeutic use in humans. By virtue of its potent replication-inducing action on activated T cells and its restricted biological activity, IL-2 has great theoretical value as a therapeutic agent to augment specific T-cell immunity. Until recently, reagents and procedures were not available for examination of the efficacy of exogenous IL-2 *in vivo*. However, recent breakthroughs in the production and purification of IL-2 now afford the opportunity to explore the capacity of IL-2 to influence immune responses *in vivo*.

In order to establish effective therapeutic regimens using IL-2, we have developed murine models in which the effect of IL-2 administration on T-cell number and function can be quantified. The results of studies in these models have shown that administration of exogenous IL-2 can induce *in vivo* growth of long-term-cultured T cells and that the magnitude of T-cell growth is proportional to the dose of IL-2 administered. Similar IL-2 regimens have been shown to induce *in vivo* growth of donor T cells activated by culture with antigen for only 5 days and not exposed to exogenous IL-2 *in vitro*: but IL-2 failed to augment the *in vivo* growth of donor T cells not activated *in vitro*. Importantly, regimens of IL-2 that were shown to induce donor T-cell growth *in vivo* were also found to augment donor T-cell function *in vivo*.

These studies highlight the potential of exogenous IL-2 to induce T-cell growth *in vivo* and suggest that therapy with IL-2 may be useful for augmenting T-cell responses that are relatively deficient in the production of endogenous IL-2. Adaptation of IL-2 administration to the therapy of human disease will require learning more about the production, consumption, and localization of IL-2 *in vivo* during normal T-cell responses, as well as identification of disease states in which the overriding problem is deficient IL-2 production. Additional obstacles to be overcome prior to effective therapeutic use of IL-2 are the lack of detailed knowledge of pharmacokinetics of IL-2 administration, *in vivo* inhibitors to IL-2 function, and the potential effect of exogenous IL-2 on normal immunoregulatory circuits.

On the basis of an overwhelming number of *in vitro* studies and several recent confirmatory *in vivo* studies, it is clear that IL-2 has great potential for stimulating specific T-cell immunity *in vivo*. Further elucidation of principles necessary for effective IL-2 administration in animal models should have dramatic implications for promoting the use of IL-2 as an agent to augment specific T-cell immunity for the therapy of immunodeficient states, infectious disease, and malignancy.

ACKNOWLEDGMENTS

This investigation was supported by grants CA 30558 and CA 33084 from the National Cancer Institute, Department of Health and Human Serivces, and

IM 304 from the American Cancer Society. Dr. Cheever is the recipient of Research Career Development Award CA 00791 from the National Cancer Institute. IL-2 for the majority of these studies was provided by the Immunex Corporation, and by F. Hoffman-La Roche, Inc.

IX. REFERENCES

Altman, A., Theofilopoulos, A. N., Weiner, R., Katz, D. H., and Dixon, F. S., 1981, *J. Exp. Med.* **154**:791–808.

Bonnard, G. D., Yasaka, K., and Jacobson, D., 1979, *J. Immunol.* **123**:2704–2708.

Cheever, M. A., Greenberg, P. D., and Fefer, A., 1981, *J. Immunol.* **126**:1318–1322.

Cheever, M. A., Greenberg, P. D., Fefer, A., and Gillis, S., 1982a, *J. Exp. Med.* **155**:968–980.

Cheever, M. A., Greenberg, P. D., Gillis, S., and Fefer, A., 1982b, in: *The Potential Role of T Cells in Cancer Therapy* (A. Fefer and A. L. Goldstein, eds.), pp. 127–146, Raven Press, New York.

Cheever M. A., Greenberg, P. D., Irle, C., Thompson, J. A., Urdal, D. L., Mochizuki, D. Y., Henney, C. S., and Gillis, S., 1984, *J. Immunol.* **132**:2259–2265.

Dennert, G., Yogeeswaran, G., and Yamagata, S., 1981, *J. Exp. Med.* **153**:545–556.

De Sousa, M. (ed.), 1981, *Lymphocyte Circulation: Experimental and Clinical Aspects*, Wiley, New York.

Donohue, J. H., and Rosenberg, S. A., 1983, *J. Immunol.* **130**:2203–2208.

Eberlein, T. J., Rosenstein, M., and Rosenberg, S. A., 1982, *J. Exp. Med.* **156**:385–397.

Fauci, A. S., Lane, H. C., and Volkman, D. J., 1983, *Ann. Intern. Med.* **99**:61–75.

Fefer, A., Einstein, A. B., Cheever, M. A., and Berenson, J. R., 1976, *Ann. N.Y. Acad. Sci.* **276**:573–583.

Gautam, S. C., Hilfiker, M. L., and Battisto, J. R., 1983, *J. Immunol.* **130**:533–537.

Gillis, S., and Smith, K. A., 1977, *Nature* **268**:154–156.

Gillis, S., Crabtree, G. R., and Smith, K. A., 1979a, *J. Immunol.* **123**:1624–1631.

Gillis, S., Crabtree, G. R., and Smith, K. A., 1979b, *J. Immunol.* **123**:1632–1638.

Gillis, S., Kozak, R., Durante, M., and Weksler, M. E., 1981, *J. Clin. Invest.* **67**:937–942.

Greenberg, P. D., and Cheever, M. A., 1983, in: *UCLA Symposia on Molecular and Cellular Biology* (R. P. Gale, ed.), pp. 255–259, Alan R. Liss, New York.

Greenberg, P. D., Cheever, M. A., and Fefer, A., 1980, *Cancer Res.* **40**:4428–4432.

Greenberg, P. D., Cheever, M. A., and Fefer, A., 1981, *J. Exp. Med.* **154**:952–963.

Grimm, E., Mazumder, A., Ahang, H., and Rosenberg, S. A., 1982, *J. Exp. Med.* **155**:1823–1841.

Hardt, C., Röllinghoff, M., Pfizenmaier, K., Mosmann, H., and Wagner, H., 1981, *J. Exp. Med.* **154**:262–274.

Hefeneider, S. H., Conlon, P. J., Henney, C. S., and Gillis, S., 1983, *J. Immunol.* **130**:222–227.

Kanagawa, O., Louis, J. A., Engers, H. D., and Cerottini, J.-C., 1983, *J. Immunol.* **130**:24–28.

Kern, D. E., Gillis, S., Okada, M., and Henney, C. S., 1981, *J. Immunol.* **127**:1323–1328.

Krammer, P. H., Dy, M., Hultner, L., Isakson, P., Kees, U, Lohmann-Matthes, M.-L., Marcucci, F., Michanay, A., Pure, E., Schimpl, A., Staber, F., Vitetta, E. S., and Waller, M., 1982, in: *Isolation, Characterization, and Utilization of T Lymphocyte Clones* (C. G. Fathman and F. W. Fitch, eds.), pp. 253–265, Academic Press, New York,

Lafferty, K. J., Warren, H. S., Woolnough, J. A., and Talmage, D. W., 1978, *Blood Cells* **4**:395–404.

Merluzzi, V. J., Faanes, R. B., and Choi, Y. S., 1980, *Int. J. Immunopharmacol.* **2**:341–344.

Merluzzi, V. J., Walker, M. M., and Faanes, R. B., 1981a, *Cancer Res.* **41**:850–853.

Merluzzi, V. J., Kenney, R. E., and Schmid, F. A., Choi, Y. S., and Fannes, R. B., 1981b, *Cancer Res.* **41**:3663–3665.

Merluzzi, V. J., Welte, K., Savage, D. M., Last-Barney, K., and Mertelsmann, R., 1983, *J. Immunol.* **131**:806–809.

Mertelsmann, R., Welte, K., Sternberg, C., O'Reilly, R., Moore, M.A.S., Oettgen, H. F., and Clarkson, B. D., 1983, *Blood* 62 (Suppl.) **1**;114a (abst.).

Mori, T., Tsoi, M.-S., Gillis, S., Santos, E., Thomas, E. D., and Storb, R., 1983, *J. Immunol.* **130**:712–716.

Nabholz, M., Engers, H. D., Collavo, D., and North, M., 1978, *Curr. Top. Microbiol. Immunol.* **81**:176–187.

North, R. J., 1982, *J. Exp. Med.* **155**:1063–1074.

Oppenheim, J. J., and Gery, I., 1982, *Immunol. Today* **3**:113–119.

Paetkau, V., Mills, G. B., and Bleackley, R. C., 1982, in: *Progress in Cancer Research and Therapy*, Vol. 22: *The Potential Role of T Cells in Cancer Therapy* (A. Fefer and A. L. Goldstein, eds.), pp. 147–159, Raven Press, New York.

Robb, R. J., 1982, *Immunobiology* **161**:21–50.

Robb, R. J., Munck, A., and Smith, K. A., 1981, *J. Exp. Med.* **154**:1455–1474.

Rosenberg, S. A., Schwarz, S., and Spiess, P. J., 1978, *J. Immunol.* **121**:1951–1955.

Rosenberg, S. A., Spiess, P. J., and Schwarz, S., 1983, *Transplantation.* **35**:631–634.

Smith, K. A., 1982, in: *Lymphokines*, Vol. 7 (M. Landy, ed.), pp. 203–211, Academic Press, New York.

Smith, K. A., Gillis, S., Baker, P. D., McKenzie, D., and Ruscetti, F. W., 1979, *Ann. N.Y. Acad. Sci.* **332**:423–432.

Smith, K. A., Lachman, L. B., Oppenheim, J. J., and Favata, M. F., 1980, *J. Exp. Med.* **151**:1551–1556.

Stötter, H., Rüde, E., and Wagner, H., 1980, *Eur. J. Immunol.* **10**:719–722.

Vose, B., and Bonnard, G., 1983, *J. Immunol.* **130**:687–693.

Wagner, H., and Röllinghoff, M., 1978, *J. Exp. Med.* **148**:1523–1538.

Wagner, H., Hardt, C., Heeg, K., Röllinghoff, M. and Pfizenmaier, K., 1980a, *Nature* **284**: 278–280.

Wagner, H. C., Hardt, K., Heeg, K., Pfizenmaier, W., Solbach, R., Bartlett, H., Stockinger, H., and Röllinghoff, M., 1980b, *Immunol. Rev.* **51**:215–255.

Wagner, H., Hardt, C., Heeg, K., Pfizenmaier, K., Stötter, H., and Röllinghoff, M., 1982a, *Immunobiology* **161**:139–156.

Wagner, H., Hardt, C., Rouse, B. T., Röllinghoff, M., Scheurich, P., and Pfizenmaier, K., 1982b, *J. Exp. Med.* **155**:1876–1881.

Zaleski, M. B., Gorzynski, T. J., and Reichner, J., 1981, *Am. J. Reprod. Immunol.* **1**:140–144.

Index